AF692093

ALLE ZEIT WACH 1842

Cardiomyopathies

Realisations and Expectations

Edited by

J. F. Goodwin and E. G. J. Olsen

With 77 Figures, Partly in Colour

Springer-Verlag

Berlin Heidelberg New York
London Paris Tokyo
Hong Kong Barcelona
Budapest

JOHN F. GOODWIN, MD, FRCP, FACP (Hon), FACC, FESC, Dr. hc. U Lisbon
Emeritus Professor of Clinical Cardiology
Royal Postgraduate Medical School, Du Cane Road,
London W12 0NN, UK

ECKHARDT G. J. OLSEN, MD, FRCPath, FACC, FESC
Consultant Histopathologist (Cardiovascular Division)
Royal Brompton National Heart and Lung Hospital London
Department of Histopathology
Fulham Road, London SW3 6HP, UK

ISBN 3-540-55608-7 Springer-Verlag Berlin Heidelberg New York
ISBN 0-387-55608-7 Springer-Verlag New York Berlin Heidelberg

Library of Congress Cataloging-in-Publication Data. Cardiomyopathies / J. Goodwin, E. Olsen (eds.). p. cm. Includes bibliographical references and index. ISBN 3-540-55608-7 (alk. paper). – ISBN 0-387-55608-7 (alk. paper) 1. Myocardium – Diseases. I. Goodwin, John F. II. Olsen, E. G. J. (Eckhardt G. J.) [DNLM: 1. Cardiomyopathy, Congestive. 2. Cardiomyopathy, Hypertrophic. 3. Cardiomyopathy, Restrictive. WG 280 C2667] RC685.M9C355 1993 616. 1'24 – dc20 DNLM/DLC for Library of Congress 92-49589

This work is subject to copyright. All rights are reserved, whether the whole or part of the material is concerned, specifically the rights of translation, reprinting, reuse of illustrations, recitation, broadcasting, reproduction on microfilm or in any other way, and storage in data banks. Duplication of this publication or parts thereof is permitted only under the provisions of the German Copyright Law of September 9, 1965, in its current version, and permission for use must always be obtained from Springer-Verlag. Violations are liable for prosecution under the German Copyright Law.

© Springer-Verlag Berlin Heidelberg 1993
Printed in

The use of general descriptive names, registered names, trademarks, etc. in this publication does not imply, even in the absence of a specific statement, that such names are exempt from the relevant protective laws and regulations and therefore free for general use.

Product liability: The publishers cannot guarantee the accuracy of any information about dosage and application contained in this book. In every individual case the user must check such information by consulting the relevant literature.

Typesetting: Thomson Press (India) Ltd., New Delhi

23/3130/SPS-543210—Printed on acid-free paper

Dedicated
to the memory of
ALAN STENHOUSE GOURLEY
1909–1991

Preface

This book reviews the basic knowledge about the cardiomyopathies and re-enforces the well-known definitions and classification of cardiomyopathies and specific heart muscle diseases, respectively. It emphasizes the importance of maintaining the classification into hypertrophic, dilated and restrictive cardiomyopathies, even though there are exceptions.

The term "realisations" in the title is used in the sense of "achievements" and alludes to the progress in the understanding of heart muscle diseases over the last three decades and also to the areas of knowledge still not fully explored, for example, the as yet unclassified putative cardiomyopathies such as arrhythmogenic right ventricular dysplasia, long QT syndrome and syndrome X. The accurate and sensitive identification of major risk factors for sudden death in hypertrophic cardiomyopathy needs further study, as do the implications of a familial basis in some patients with dilated cardiomyopathy.

The "expectations" mentioned in the title centre around the molecular biological aspects of viral myocarditis and dilated cardiomyopathy and their relationship to each other; around the autoimmune basis for dilated cardiomyopathy and its implications for drug therapy and cardiac transplantation; and around molecular genetic techniques for identifying the genes involved in hypertrophic cardiomyopathy that will be developed further. These will have implications for pre-natal recognition and for diagnosis in early life in apparently fit and active persons, and offer better prospects of prevention and cure.

The prospects for realising these expectations are bright, and many of the outstanding problems should be resolved in the near future. The availability of refined clinical investigation techniques, such as echocardiography and Doppler methods, and the development of molecular biological testing have provided vital additions to the tools for clinical assessment. Thus the prospects of unravelling the mysteries of the cardiomyopathies are challenging and exciting.

Finally, it is imperative to maintain the crucial clinical skills and approach to guide, advise and treat patients: this book therefore emphasises the clinician's vital role in managing these life-threatening conditions.

London, August 1992

J. F. Goodwin
E. G. J. Olsen

Contents

Part I. Introduction

Part II. Dilated Cardiomyopathy

Part III. Hypertrophic Cardiomyopathy

List of Contributors

ACQUATELLA, H., Centro Medico 275, San Bernardino, Caracas 1011, Venezuela

ARCHARD, L. C., Department of Biochemistry, Charing Cross & Westminster Medical School, London W6 8RF, UK

CUNNINGHAM, L., Department of Biochemistry, Charing Cross & Westminster Medical School, London, UK

GILBERT, E. M., Division of Cardiology, 4A-100 University of Utah Medical Centre, 50 North Medical Drive, Salt Lake City, UT 84132, USA

GOODWIN, J. F., Department of Cardiology, Royal Postgraduate Medical School, Du Cane Road, London W12 0NN, UK

HERZUM, M., Department of Internal Medicine and Cardiology, Philipps-University Marburg, W-3550 Marburg, Germany

LENARDA, A. Di, Division of Cardiology, 4A-100 University of Utah Medical Centre, 50 North Medical Drive, Salt Lake City, UT 84132, USA

MAISCH, B., Department of Internal Medicine and Cardiology Philipps-University Marburg, W-3550 Marburg, Germany

MCKENNA, W. J., Department of Cardiological Sciences, St. George's Hospital Medical School, Cranmer Terrace, London SW17 0RE, UK

OAKLEY, C. M., Department of Cardiology, Royal Postgraduate Medical School, Hammersmith Hospital, Du Cane Road, London W12 0NN, UK

O'CONNELL, J. B., Department of Medicine, University of Mississippi Medical Center 2500 North State Street, Jackson, MS 39216 4505, USA

OLSEN, E. G. J., Consultant Histopathologist (Cardiovascular Division) Royal Brompton National Heart and Lung Hospital London, Department of Histopathology, Fulham Road, London SW3 6HP, UK

RICHARDSON, P. J., Department of Cardiology, King's College Hospital, Denmark Hill, London SE5, UK

SCHULTHEISS, H.-P., Medical Clinic, Department of Cardiology, Pneumology, Angiology, Heinrich-Heine-University Düsseldorf, Moorenstrasse 5, W-4000 Düsseldorf, Germany

SEIDMAN, C. E., Department of Genetics, Havard Medical School, Thorn Building, Room 509, 25 Shattuck Street, Boston, MA 02115, USA

STEWART, J. T., Department of Cardiological Sciences, St. George's Hospital Medical School, Cranmer Terrace, London SW17 0RE, UK

TROTTER, S. E., Department of Histopathology, Brompton Hospital, Fulham Road, London SW3 6HP, UK

WATKINS, H., Department of Cardiological Sciences, St. George's Hospital Medical School, Cranmer Terrace, London SW17 0RE, UK

WHY, H. J. F., Department of Cardiology, King's College Hospital, Denmark Hill, London SE5, UK

Part I
Introduction

CHAPTER 1

Definition, Classification and Terminology

E. G. J. Olsen and J. F. Goodwin

In the 1950's workers in the United States of America (Mattingly, Burch and Proctor Harvey) were studying cases of heart muscle disease. Brigden in 1957 [1] published his St. Cyres lecture on "Uncommon myocardial diseases: the non-coronary cardiomyopathies". It seems likely that this was the first time the term "cardiomyopathy" had been used in this sense, though workers in continental Europe often referred to "myocardopathies" and used the term "cardiopathy" or "cardiomyopathy" to denote any form of heart disease affecting heart muscle—for example "congenital cardiopathies".

In 1961, 1964 and 1970 Goodwin [2–4], proposed a somewhat unwieldy definition of cardiomyopathies which was subsequently shortened to "Heart muscle disease of unknown cause" [4] and separated from heart muscle disease due to conditions involving organs other than the heart: the "specific heart muscle diseases" (Table 1.1). The cardiomyopathies thus defined were divided into Hypertrophic, Dilated and Restrictive types and their classification was confirmed by the WHO/ISFC Task Force [5] and the report of the WHO Expert Committee on cardiomyopathies in 1984 [6]. The classification into hypertrophic, dilated and restrictive has been used throughout this book, as it has stood the test of time so far, but increasing knowledge and advanced medical investigation have indicated that all types of cardiomyopathy cannot be covered completely by this simple classification, which is, like all classifications, a bridge between ignorance and knowledge. The cardiomyopathies are in a watershed now between clinical identification and basic scientific advances. They must not be frozen in a time warp. Conditions difficult to place in the "cardiomyopathy" or "specific heart muscle disease" classification include (see Chap. 13):

1. Takayasu's syndrome
2. Kawasaki disease
3. Long Q-T syndromes
4. Syndrome "X"
5. Congenital heart block syndromes
6. Endocardial fibroelastosis
7. Right ventricular dysplasia

New techniques of investigation, especially in the field of immunology and molecular biology, are opening up fresh avenues of study and further understanding of the problems of causation, genetics and management of the main

Table 1.1. Specific heart muscle disease

General class	Specific example(s)
Infective	*Borrelia*
	HIV
	Coxsackie
	Chagas myocarditis
Connective tissue disorder	Diffuse systemic sclerosis
Metabolic	
Endocrine causes	Thyrotoxicosis
Familial storage diseases and infiltration	Haemochromatosis
	Glycogen storage disease
Deficiency diseases	Selenium; Kashin disease
Amyloid	
General system diseases	
Infiltrations, granulomas and neoplasms	Sarcoidosis
	Phaeochromocytoma
	Secondary neoplasm
Heredo-familial muscular dystrophies	
Muscular dystrophies	Duchenne muscular dystrophy
Neuromuscular disorders	Friedreich's ataxia
Sensitivity and toxic reactions	Adriamycin
	Penicillin
Poisonings	Alcohol
	X-radiation

Though no classification is perfect the above has proved to be a good working model. This list is necessarily incomplete [8] but indicates the main principles. Most specific heart muscle diseases cause a dilated form of heart muscle disease, with certain exceptions (see Chap. 10). Amyloid disease represents a link between cardiomyopathy and specific heart muscle disease (see Chaps. 10, 13). Friedreich's ataxia and glycogen storage disease can be associated with hypertrophic cardiomyopathy (see Chap. 6).

groups of cardiomyopathies. Of particular importance are the discoveries by new techniques of the gene for familial hypertrophic cardiomyopathy [7] and the much higher familial incidence of dilated cardiomyopathy than was previously thought. Molecular genetics and biological techniques are also exploring the problems of myocarditis and its relation to dilated cardiomyopathy.

The question of whether true outflow tract obstruction occurs in hypertrophic cardiomyopathy is now solved. The answer is that in 70% or more of cases true obstruction does not occur; pressure gradients are due to powerful ventricular contraction, overemptying and turbulence. Gradients may be created by high flow velocity without true obstruction [9, 10], as may occur in atrial septal defect. But in a minority of cases true obstruction does occur due to massive ventricular hypertrophy, small ventricular cavity, huge papillary muscles and mitral valve/septal contact (see Chap. 9).

The object of this book is to review the known aspects of cardiomyopathies, to emphasise the unknown, to point out the uncertainties and indicate the way ahead by present and future research. Whenever possible, cross-referencing to appropriate parts of the book has been used to emphasise the important areas of discovery and controversy. The essential contribution of the clinical approach to the understanding and management of the cardiomyopathies is stressed throughout.

Terminology

The following terms are considered by the editors to be helpful in clarifying disorders of function [11]:

Elimination: the disappearance of the ventricular cavity in systole by apposition and compression on its walls in hypertrophic cardiomyopathy.
Obstruction: organic physical obstruction to ventricular outflow.
Restriction: organic interference as a result of endomyocardial disease with rapid early ventricular filling and slow reduced late ventricular filling.
Resistance: hindrance to ventricular filling caused by stiff irregularly relaxing poorly compliant ventricles.
Obliteration: organic blockage of the ventricular cavities by fibrotic material and thrombosis [8].

References

1. Brigden W (1957) Uncommon myocardial diseases: the non- coronary cardiomyopathies. Lancet 2: 1179, 1243
2. Goodwin JF, Hollman A, Bishop MB (1961) Clinical aspects of cardiomyopathy. Br Med J 1: 69
3. Goodwin JF (1964) Cardiac function in primary myocardial disorders. Br Med J 1: 1527, 1595
4. Goodwin JF (1970) Congestive and hypertrophic cardiomyopathy: a decade of study. Lancet 1: 731
5. WHO/ISFC Task Force (1980) Report on the definition and classification of cardiomyopathy. Heart J 44: 672
6. WHO Expert Committee (1984) Cardiomyopathies. WHO Tech Rep Ser 697
7. Jarcho JA, McKenna W, Pare JAP, Solomon SD, Holcombe RF, Dickie S, Levi T, Donis-Keller H, Seidman JG, Seidman C (1989) Mapping a gene for familial cardiomyopathy to chromosome 14q1. N Engl J Med 321: 1372–1378
8. Goodwin JF (1983) Terminology of disorders of cardial muscle. In: Symons C, Evans T, Mitchell AG (eds) specific heart muscle disease. Wright, Bristol, p 1
9. Criley JM, Siegel RJ (1985) A non-obstructive view of hypertrophic cardiomyopathy. In: Goodwin JF (ed) Heart muscle disease. MTP Press, Lancaster, p 157
10. Murgo JP, Miller JW (1985) Haemodynamic, angiographic and echocardiographic evidence against inpeded ejection in hypertrophic cardiomyopathy. In: Goodwin JF (ed) Heart muscle disease. MTP Press, Lancaster, p 187
11. Goodwin JF (1985) Cardiomyopathies and specific heart muscle diseases: definition, classification and terminology. In: Goodwin JF (ed) Heart muscle disease. MTP Press, Lancaster, p 1

Part II
Dilated Cardiomyopathy

CHAPTER 2

Clinical Aspects

J. F. Goodwin

Dilated (previously known as congestive) cardiomyopathy is essentially a disorder manifest by heart failure of unknown origin. It may be defined as a myocardial disorder with ventricular dilatation and reduced systolic function. In early studies [1] the diagnosis was not appreciated until congestive signs had appeared, but now, because of improved knowledge, better technology and diagnostic advances, diagnosis can be made at an earlier stage. The descriptive title of "dilated" [2] is appropriate, since ventricular dilatation is the most striking pathological feature.

Incidence

The incidence is world-wide, affecting males more than females and the middle-aged more than children and the elderly [3]. Dilated cardiomyopathy seems to be more frequent in developing than developed countries. In Ceylon it was the cause of heart failure in 26% of patients [4], whereas in Sweden it has been reported to have an incidence of 7–10 cases per 100 000 inhabitants [5]. Similar figures have been estimated for the east of England [6].

Symptoms and Presentation

Since reduction of systolic function is the principal feature, early symptoms tend to reflect reduced cardiac output and failure of minute volume and stroke volume to rise appropriately on effort. Thus, tiredness with undue fatigue on effort are usually the first symptoms, and may be quite mild for a considerable period of time. As the disease advances, the symptoms become more severe. Usually dyspnoea dominates, but since the right ventricle is usually involved as well as the left, tiredness tends to increase and some swelling of the ankles at the end of the day may occasion anxiety. Paroxysmal nocturnal dyspnoea often develops ushered in by an irritating dry cough and orthopnoea. In the late phases frank right ventricular failure occurs with complaints of swelling of the ankles and of the abdomen, with tenderness in the right hypochondrium due to lymphatic congestion.

The development of arrhythmia may add palpitations to the other symptoms. Chest pain of anginal type is well recognised but rare. Pleuritic pain may be intense if peripheral pulmonary infarction has occurred, which may be accompanied by haemoptysis. In some patients the early symptoms may be introduced by fever and upper respiratory tract infection, suggesting the possibility of an underlying viral myocarditis.

The history, although often prolonged, may be quite short—even a few weeks. This also suggests a viral origin.

There is usually no history of addiction of note. Alcohol is often taken in moderate amounts and tends to damage the heart further. Intake of large amounts of alcohol (40 g daily for 10 years or more) may cause severe myocardial disease and dilated ventricles with greatly impaired systolic function [7]. The diagnosis is then alcoholic heart muscle disease as distinct from dilated cardiomyopathy. There is nothing in the history of patients with dilated cardiomyopathy to suggest any dietary deficiency. Selenium deficiency occurs in China, while genetically determined carnitine deficiency may cause a syndrome similar to specific heart muscle disease. Most patients who develop dilated cardiomyopathy have previously been healthy, active or even athletic individuals, without any exposure to toxic substances or radiation.

Clinical Examination

Clinical signs may be few even when quite extensive myocardial damage has already occurred. The clinical signs of congestive heart failure represent a late stage of the disease. Nevertheless, important clues to the diagnosis of myocardial failure can often be elicited early. The most important of these are added heart sounds: a fourth sound due to increased left atrial pressure secondary to raised left ventricular end-diastolic pressure, and a third heart sound due to rapid filling of the dilated ventricle. Not infrequently both third and fourth heart sounds may be present; this, if there is tachycardia, produces a summation gallop that is highly suggestive of a poorly contracting dilated left ventricle. The echocardiogram will usually show, before any signs of congestive failure are apparent, increased ventricular dimensions, impaired contraction and ventricular hypertrophy (see Chap. 4). Other clues are: inappropriate tachycardia at rest, low blood pressure and poor left ventricular cardiac impulse. According to Laplace's law, the dilated ventricles are able to achieve a reasonable stroke volume, while cardiac output is maintained by tachycardia, but eventually the overloaded ventricles generate an end-diastolic pressure high enough to cause venous congestion in lungs and body tissue. If cardiac function further diminishes, the jugular venous pressure rises and evidence of tricuspid regurgitation may appear with the development of a systolic venous wave.

In the fully developed picture there will be hepatomegaly (often with ascites), oedema of the lower extremities and crepitations at the bases of the lungs;

pleural effusions often occur. Ventricular dilatation is often accompanied by atrioventricular valvar regurgitation. Mitral and tricuspid regurgitation develop as papillary muscle function deteriorates and loud systolic murmurs (occasionally mid–late in time) appear in mitral and tricuspid areas. The dangerously low cardiac output is manifest by cold, blue extremities, a thready arterial pulse, and a trace of icterus, due usually to hepatic congestion but occasionally to pulmonar infarction.

Arrhythmias are common; atrial fibrillation occurs in around 20% of patients and reduces cardiac function further. The incidence of ventricular arrhythmias varies from 77% to 36% for complex arrhythmias and from 60% to 15% for non-sustained ventricular tachycardia. Ventricular tachycardia with symptoms may be a presenting feature of dilated cardiomyopathy. Complex ventricular arrhythmias occur in 49% of cases, less complex ones in 95%. Patients are often asymptomatic in recorded episodes of non-sustained ventricular tachycardia [8]. Twenty-four hour or, better, 48 ECG tape monitoring in an essential investigation in dilated cardiomyopathy (see Chap. 5 for risk assessment).

Blood Investigations

In the early stages of dilated cardiomyopathy the results of full blood count and biochemical studies are normal, and no significant abnormalities have been identified or regarded as a cause of the disease. In the late stages hepatic function deteriorates and liver function tests show abnormalities.

Electrocardiography

The electrocardiographic changes are frequently non-specific: tachycardia, low voltage with flattening or inversion of T waves over the left precordium (Fig. 2.1). The P waves may suggest left or right atrial enlargement if atrial fibrillation is absent. High-voltage R waves indicate the left ventricular hypertrophy that is always present in some degree. The frontal plane axis is usually neutral unless pulmonary embolism has deviated it to the right or there is an atrioventricular conduction defect. Left bundle branch block (but rarely right bundle branch block) is a well-recognised feature. Occasionally prominent Q waves are seen, suggestive of anterior myocardial infarction, but there is usually no ST segment elevation. The explanation is either diffuse myocardial damage leading to loss of positive vector forces or anterior regional necrosis produced by viral myocarditis. In spite of the frequency of ventricular arrhythmias, these are rarely seen on standard resting electrocardiograms.

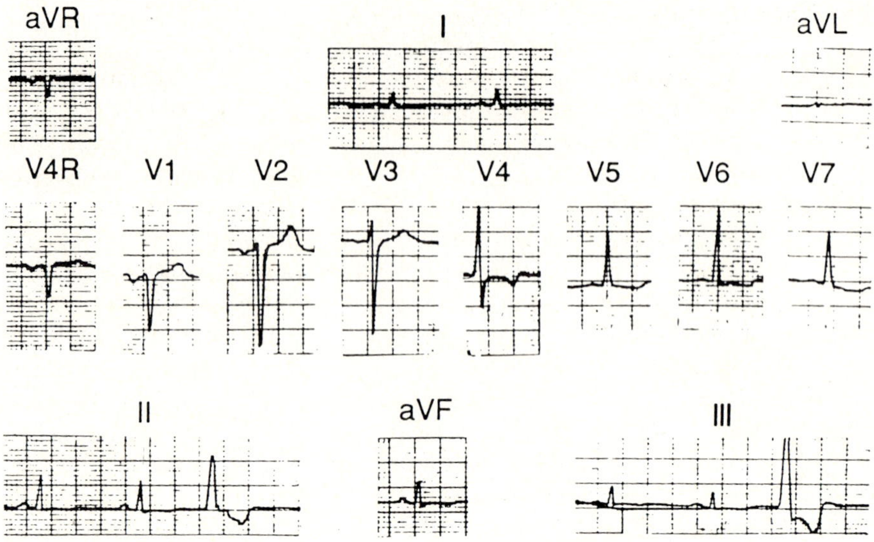

Fig. 2.1. Electrocardiogram in dilated cardiomyopathy. There is low voltage of QRS in limb leads, inversion of T in V_4 and flattening of T in V_5–V_7 and limb leads. Two ventricular ectopic beats are seen

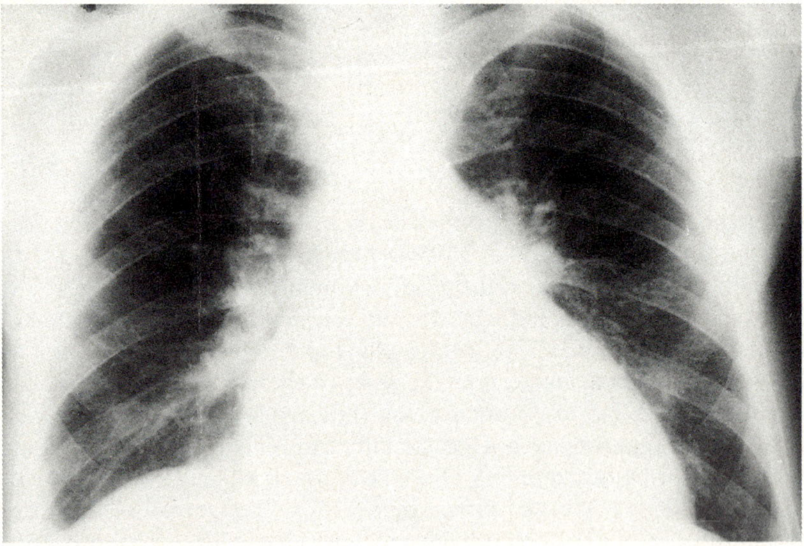

Fig. 2.2. Six-foot posture anterior chest radiograph in dilated cardiomyopathy showing massive generalised cardiac enlargement and enlarged main pulmonary arteries

Chest Radiography

The cardiac silhouette may not be enlarged on the chest radiograph in the early stages and the lung fields are normal. Later, the heart is enlarged (Fig. 2.2) and there may be evidence of pulmonary venous hypertension with dilatation of upper lobe vessels, narrowing of lower lobe vessels and horizontal costophrenic lines. If pulmonary embolism has occurred there will be distension of the main pulmonary arteries and areas of reduced vascularity alternating with increased transradiancy in the lung fields. Pulmonary infarcts can produce any type of localised opacity including interlobular effusions, linear atelectasis and wedge-shaped areas of consolidation.

Complications

The commonest complication is *embolism* arising from a thrombus in one of the cardiac chambers. Intraventricular thrombosis is favoured by dilatation of the cavity and poor contractility, while atrial thrombus is encouraged by atrial fibrillation which greatly increases the risk of embolism.

Both pulmonary embolism and systemic embolism may occur. The former tends to cause brief attacks of dyspnoea due to hyperventilation, spikes of fever and short episodes of impairment of consciousness. Systemic embolism is commonly cerebral but may be directed to limb, mesenteric, renal or other arterial distributions with appropriate symptoms. An acute abdominal emergency in a patient with dilated cardiomyopathy who is in atrial fibrillation should prompt consideration of this diagnosis.

Infective endocarditis is rare in dilated cardiomyopathy but can occur on mitral or tricuspid valves. Symptoms begin insidiously with low fever, lassitude, general malaise and anaemia. Infective endocarditis may precipitate or aggravate heart failure, and can cause acute valve failure with resultant pulmonary oedema. Mycotic arterial aneurysms as a result of infected embolism can rupture, but rarely do so when the infection is controlled.

Deep venous thrombosis of the lower extremity is a complication due to the continued effects of congestive heart failure and immobilisation. It is an important cause of pulmonary embolism, but probably less frequent than thrombus in the right heart. Valvular lesions, apart from mitral and tricuspid dilatation, are unusual, but aortic regurgitation is a well-recognised complication, the cause of which is obscure.

Differential Diagnosis

The differential diagnosis is mainly from coronary heart disease and from specific heart muscle disease producing a syndrome similar to dilated cardiomyopathy. Of particular importance is thyrotoxicosis which, in older patients, may give rise to heart failure with rapid atrial fibrillation but without overt signs of thyrotoxicosis. In such patients an important clue is the warmth and vasodilatation of the extremities, suggesting a high rather than a low cardiac output with its accompanying vasoconstriction. Less common conditions that must be distinguished from dilated cardiomyopathy are silent aortic stenosis and mitral stenosis in patients when heart failure and low cardiac output conceal the signs of severe valve disease. The late stage of hypertrophic cardiomyopathy with ventricular dilatation and congestive heart failure may present a picture closely similar to dilated cardiomyopathy. Finally, amyloid disease is an important though rare cause of congestive heart failure (see Parts II, III and IV).

Specific Heart Muscle Disease

Myocardial disorders which are part of a general system disease fall into the category of specific heart muscle disease. Most produce a dilated poorly contracting, moderately hypertrophied cardiac state with progressive congestive heart failure and low cardiac output. Specific heart muscle disease may be grouped into infiltrative disease, connective tissue disorders, granulomas, infection, poisons, allergic phenomena, metabolic disorders, and neuromuscular and endocrine conditions [2, 9]. Myocarditis will be mentioned later. In assessing any patient with congestive heart failure of obscure cause, it is important to enquire carefully about exposure to toxic substances, alcohol intake and drug abuse, in addition to eliciting symptoms of heart failure and cardiac abnormalities. On examination, signs of specific heart muscle disease should be sought specifically, such as glycosuria, skin lesions, pigmentation, arthritic changes, splenomegaly, lymphadenopathy, salivary gland enlargement, sicca syndrome, neurological abnormalities, muscle wasting or fibrillation, ocular abnormalities, signs of thyroid dysfunction and anaemia. A diagnosis of hyperthyroidism requires exclusion of a phaeochromocytoma.

Late Stage of Hypertrophic Cardiomyopathy

When heart failure has developed in hypertrophic cardiomyopathy the ventricles may dilate and the clinical picture, especially if there is atrial fibrillation, is indistinguishable from dilated cardiomyopathy. A strong family history of hypertrophic cardiomyopathy and a poorly contracting (though dilated) left ventricle may provide clues, but the diagnosis usually depends on further investigation.

Coronary Heart Disease

The main points that differentiate coronary heart disease from dilated cardiomyopathy are evidence of arterial disease elsewhere (peripheral or carotid), abnormal carbohydrate tolerance, and evidence of abnormal lipid metabolism, such as cholesterol deposits on the skin. However, many patients with coronary heart disease do not have definite signs of the disease and diagnosis may be extremely difficult without coronary arteriography. In the syndrome inaccurately known as "ischaemic cardiomyopathy" (in which severe coronary artery disease masquerades as dilated cardiomyopathy because of lack of history of angina or myocardial infarction) coronary arteriography shows severe coronary artery disease. Diabetes mellitus may be associated.

Amyloid Heart Disease

Amyloid heart disease can resemble hypertrophic or dilated cardiomyopathy or coronary heart disease. Chest pain is not uncommon in amyloid disease, congestive heart failure occurs and the ECG may show q waves. Clinical examination (supported by echocardiography) indicates diastolic faults, notably signs suggesting a restrictive state with the jugular venous pulse showing prominent a and v waves with sharp x and y descents. But a third heart sound, so common in restrictive cardiomyopathy and constrictive pericarditis, is usually absent [10] (see part IV).

Hypertension

Slight elevation of blood pressure is common in dilated cardiomyopathy; repeatedly high levels and evidence of hypertensive complications (retinopathy, stroke and renal impairment) suggest a diagnosis of hypertensive heart disease rather than dilated cardiomyopathy. Dilatation of the left ventricle tends to be greater, and hypertrophy less, in dilated cardiomyopathy than in hypertensive heart disease. Phaeochromocytoma should be excluded if there is hypertension.

Myocarditis

Viral myocarditis and its relation to dilated cardiomyopathy will be fully covered in Chap. 3 and Part VI.

From the clinical aspect, the differentiation between dilated cardiomyopathy and myocarditis may be more apparent than real, since the evidence suggests that up to 50% of cases of dilated cardiomyopathy can be due to preceding viral myocarditis, and that an episode of acute viral myocarditis may lead to the clinical and haemodynamic syndrome of dilated cardiomyopathy. From the aspect of clinical diagnosis, a short history and symptoms suggestive of a virus infection followed by heart failure suggest that dilated cardiomyopathy has been caused by or precipitated by a virus. Confirmation can only be obtained by special tests and viral studies; endomyocardial biopsy is a crucial investigation (see Chaps. 1 and 15).

There are several pathways that acute viral myocarditis may take [11]: complete recovery (95+%); rapid death from circulatory collapse and heart failure; progression to dilated cardiomyopathy within a matter of months; and apparent recovery followed by a latent period and then slow development of dilated cardiomyopathy due to an immunological syndrome set up by the infection [12–15].

Acute Viral Myocarditis (see part VI, Chaps. 1–3)

Symptoms of acute viral myocarditis are commonly those of influenza: upper respiratory tract infection, aching muscles, general malaise. The Coxsackie group of viruses is probably the commonest to be involved in myocarditis/dilated cardiomyopathy, and produces symptoms of encephalitis with headache or gastrointestinal disturbance also. In fulminant cases there is circulatory failure with hypotension, dyspnoea and chest pain, the last sometimes due to associated pericarditis. Physical signs are those of tachycardia out of proportion to the fever, thready arterial pulse of small volume, raised jugular venous pressure, hepatomegaly and rales at the bases of the lungs. Pulmonary oedema may occur. Auscultation usually reveals summation gallop and often there is a pericardial friction rub. Cardiac tamponade is suggested if the jugular venous pressure rises and the arterial pressure falls on inspiration, the heart sounds are faint and the cardiac impulse feeble with displacement of the apex beat outside the left mid-clavicular line. Atrial fibrillation, supraventricular tachycardia, ventricular tachycardia and occasionally complete heart block may occur. Death is often sudden.

The Electrocardiogram shows flat or inverted T waves, and ST elevation if pericarditis is present. T wave changes do not necessarily imply myocarditis and may be due to pericarditis alone.

Chest radiography shows cardiomyopathy, which can be due either to dilatation of the heart or pericardial effusion or both. Evidence of a raised left atrial pressure or shadows of pulmonary oedema may be present.

Virus Myocarditis and Myocardial Infarction

Occasionally acute myocarditis produces regional left ventricular involvement rather than diffuse myocardial damage and gives a picture akin to acute myocardial infarction [16] with appropriate symptoms and electrocardiographic and enzyme changes. Diagnosis depends upon confirmation of a virus infection and demonstration of normal coronary arteries on angiography.

Dilated Cardiomyopathy in Children

Although rare, dilated cardiomyopathy in children is a serious problem. The usual presentation is heart failure which may follow an upper respiratory tract infection. Some patients are detected earlier because of unexpected cardiomegaly on radiography or an abnormal ECG. About 80% present with heart failure, 5% with arrhythmia and 5% with asymptomatic cardiac enlargement [17, 18]. The disease in children is similar to that in adults with survival at 1 year of 57% and 5 years of 47%. Children under 2 years may have a worse prognosis than older children.

Right Ventricular Dysplasia, Arrhythmogenic Right Ventricular Cardiomyopathy, Right Ventricular Arrhythmic Dysplasia

These terms are commonly employed synonymously (though not always correctly) to denote a syndrome of dilated fibrotic right ventricle (which may or may not be atrophied), and fibrolipomatous degeneration and changes in myocytes. The principle clinical feature is repetitive malignant ventricular arrhythmia, although heart failure and sudden death are well recognised [19, 20], The left ventricle is in some cases slightly involved (see Chap. 13).

References

1. Goodwin JF (1970) Congestive and hypertrophic cardiomyopathies: a decade of study. Lancet 1:731
2. WHO/ISFC Task Force (1980) Report on the definition and classification of cardiomyopathies. Br Heart J 44:672
3. Brandenburg RO (1985) Dilated (congestive) cardiomyopathy: clinical aspects, treatment and prognosis. In: Goodwin JF (ed) Heart muscle disease. MTP Press, Lancaster, pp 75–86
4. Obesekere I (1968) Idiopathic cardiomegaly in Ceylon. Br Heart J 30:226–235
5. Torp A (1978) Incidence of congestive cardiomegaly. Postgrad Med J 54:435–439
6. Williams DG, Olsen EGJ (1985) Prevalence of overt dilated cardiomyopathy in two regions of England. Br Heart J 54:153–155
7. Richardson P, Wodak AA (1983) Alcohol-induced heart muscle disease. In: Symons C, Evans T, Mitchell AG (eds) Specific heart muscle disease. Wright, Bristol, p 99
8. Gavazzi A, de Maria R, Caralli A, di Lenarda A, Veritti U, Miami D, Sinagra G, Luvini M, Ometto R, Borgia M, Ciaccheri M, Campana C, Graziano G, Lanzareni L, Gronda E, Camerini F (1990) Complex ventricular arrhythmias in dilated cardiomyopathy: a multicentre Italian experience. In: Baroldi G, Camerini F, Goodwin JF (eds) Advances in cardiomyopathy. Springer Berlin Heidelberg New York, pp 354–367
9. Wengger NK (1985) Specific heart muscle disease. In: Goodwin JF (ed) Heart muscle disease. MTP Press, Lancaster, pp 95–122
10. Oakley CM (1985) Amyloid Heart disease. In: Goodwin JF (ed) Heart muscle disease. MTP Press, Lancaster, pp 141–153
11. Goodwin JF (1983) Myocarditis as a possible cause of cardiomyopathy. In: Just H, Schuster HP (eds) Myocarditis and cardiomyopathies. Springer, Berlin Heidelberg New York, pp 7–11
12. Kawai C (1971) Idiopathic cardiomyopathy: A study on the infection–immune theory as a cause of the disease. Jpn Circ J 33: 765–770

13. Goodwin JF (1988) Virological, immunological and clinical features of myocarditis and dilated cardiomyopathy. In: Schultheiss H-P (ed) New concepts in viral heart disease. Springer, Berlin Heidelberg New York
14. Miklozek Cl, Come TC, Royal HD, Crumpacker CS, Abelman WH (1984) Viral heart disease: a precurser of congestive cardiomyopathy. In: Bolte H-D (ed) Viral heart disease. Springer, Berlin Heidelberg New York, pp 95–98
15. Sekiguchi M, Hiroe M, Nunoda S, Hongo M, Misawa T (1990) Natural history of viral myocarditis: critical viewpoints. In: Baroldi G, Camerini F, Goodwin JF (eds) Advances in cardiomyopathies. Springer, Berlin Heidelberg New York, pp 302–315
16. Thomas M, Slocum N, Nichols AC (1984) Relations between virus infections and coronary artery disease. In: Bolte H-D (eds) Viral heart disease. Springer, Berlin Heidelberg New York, pp 217–222
17. Taliercio CP (1990) Dilated cardiomyopathy in children. In: Baroldi G, Camerini F, Goodwin JF (eds) Advances in cardiomyopathies. Springer, Berlin Heidelberg New York, pp 391–396
18. Fuster V, Gersh BJ, Guillani ER, Tajik AJ, Brandenburg RO, Frye RL (1981) The natural history of idiopathic dilated cardiomyopathy. Am J Cardiol 47: 525–531
19. Thiene G, Nava A, Angelini A, Daliento L, Scognamiglio R, Corrada D (1990) Anatomoclinical aspects of arrhythmogenic right ventricular cardiomyopathy. In: Baroldi G, Camerini F, Goodwin JF (eds) Advances in cardiomyopathies. Springer, Berlin Heidelberg New York, pp 397–408
20. Dalla-Volta S (1990) Right ventricular arrhythmogenic cardiomyopathy: the clinical point of view. In: Baroldi G, Camerini F, Goodwin JF (eds) Advances in cardiomyopathies. Springer, Berlin Heidelberg New York, pp 409–415

CHAPTER 3

Pathology

E. G. J. Olsen and S. E. Trotter

The term "dilated cardiomyopathy" is preferable to the previously used term, "congestive cardiomyopathy", because dilatation may be present for many years without patients having signs and symptoms of congestion.

Macroscopic Appearance

Classically, the heart weight is occasionally double the normal value for the patient's sex and height [1]. All chambers are severely dilated and measurements of ventricular (and atrial) walls frequently fall within normal limits, despite the hypertrophy which is invariably present, the dilatation masking the degree of hypertrophy. Caution should therefore be exercised in recording and interpreting degrees of hypertrophy in the presence of chamber dilatation. The heart muscle is often pale and flabby and scarring of the ventricular walls may not infrequently be observed [2].

The endocardium is frequently thickened and has a white appearance. Normally, the endocardium gives the cavities a glossy appearance, due to the fact that the ventricular endocardium is, at its thickest, 20 μm. Any whiteness in the ventricular chambers indicates abnormal thickening, which in dilated cardiomyopathy is haphazardly distributed.

Not infrequently thrombus is superimposed due to the poorly contracting ventricles. Thrombi are usually in the apex, but may be encountered anywhere else in the ventricles (and atria) [3, 4]. Extramural coronary arteries are usually free from atherosclerotic plaques or narrowing but, with rare exceptions, some coronary arterial disease may be encountered [5].

The morphological diagnosis of dilated cardiomyopathy can only definitely be made at post-mortem, having excluded all possible entities that may give rise to a hypertrophied, dilated myocardium.

Histology

The myocardial fibres are in normal regular alignment. Nuclear changes of hypertrophy exemplified by pyknosis or vesicular changes and blunting of the nuclear poles are often striking. Despite these clear nuclear changes, the myocardial fibres may be of normal, or less than normal, diameter (up to 14 μm) due to their being stretched. That stretching does occur has been well documented by Hort [6]. The interstitium is frequently widened, predominantly due to an increase in collagen fibres, which may vary from mild to severe, is frequently focal in distribution and most prominent in the subendocardial regions. Not uncommonly, lymphocytes are found in these areas, but may also be seen in the widened interstitium without evidence of fibrosis. The increase in collagen tissue may be so severe as to replace groups of myocytes following necrosis of these cells.

Intramural vessels are usualy normal, but there are well-documented reports of small vessel involvement [7, 8]; however, apart from some increase in thickening of the wall and intimal thickening not obstructing the lumen, this is all that has been personally observed, particularly in areas of fibrosis. These statements are based on examination of hearts post-mortem or on tissue obtained by bioptome (personal observation). The thickened endocardium is due to an increase in collagen and elastic fibres, but if dilatation has been present for some time (more than 6 weeks) there is an increase in the smooth muscle component and this finding may occasionally be striking in long-standing cases.

Histochemistry

Substances such as glycogen and succinic dehydrogenase are usually reduced, but this is dependent on the degree of dilatation and/or heart failure.

Ultrastructure

At the ultrastructural level of investigation, which usually requires fresh tissue acquired by biopsy for best results, the description will be based on the tissue thus obtained. In post-mortem tissue, autolytic changes may distort the appearance. Essentially, the myofibrils are in parallel alignment. There is an increase in the numbers of mitochondria, which may be smaller than normal, to more than one mitochondrion per two sarcomeres; depending on the degree of hypertrophy, three or four mitochondria per two sarcomeres is not unusual. Folding of the nuclear membrane is found as well as degenerative changes, exemplified by myelin bodies, membrane-bound vesicles and focal dissolution of actin ad myosin, together with widening of the intercalated discs. Dilatation of the transverse tubular system and sarcoplasmic reticulum together with an increase in lipofuscin granules are typical findings. Capillaries are normal, but oedema in their walls may occasionally be observed, interpreted as a non-specific finding. The interstitium is widened and shows oedema, and an increase in collagen fibrils and cellular elements (including macrophages and lymphocytes) may be encountered [9–11].

This description applies to severely dilated hearts. Unfortunately, patients may die at any stage and therefore may show hypertrophy alone or accompanied by some mild degree of dilatation. In these cases attenuation of myofibres may be absent or minimal. Interstitial collagen tissue may also not be increased and endocardial changes may be absent or mild. Histochemically, an increased normal distribution of substances examined, such as glycogen and succinic dehydrogenase, and ultrastructural changes of mild hypertrophy without degenerative changes is all that may be discerned.

Morphometric Studies

Assessment of hypertrophy has included experimental studies of hypertrophy obtained by stenosing the ascending or abdominal aorta, banding of the suprarenal abdominal aorta, banding of the pulmonary artery, swimming tests, treadmill exercises, aorto-caval fistula, induction of renal hypertension, administration of hormones such as thyroxine and triiodothyroacetic acid, and the production of anaemia. These various studies have previously been summarised [1–2]. Measurements of wall thickness in humans are unreliable in view of dilatation. Total heart weight is also not an accurate assessment because of varying degrees of epicardial fat, and more reliable information can be obtained by separating the right ventricular free wall and expressing the weights in relation to both that chamber and the left ventricle, including the interventricular septum. These weights are recorded after removing the valves, aorta, pulmonary trunk and atria, as well the epicardial fat [13].

Attempts to relate morphological changes to clinical parameters such as length of history, left ventricular end-diastolic pressure and ejection fraction have yielded contradictory results from various workers. Some studies have yielded no correlations, others have found excellent correlation [14–16]. Assessment of myofibres has shown only partial correlation [17]. As far as prognosis is concerned both light and electron microscopy have yielded useful information. Tangenelli et al. [18] noted that the area of myocardial cells was prognostically significant on light microscopy, whilst Hammond et al. [19] recorded that myofibrillar loss ultrastructurally was a helpful finding in predicting the clinical outcome.

Biopsy Examination and Differential Diagnosis

Morphological parameters have been assessed in endomyocardial biopsy samples. Endomyocardial biopsies from over 2000 patients (average 2.8 biopsies per patient) with a presumptive diagnosis of dilated cardiomyopathy have been personally examined (EGJO). Diseases mimicking dilated cardiomyopathy, such as heart failure due to alcohol abuse and other specific heart muscle diseases characterised by heart failure, can be excluded by additional investigations on the same tissue samples.

One other important morphological change, namely that due to myocarditis, can also be recognised. The reported incidence of myocarditis varies greatly (3%–65%) [20]. This wide range has been variously attributed to the timing of the biopsy, seasonal variation and also to the interpretation of morphological changes. Lymphocytes per se do not necessarily indicate myocarditis as lymphocytes have been found in normal hearts. It is the presence of lymphocytes and the proximity of these cells to adjacent myocytes, as well as changes in the interstitium, which together permit a diagnosis of myocarditis to be made. Furthermore, one of us (EGJO) has developed a categorisation of these stages of inflammation into "acute healing" and "healed" [21]. The latter categorisation could only be used if a previous biopsy showing more active stages of myocarditis had been found. In view of the variety of interpretation exemplified by interchange of biopsies between experienced pathologists [22], a group of pathologists was called to Dallas, Texas, to lay down criteria and to ensure uniformity in interpreting endomyocardial biopsies and myocarditis for a multicentre National Institutes of Health myocarditis treatment trial. The criteria that were laid down are now referred to as the Dallas criteria [23]; they are based on the criteria previously defined, but with minor alterations [24].

Definition of Myocarditis

Myocarditis is characterised by an inflammatory infiltrate of the myocardium with necrosis and/or degeneration of adjacent myocytes, not typical of ischaemic damage due to coronary arterial disease, and classified into the following categories:

First Biopsy

1. *Myocarditis with/without fibrosis.*
2. *Borderline (repeat biopsy may be advisable).* This category is applied when the changes are sparse.
3. *No mycarditis.*
4. *Acute myocarditis.* This consists of an often intense, chronic inflammatory cell infiltrate with the inflammatory cells in intimate contact with adjacent myocytes and producing an irregular outline of their contours due to necrotic changes. Occasionally, the cells may be entirely necrotic. The distribution of the inflammatory cells may be confluent or focal and, usually, interstitial collagen tissue is not increased.

Subsequent Biopsies

1. *Ongoing (persistent) myocarditis.* This term implies that the biopsy under investigation shows at least as much damage to myofibrils and an equal severity of inflammatory cell infiltrate as the most recent biopsy.

2. *Resolving (healing) myocarditis.* The inflammation has been greatly reduced in severity and inflammatory cells are not in intimate contact with adjacent myocytes. In the early phases of this stage a few areas of necrosis could still be observed.
3. *Resolved (healed) myocarditis.* The cellular infiltrate has almost disappeared, although a few chronic inflammatory cells may still be identified, usually confined to areas of fibrosis. This varies in degree and distribution. Fibrosis may accompany any stage of the inflammatory process but is most frequently seen in the healed stage. The cellular infiltrate consists predominantly of chronic inflammatory cells, especially lymphocytes, but neutrophils, eosinophils and macrophages may dominate the morphological picture.

It was initially suggested that myocarditis should only be diagnosed in the acute phase. Whereas this applied to the entry for the multicentre study, experience has shown that even if the first biopsy is in the healing phase diagnosis can confidently be made. Once the healed stage is reached, however, myocarditis cannot be diagnosed despite persistence of a few chronic inflammatory cells. *This stage can only be accurately categorised if a previous biopsy showing an earlier stage has been examined.* Despite the criteria laid down may pitfalls remain, including interpretation of the site of a previous biopsy, and the examiner, however experienced, should be aware of the difficulties [24].

Categorisation of myocarditis is important for it has therapeutic implications that are discussed elsewhere (see Chaps. 1, 4 and 14–16). Inflammatory cellular infiltrates occur in a number of other disease processes, such as drug-related hypersensitivity, toxicity and organising infarction [25]. The differential diagnosis in the latter is usually easy. In myocarditis the lymphocytes are in contact with adjacent myofibrils showing nuclei, whereas in coronary heart disease, by the time the lymphocytes make their appearance the nuclei of the myocytes are absent. Though morphological interpretation is often made without referring to the clinical history, full detailed clinical information, including therapy, should always be available. Evidence continues to accumulate on the relationship between viral myocarditis and dilated cardiomyopathy at experimental level and in man [26–28] (see Chap. 15). It was not until the hybridisation probe was applied to endomyocardial tissue obtained by bioptome (see Chap. 15) [29, 30] that association with virus could be documented clearly.

Differential Diagnosis

Alcoholic Heart Muscle Disease

The morphological changes described above apply in every detail to both myocarditis and heart failure attributable to high alcohol intake. In a series of previous reports, in 21% of 104 clinical cases a history of alcoholism could be obtained [31]. This emphasises again the necessity of a detailed clinical history. In an autopsy series of 128 cases a history of alcohol was present in 45% [2].

There are several pathways of alcohol abuse affecting the heart, among which the direct toxic effect [32], metabolism of alcohol in the form of acetaldehyde and associated nutritional factors may all play a role. The amount of alcohol imbibed also varies with individuals. It has been suggested that if 7 g/day were imbibed heart failure may result [33]. As far as morphology is concerned the changes are identical at all levels of investigation, including ultrastructural changes. Though differences between dilated cardiomyopathy and heart failure due to alcohol abuse have from time to time been described in the past, differentiation is, in our opinion, impossible. It may be mentioned that toxic additives, such as cobalt to beer, may have invoked cardiac disease [34]. (see Chaps. 1, 2 and 4).

Peripartal Heart Disease

Peripartal heart disease usually occurs during the third trimester or at any stage following delivery up to 3 months [35]. Cardiac changes identical to dilated cardiomyopathy occur. The aetiology is unknown, and it may be that pregnancy unmasks a pending cardiomyopathy. This condition should only be diagnosed if eclampsia, post-partum hypertension and tribal customs can be excluded. Myocarditis, similar to that found in dilated cardiomyopathy, plays a role in a substantial number of cases as, for example, reported in a joint study with cases from East Africa [36] (see Chap. 13).

In conclusion, the term dilated cardiomyopathy should only be used if causal agents cannot be identified and, although the changes are non-specific, a morphological diagnosis can be achieved in conjunction with either a full post-mortem examination or a clinical evaluation. Causal agents may not always be recognised initially; a good example is Kashan disease, where selenium deficiency causes changes similar to dilated cardiomyopathy [37].

References

1. Zeek PM (1942) Heart weight. I. The weight of the normal human heart. Arch Pathol 34: 820–832
2. Roberts WC, Siegel RJ, McManus BM (1987) Idiopathic dilated cardiomyopathy: analysis of 152 necropsy patients. Am J Cardiol 60: 1340–1355
3. Olsen EGJ (1972) Cardiomyopathies. Cardiovasc Clin 4: 240–261
4. Olsen EGJ (1981) Pathology of congestive cardiomyopathy. In: Goodwin JF, Hjalmarson A, Olsen EGJ (eds) Congestive cardiomyopathy, Hassle, Molndal, pp 66–74
5. Gau GT, Goodwin JF, Oakley CM, Olsen EGJ, Rahimtoola SH, Raphael MJ, Steiner RE (1972) Q waves and coronary arteriography in cardiomyopathy. Br Heart J 34: 1034–1041
6. Hort W (1967) Funktionelle Morphologie der akuten Herzinsuffizienz. Verh Dtsch Ges Pathol 51: 114–124
7. James TN (1964) An aetiologic concept concerning the obscure cardiomyopathies. Prog Cardiovasc Dis 7: 43–64

8. Factor SM, Cho S, Sonnenblick EH (1981) Verapamil treatment of cardiomyopathic Syrian hamsters: effects on the microcirculation and the extent of myocardial necrosis. Fed Proc 40: 758
9. Olsen EGJ (1978) Special investigations of COCM: endomyocardial biopsies (morphological analysis). Postgrad Med J 54: 486–490
10. Kunkel B, Lapp H, Kober G, Kaltenbach M (1978) Ultrastructural evaluation in early and advanced congestive cardiomyopathies. In: Kaltenbach M, Loogen F, Olsen EGJ, Bussman W-D (eds) Cardiomyopathy and myocardial biopsy. Springer, Berlin Heidelberg New York, pp 87–99
11. Ferrans VJ (1989) Pathological anatomy of dilated cardiomyopathies. Am J Cardiol 64: 9c–11c
12. Olsen EGJ (1980) The pathology of the heart 2nd edn. Macmillan, Basingstoke, pp 41–55
13. Fulton RM, Hutchinson EC, Morgan Jones A (1952) Ventricular weight in cardiac hypertrophy. Br Heart J 14: 413–420
14. Baandrup U, Florio RA, Rehahn M, Richardson PJ, Olsen EGJ (1981) Critical analysis of endomyocardial biopsies from patients suspected of having cardiomyopathy. II. Comparison of histological clinical haemodynamic information. Br Heart J 45: 487–493
15. Baandrup U, Florio RA, Roter, Olsen EGJ (1981) Electron microscopic investigation of endomyocardial biopsy samples in hypertrophy and cardiomyopathy: a semiquantitative study in 48 Patients. Circulation 63: 1289–1298
16. Kunkel B, Schneider M, Kober G, Bussman WD, Hopf R, Kaltenbach M (1982) Myocardial biopsy: morphological analysis and clinical implications. Z Kardiol 71: 787–794
17. Figulla HR, Rahlf G, Nieger M, Luig H, Kreuzer H (1985) Spontaneous hemodynamic improvement or stabilization and associated biopsy findings in patients with congestive cardiomyopathy. Circulation 71: 1095–1104
18. Tangenelli P, di Lenarda A, Bianciardi G, Salvi A, Silvestri F, Mestroni L, Camerini F (1989) Correlation between histomorphometric findings on endomyocardial biopsy and clinical findings in idiopathic dilated cardiomyopathy. Am J Cardiol 64: 504–506
19. Hammond EH, Menlove RL, Anderson JL (1987) Predictive value of immunofluorescence and electron microscopy in the diagnosis and prognosis of myocarditis and idiopathic dilated cardiomyopathy. Am Heart J 114: 1055–1065
20. Olsen EGJ, Meany BT, Richardson PJ (1988) The role of biopsy in the diagnosis and follow-up of myocarditis: a critical review. In: Schultheiss H-P (ed) New concepts in viral heart disease. Springer, Berlin Heidelberg New York, pp 285–294
21. Olsen EGJ (1981) Panel discussion. In: Goodwin JF, Hjalmarson A, Olsen EGJ (eds) Congestive cardiomyopathy. Hassle, Molndal, p 122
22. Shanes JG, Ghali J, Billingham ME et al. (1987) Interobserver variability in the pathologic interpretation of endomyocardial biopsy results. Circulation 75: 401–405
23. Aretz HT, Billingham ME, Edwards WD, Factor SM, Fallon JT, Fenoglio JJ, Olsen EGJ, Schoen FJ (1987) Myocarditis: a histopathologic definition and classification. Am J Cardiovasc Pathol 1: 3–13
24. Atkinson JB, Virmani R (1991) The endomyocardial biopsy: techniques, indications and limitations. In: Virmani R, Atkinson JB, Fenoglio JJ (eds) Cardiovascular pathology. Saunders, London, pp 203–219 (Major problems in pathology, Vol 23)
25. Aretz T (1991) Myocarditis: the Dallas criteria. In: Virmani R, Atkinson JB, Fenoglio JJ (eds) Cardiovascular pathology. (Major problems in pathology, vol 23) Saunders, London, pp 246–256
26. Sekiguchi M, Hiroe M, Hiramitusu S, Izumi T (1988) Natural history of acute viral or idiopathic myocarditis: a clinical and endomyocardial biopsy follow-up. In: Schultheiss H-P (ed) New concepts in viral heart disease. Springer, Berlin Heidelberg New York, pp 33–50
27. Kawai C, Matsumori A, Fujiwara H (1987) Myocarditis and dilated cardiomyopathy. Annu Rev Med 38: 221–239
28. Matoba Y, Matsumori A, Ohtani H, Tominaga M, Fujiwara H, Toyokuni S (1990) A case of biopsy proven myocarditis progressing to autopsy proven dilated cardiomyopathy. Clin Cardiol 13: 732–737

29. Bowles NE, Richardson PJ, Olsen EGJ, Archard LC (1986) Detection of Coxsackie B virus specific RNA sequences in myocardial biopsy samples from patients with myocarditis and dilated cardiomyopathy. Lancet 1: 1120–1122
30. Lansdown ABG (1978) Viral infections and diseases of the heart. Prog Med Virol 24: 70–113
31. Fuster V, Gersh BJ, Guiliani ER et al. (1981) The natural history of idopathic dilated cardiomyopathy. Am J Cardiol 47: 525–531
32. Klein H, Harmjanz D (1975) Effect of ethanol on the ultrastructure of human myocardium. Postgrad Med J 51: 325–329
33. Richardson PJ, Atkinson L (1981) The aetiological separation of the congestive cardiomyopathies using the measurement of myocardial enzyme activities in biopsy samples. In: Goodwin JF, Hjalmarson A, Olsen EGJ (eds) Congestive cardiomyopathy. Hassle, Molndal, pp 103–110
34. Rona G, Chappel C (1973) Pathogenesis and pathology of cobalt cardiomyopathy. Recent Adv Stud Cardiac Struct Metab 2: 407–422
35. WHO Expert Committee (1984) Peripartal heart disease. WHO Tech Rep Ser 697: 47–50
36. Sanderson JE, Olsen EGJ, Gatei D (1986) Peripartum heart disease. An endomyocardial biopsy study. Br Heart J 56: 285–291
37. WHO Expert Committee (1984) Keshan disease (in China). In: WHO Tech Rep Ser 697: 55–57

CHAPTER 4

Clinical Investigation: New Approaches

P. J. Richardson and H. J. F. Why

Introduction

In dilated cardiomyopathy there is impairment of systolic function, ventricular dilatation and myocardial hypertrophy [1]. Following the first use of the term "cardiomyopathy", the investigation of the patient has become increasingly sophisticated. The initial classification was based on the ability of the clinician to define the anatomical structure and function following routine cardiac catheterisation including coronary arteriography. This level of investigation has now been enhanced by the development of newer techniques such as echocardiography, endomyocardial biopsy (enabling histopathological examination of the myocardium) and radionuclide techniques enabling assessment of myocardial perfusion and ventricular function. The most recent technique being applied to the heart muscle diseases is MRI (magnetic resonance imaging). Recent advances in research have contributed to our understanding of the pathogenetic mechanisms of dilated cardiomyopathy by the examination of myocardial tissue obtained at catheter biopsy. In particular the application of biochemical (myocardial enzyme assay and assessment of receptor structure and function), molecular biological (enterovirus RNA probes and the polymerase chain reaction) and immunological (detection of specific antimyocardial antibodies and altered immune responses) techniques have contributed greatly to our understanding. Against this background there are, therefore, differing levels of investigation that can now be undertaken, but from the practical point of view the physician should understand the nature and limitations of these techniques in contributing to the final diagnosis.

Clinical Aspects (see Chap. 2)

The major diagnostic hurdle is to decide whether the patient may be suffering from a systemic disease which is known to involve the myocardium. Should such a condition be present then clearly the diagnosis is that of specific heart muscle disease rather than dilated cardiomyopathy (see Chap. 1). The clinical presentation in most cases of specific heart muscle disease and all cases of dilated cardiomyopathy, however, may be identical, although the precise form may differ, encompassing congestive cardiac failure, arrhythmias, embolic episodes or even sudden death. The degree of myocardial involvement in specific heart muscle disease differs considerably, and may be diffuse or localised; in some cases there may be associated valvar and/or pericardial disease. A careful history may provide evidence of nutritional deficiency, exposure to toxic agents such as the amphetamines, or treatment with the anthracycline drugs. The most commonly encountered problems relate to exposure to recent viral illness or to alcohol abuse. It is increasingly recognised, however, that infectious agents other than viruses may be responsible for the development of dilated heart muscle disease. Of particular interest in Europe (but not so far reported from the United States), is the possibility that infection with the spirochaete *Borrelia burgdorferi*, the aetiological agent of Lyme disease, may also produce a dilated and poorly contracting ventricle. Evidence for this hypothesis has been provided by serological tests [2, 3], histological examination [4, 5], and, in one case, culture of the spirochaete from an endomyocardial biopsy specimen [4]. Infection with HIV, the virus which produces AIDS, is also known to affect the heart in various ways. It may be associated with Kaposi's sarcoma or produce a direct myocarditis eventually progressing to dilated cardiomyopathy. In addition to myocarditis due directly to HIV infection, opportunistic infection with *Toxoplasma gondii* can occur [6]. Table 1.1 lists the commoner forms of specific heart muscle disease from which dilated cardiomyopathy needs to be differentiated.

The problem of the differentiation of myocarditis and dilated cardiomyopathy remains a difficult one, and consideration must be given to the role that myocarditis plays as a precursor to dilated cardiomyopathy. Over the last decade an increasing body of evidence has been published supporting a transition from myocarditis to dilated cardiomyopathy. This possibility is supported by work indicating a substantial incidence of myocarditis in patients with the clinical features of dilated cardiomyopathy in whom no history of viral or other illness is obtained; indeed, relatively poor correlation exists between clinically diagnosed myocarditis and the histological findings at endomyocardial biopsy [7–9]. The incidence of histologically proven myocarditis in reported series varies according to the criteria used to select patients for investiation, but ranges from 4.4% in one series [10] to over 60% in two others [11, 12]. In our own series the rate has varied from less than 5% in the 1970's to around 20% in the early 1980's and 35% in the period between 1985 and 1989. This variation reflects not only an alteration in the clinical indications for endomyocardial biopsy but also a variation in the incidence of viral illness within the community.

The long-term clinical follow-up of myocarditis provides evidence that dilated cardiomyopathy may often represent the end-stage of this condition. Levi et al. followed for a 15-year period a group of 68 patients who had been admitted to hospital with clinical myocarditis [13]. In 42 cases where some confirmation of the diagnosis had been provided by a fourfold rise in Coxsackie virus complement fixing antibody titre, 7 deaths with complications of dilated cardiomyopathy were recorded. In addition, a further 3 patients died of chronic myocarditis. In contrast, of the 23 patients where serological evidence of Coxsackie virus infection was lacking, no patients were shown to have evidence of dilated cardiomyopathy at follow-up. This comparison suggests that viral myocarditis may well result in dilated cardiomyopathy in a proportion of cases.

There is much evidence suggesting that an autoimmune disorder is implicated in dilated cardiomyopathy, probably as a result of previous virus myocarditis (see Part VI). A recent study by Caforio et al. [13a] demonstrated organ-specific cardiac antibodies in dilated cardiomyopathy with far greater frequency than in other forms of heart disease, lending further support to the infective–immune theory of causation in some cases.

More direct histological evidence for this disease progression is provided by a study of 23 patients with biopsy-proven acute myocarditis followed up over a 4-year period [14]. Twelve patients progressed to dilated cardiomyopathy and 4 of these 12 died. Even in those who appeared to recover, radionuclide exercise ejection fractions remained impaired in the majority, whilst the minority who regained a normal ejection fraction appeared to do so at an early stage. Thus serial biopsy and assessment of left ventricular function 6 months after presentation with acute myocarditis may distinguish those patients in whom dilated cardiomyopathy is likely to be the end result. Although it was hoped that the early histological evaluation of endomyocardial tissue might enable the prediction of the outcome, this has not proved possible in practice. In those patients where ventricular impairment remains, the healed phase of myocarditis can be histologically indistinguishable from dilated cardiomyopathy [15]. The variable haemodynamic and histological outcome of myocarditis is summarised in Fig. 4.1. There may be a progression (via a healing phase) to histological and clinical normality or to histological appearances compatible with dilated cardiomyopathy.

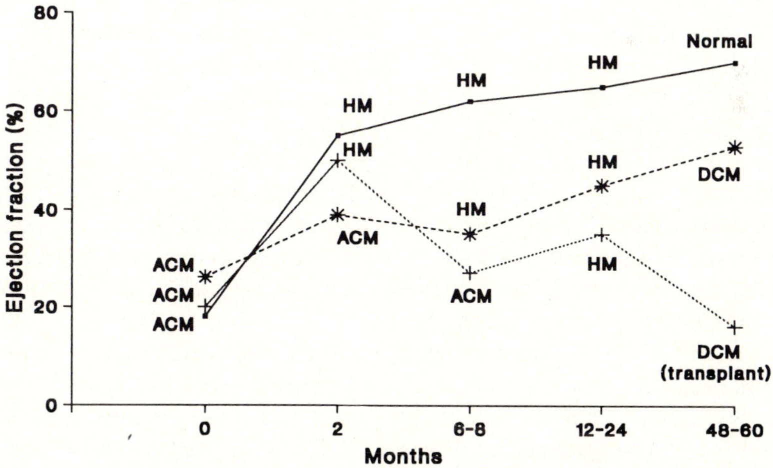

Fig. 4.1. Stylised diagram to illustrate the natural history of acute myocarditis: serial biopsy results correlating histological findings with ejection fraction and time course of the disease. *ACM*, acute myocarditis; *HM*, healing myocarditis; *DCM*, dilated cardiomyopathy

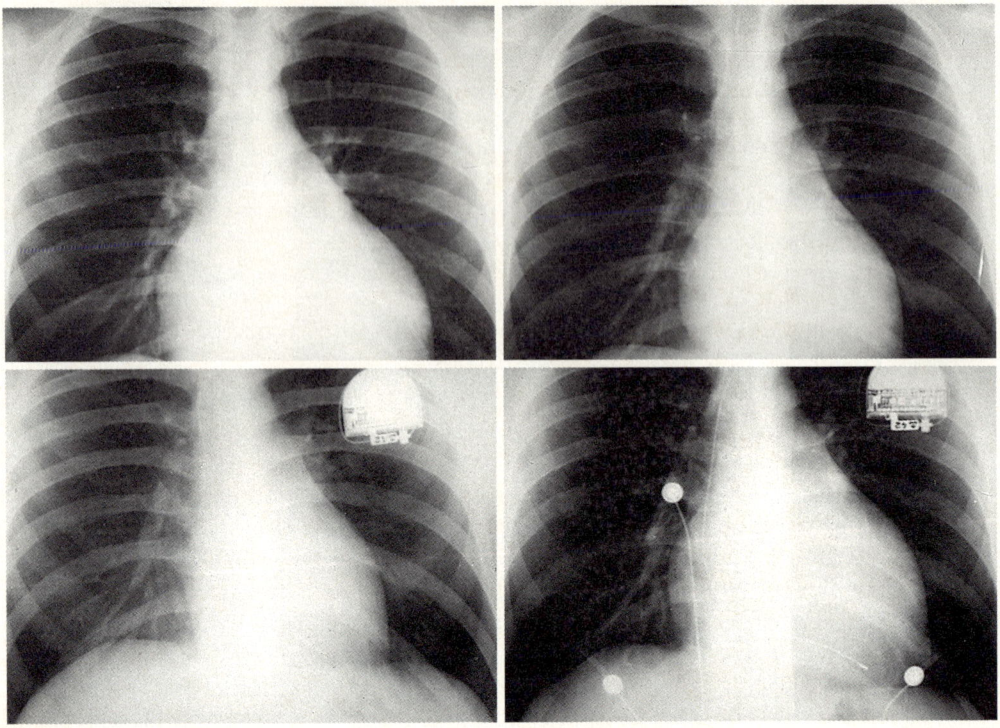

Fig. 4.2. Sequential chest radiographs from a patient with acute myocarditis.
Upper left: grossly enlarged heart at time of presentation. Histological changes of acute myocarditis were found on endomyocardial biopsy.
Upper right: repeat radiograph 2 months later showing a reduction in heart size. Repeat biopsy at this stage showed healing myocarditis.
Lower left: re-presentation with fast atrial fibrillation and ventricular tachycardia at 3 months. Histology revealed a relapse to acute myocarditis. The patient was treated with amiodarone and a ventricular pacemaker inserted.
Lower right: at 6 months in spite of a reduction in heart size left ventricular function remained impaired. Histology was compatible with a diagnosis of dilated cardiomyopathy

In these circumstances the degree of abnormality of left ventricular function may vary between moderate impairment with stable symptoms to severe, continuing dilatation and left ventricular failure requiring transplantation. It is of note that progression to the healing phase does not preclude relapse of acute myocarditis at a later date. Figure 4.2 demonstrates this pattern of natural history in a 16-year-old patient who did not receive immunosuppression.

The link between myocarditis and dilated cardiomyopathy has been further strengthened by the development of advanced molecular biological techniques for the detection of enteroviral RNA sequences within myocardial biopsy tissue samples. The application of cDNA hybridisation probes [16, 17] has enabled the detection of enterovirus in endomyocardial biopsy tissue from patients with all

Table 4.1. Incidence of enterovirus RNA in endomyocardial biopsies from patients ($n = 193$) with heart muscle disease

	Myocarditis	Dilated cardiomyopathy	Controls
RNA +ve	23 (43%)	40 (41%)	2 (5%)
RNA −ve	31	57	40
Total	54	97	42

stages of myocarditis and dilated cardiomyopathy. The results of our total experience with this technique to date are shown in Table 4.1 (see also Chap. 16).

Methods of Investigation

The routine clinical assessment of the patient with dilated cardiomyopathy, including electrocardiography, chest radiograph and routine haematological and biochemical screening has been dealt with in Chap. 2.

Echocardiography

Echocardiography has proved a valuable non-invasive tool for the detection of all degrees of myocardial involvement in patients with either dilated cardiomyopathy or specific heart muscle disease. Whilst initially echocardiography was confined to M-mode allowing the measurement of ventricular dimensions and the relatively crude exclusion of rheumatic valvar disease, the subsequent development of 2D sector echo, Doppler studies, and more recently colour flow imaging,

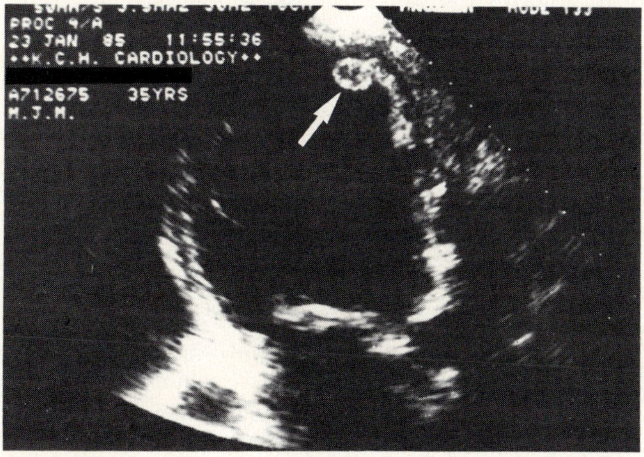

Fig. 4.3. 2D sector echocardiogram showing dilated left ventricle with an apical thrombus indicated by *arrow*

has permitted the more accurate diagnosis of dilated cardiomyopathy and its differentiation from restrictive cardiomyopathies, endomyocardial fibrosis and amyloid. Currently the limitations of echocardiography include its inability to define the coronary anatomy or to enable precise myocardial tissue characterisation. Studies have, however, drawn attention to the potential for the assessment of fibrosis in the cardiomyopathic heart. Ultrasonic tissue characterisation has been applied experimentally to the differentiation of calcification and fibrosis [18], and in vivo quantification of myocardial fibrosis has been assessed in patients with dilated cardiomyopathy [19].

The ease of use and sophistication of echocardiography are now such that this investigation is mandatory before the clinician takes the decision to proceed to invasive studies. In addition, because of its non-invasive nature, echocardiography can be used as a means of serially assessing the progress of the patient with dilated cardiomyopathy or myocarditis. Changes in ventricular dimensions and function can be monitored in response to treatment, and serial pulmonary pressures can be measured by Doppler techniques.

The typical findings on echocardiography in dilated cardiomyopathy are those of a globally dilated left ventricular cavity with overall reduction of systolic contraction. The left ventricular dimensions in both systole and diastole are markedly increased. Intracavity thrombus may be detected occasionally not only as mural thrombus but also as a pedunculated lesion. These are often situated at the apex. The advent of transoesophageal echocardiography has enhanced the detection of thrombus in the left atrium [20]. The further development of this technique with biplane and multiplane transducers may improve the imaging of left ventricular mural clot.

In some patients who have had a focal myocarditis there may be only segmental reduction of wall motion with relatively minor dilatation of the left ventricular cavity size. The very occasional patient may have a localised ventricular aneurysm. Regional left ventricular wall motion abnormalities are not confined to patients with focal disease but have been found to be frequently present in dilated cardiomyopathy in spite of the diffuse nature of the left ventricular involvement [21]. The typical M-mode findings are shown in Fig. 4.4. Doppler examination enables assessment of diastolic function [22] and documentation of regurgitation of the atrioventricular valves which may be enhanced by the use of colour flow imaging. The altered diastolic function may resemble that seen in hypertensive heart disease where there is reversal of the E/A ratio of diastolic transmitral filling velocities and reduction of the E-F slope.

Whilst echocardiography will allow differentiation of dilated from hypertrophic cardiomyopathy and the identification of certain forms of restrictive cardiomyopathy and of amyloid heart disease, the technology currently is not sufficiently refined to permit diagnostic tissue characterisation. This may be possible in the future. MRI scanning, which is a sophisticated technology, is already producing high-quality myocardial images but it remains to be seen whether these wil prove sufficiently specific and sensitive to provide diagnostic information in specific heart muscle disease. The potential for this has been

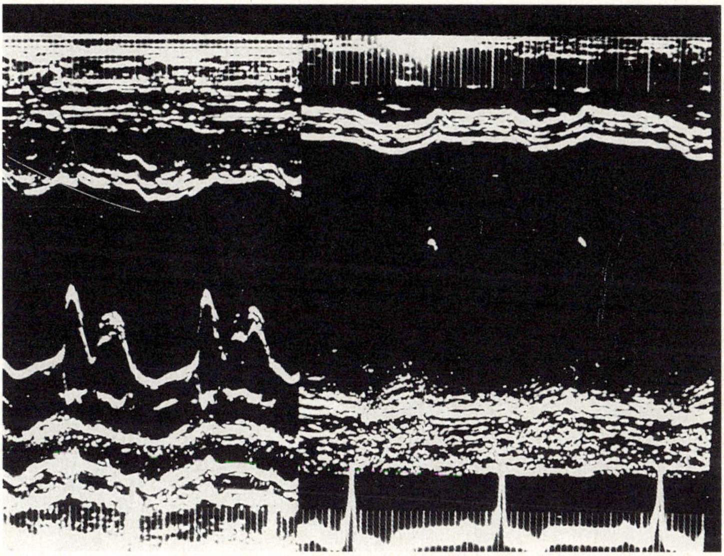

Fig. 4.4. M-mode echocardiogram illustrating a dilated, poorly contracting left ventricle

suggested by its application in the detection of acute myocarditis [23]. At the present time histopathological classification can only be achieved by microscopic examination of myocardial tissue obtained by endomyocardial biopsy.

Radionuclide Techniques

The initial application of radionuclide scanning in experimental virus perimyocarditis demonstrated the possibility of detecting myocardial inflammation using technetium-99m pyrophosphate uptake [24]. More recent studies have used gallium-67 imaging to predict myocarditis which was subsequently correlated with the biopsy findings in patients with clinical dilated cardiomyopathy [25]. Indium-111 radiolabelled monoclonal antimyosin antibodies have been shown to be promising, with a specificity of 58% and a sensitivity of 100% [26, 27]. This technique has also been undertaken in patients with dilated cardiomyopathy. Three groups were studied: 17 patients with dilated cardiomyopathy, 12 controls with poorly contracting left ventricles not due to cardiomyopathy and 8 normals. The degree of ventricular impairment was similar in the dilated cardiomyopathy and control groups. The heart/lung ratio of antimyosin uptake was significantly higher in those with dilated cardiomyopathy as compared with the controls and normals. Abnormal antimyosin uptake was seen in 12 (70%) of 17 patients with cardiomyopathy compared with 1 (8%) of 12 controls [28]. Monoclonal antimyosin antibody detection in dilated cardiomyopathy and myocarditis suggests a continuing process of active myocyte damage. The correlation of these changes with myocardial biopsy histology and the detection of enteroviral RNA may in the future provide further insight into the pathogenetic mechanisms operative in dilated cardiomyopathy.

Radionuclide ventriculography is frequently used to assess left ventricular systolic function, with ejection fraction being a predictor of survival in dilated cardiomyopathy (see Chap. 5). Recently diastolic function has been examined by radionuclide techniques in a group of patients with impaired systolic function from a number of causes including dilated cardiomyopathy. The study indicated that patients with short times to peak filling rate, or increased peak filling velocities, had a poorer prognosis. As independent predictors of prognosis both factors were statistically more significant ($p < 0.005$ and $p < 0.02$ respectively) than ejection fraction ($p < 0.05$) [29]. It remains to be seen whether this finding will be confirmed in a cohort of patients with dilated cardiomyopathy.

Cardiac Catheterisation and Endomyocardial Biopsy

Severe or end-stage coronary artery disease with extensive myocardial damage cannot be differentiated by non-invasive techniques from dilated cardiomyopathy [30] and therefore for the correct diagnosis to be made with certainty it is appropriate for diagnostic coronary arteriography to be performed. Risk factors such as family history, smoking, hypertension, hyperlipidaemia and diabetes mellitus may increase the probability of finding coronary arterial disease. Left ventriculography with measurement of the haemodynamic indices (e.g. ejection fraction, left ventricular end-diastolic filling pressure and pulmonary artery wedge pressure) provides further evidence of the degree of impairment of left

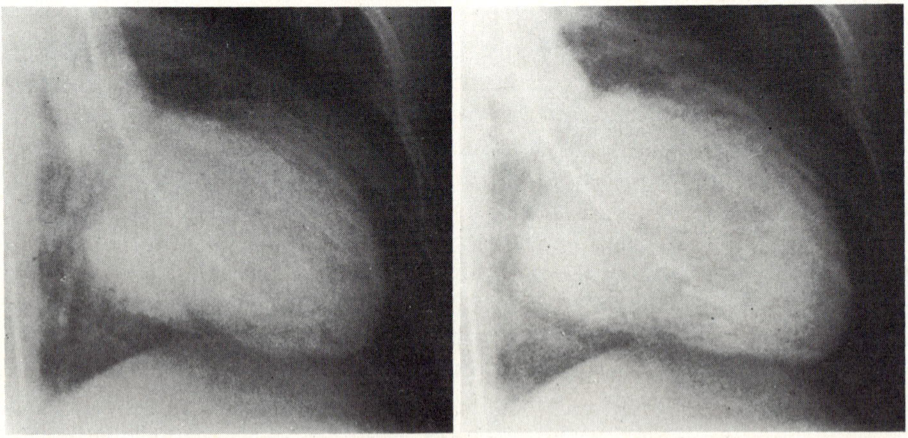

Fig. 4.5. Left ventricular angiogram showing systolic (left) and diastolic (right) frames in dilated cardiomyopathy. See text for details

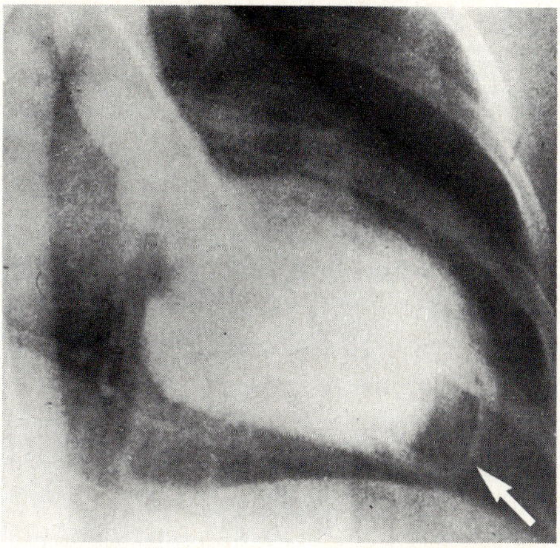

Fig. 4.6. Left ventricular angiogram in a patient with dilated cardiomyopathy showing thrombus in the ventricular apex

ventricular function and is guide to prognosis (Fig. 4.4). Intracardiac thrombus may have been detected previously by echocardiography but angiographic delineation of thrombus in the left ventricle can also be achieved (Fig. 4.5). It is clearly important to differentiate organic valvar disease from the functional regurgitation of the atrioventricular valves that is frequently observed in dilated cardiomyopathy. The haemodynamic data and full angiographic visualisation of the cardiac anatomy are also appropriate, particularly in view of the increasing application of heart transplantation as a means of treating patients with intractable cardiac failure.

Endomyocardial Biopsy

Since endomyocardial biopsy was first described in 1962 by Sakakibara and Konno [31] the initial difficulties encountered with the technique and instrument have been overcome. The development of percutaneous long sheaths for either right or left ventricular biopsy together with the appropriate biopsy forceps [32] has facilitated the histopathological classification of the dilated cardiomyopathies and specific heart muscle diseases [33]. In particular the frequency with which myocarditis in its various forms is diagnosed has increased and in addition the realisation of a progression from myocarditis to dilated cardiomyopathy has been documented [14]. The interest in myocarditis was further enchanced by the observations of Mason and colleagues [34, 35] who used immunosuppressive therapy in a similar way to that employed in reducing the frequency and severity of rejection of the transplanted heart (see Chap. 5).

In experienced hands the complications of endomyocardial biopsy are no greater than those of cardiac catheterisation; it is therefore sensible to combine biopsy with angiography to obtain maximum information. It is also important to consider the contra-indications, which include prolonged bleeding states, the presence of left ventricular intracavitary thrombus for left ventricular biopsy, and usually hypertrophic cardiomyopathy. The complications of endomyocardial biopsy are further discussed below.

The clinical indications for endomyocardial biopsy in general are summarized as follows:

1. To detect and confirm the histopathological changes of rejection in patients who have undergone, recent heart transplantation.
2. To diagnose both clinically suspected and unsuspected myocarditis, and to detect virus RNA sequences by molecular probes (see Chap. 15). Serial biopsy enables the study of the natural history of myocarditis to the healed phase. The persistence of inflammatory myocarditic changes suggests caution in predicting outcome, but does not exclude the possibility of subsequent clinical improvement if complete healing takes place. Serial biopsy is also useful in evaluating the response to immunosuppressive therapy (see Chap. 5).
3. To investigate the cause of heart failure when this is not clinically apparent and to diagnose myocarditis or specific heart muscle disease. A clinical diagnosis of dilated cardiomyopathy is confirmed when these diagnoses have been excluded. This can have prognostic implications although no precise index of prognosis on histopathological criteria has been achieved (see Chap. 3).
4. To diagnose restrictive cardiomyopathy such as endomyocardial disease (including eosinophilic and fibrotic forms) and differentiate this from specific heart muscle disease and amyloid (see Chaps. 10 and 12).
5. To investigate patients with arrhythmia to exclude myocardial disease affecting either ventricle. The diagnosis of arrythmogenic right ventricular dysplasia (ARVD) is increasingly recognised (see Chap. 13). The normality of the coronary vessels should be confirmed, however, before biopsy.
6. To assess and monitor myocardial damage secondary to cytotoxic medications such as the anthracyclines (e.g. adriamycin) (see Chap. 1).
7. To exclude myocardial disease as a specific cause for angina-like chest pain with angiographically normal coronary arteries (syndrome X).

Biopsy Technique

The major improvement in the endomyocardial technique came about with the realisation that bioptomes could be introduced using a percutaneous sheath technique (Fig. 4.6). Whilst Sakakibara and Konno [31] had pioneered the technique of catheter myocardial biopsy and shown its potential, difficulties were encountered both by the group at Stanford and by ourselves with regard to the mechanical reliabiltiy of the instrument as well as the size of the jaws, which precluded percutaneous introduction and necessitated either a venous cutdown or an arteriotomy. The Stanford group developed the Caves Schultz bioptome which could be introduced percutaneously via the jugular vein with a short sheath, enabling right ventricular biopsy [36]. This route has proved very useful for the routine monitoring of heart transplant rejection [37]. The King's endomyocardial bioptome [38] was suitable for percutaneous introduction via the transfemoral route and, with the development of a sheath technique, we were able to perform either right or left ventricular biopsy. The long sheaths which we developed for this route of biopsy have been further refined [32]. Provided left ventricular cavity thrombus has been reasonably excluded prior to sampling, the risk of embolisation is low. Routine heparinisation to minimise the risk of clot formation within the long sheath is always advisable, however, especially when sampling from the left ventricle.

Access to the vascular system for either method is by the Seldinger technique under local anaesthesia; no general anaesthesia is employed except in young children. In the case of biopsy by the Stanford technique, the bioptome is passed through a short sheath inserted into the internal jugular vein and into the right ventricle via the superior vena cava, allowing biopsy of the right ventricular surface of the interventricular septum. Biopsy using the Kings's bioptome, or the disposable Cordis modification [32], is usually performed through a long sheath inserted into either the right or left ventricle over a pigtail or multipurpose catheter from the femoral vein or artery [39]. The advantage of this is that the bioptome remains guarded until it is within the ventricular cavity. This obviates the need to recross the valve repeatedly, thus diminishing the risk of valvar perforation. Right ventricular samples are again obtained from the interventricular septum, whilst left ventricular samples are taken from the septum and apex (Fig. 4.7). Biopsy of the free wall of either ventricle should be avoided if possible in order to make haemopericardium and cardiac tamponade less likely should the bioptome penetrate the heart muscle.

Once the bioptome is within the ventricular chamber the jaws are opened, ensuring that the instrument is well away from the ventricular wall. It is then

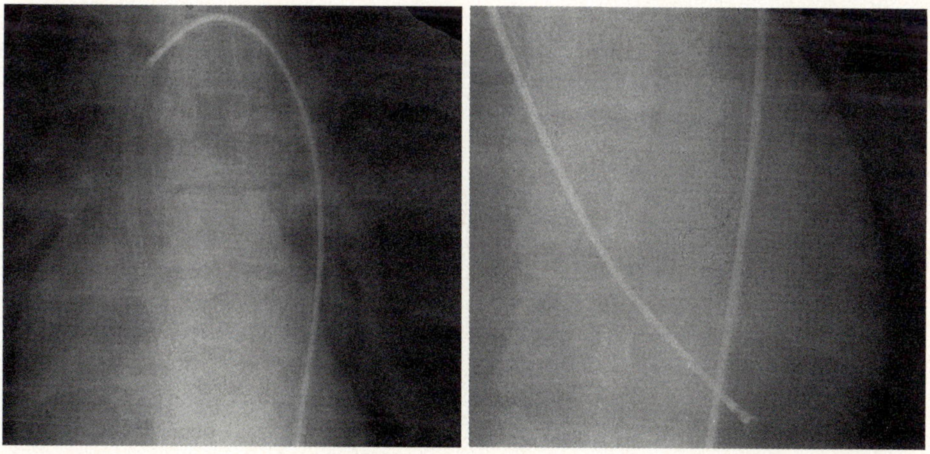

Fig. 4.7. Endomyocardial biopsy of the left ventricle by the long sheath technique. *Left*: long sheath situated within the left ventricle with bioptome advanced as far as the aortic arch. *Right*: bioptome (with jaws open) advanced against the apical wall of the left ventricle

advanced with the jaws open until contact with the muscle is made, minimising the risk of ventricular perforation with the blunt closed jaws of the bioptome. Once contact is made with the endomyocardium the jaws are closed and the bioptome is promptly withdrawn through the sheath. For right ventricular biopsies no special precautions are required at this stage; during left ventricular biopsy, however, we routinely ensure that a constant flush is maintained through the sheath during bioptome withdrawal, the positive pressure preventing air entry through the haemostatic valve and reducing stasis within the sheath. Tissue samples are removed from the jaws of the bioptome with a needle to avoid crush artefact and are then processed immediately or snap frozen to avoid deterioration or desiccation.

Although both techniques are suitable for obtaining multiple biopsies, it is important that the site of muscle biopsied is varied in order to obtain as representative a picture of the myocardium as possible [40] and to minimise the risk of cardiac perforation by repeatedly taking biopsies from the same site. This is achieved by repositioning the sheath between biopsies and/or applying a bend to the end of the bioptome.

Complications

The common complications of biopsy are shown in Table 4.2. Despite these, it remains a safe procedure in experienced hands with morbidity $<1\%$ and no mortality in two recent large series [37, 41]. It is apparent that certain complications are specific to the route of biopsy; thus pneumothorax occurs only with biopsy via the jugular approach whilst cerebral embolism is specific to left venticular biopsy.

Limitations of Biopsy

One of the principal limitations of endomyocardial biopsy lies in the apparently random sampling of the myocardium. This is especially true when considering the focal nature of certain heart muscle diseases and myocarditis in particular [40]. This limitation may be overcome by guiding the bioptome to areas of abnormal tissue. This has traditionally been achieved by performing endomyocardial biopsy using 2D sector echocardiography to visualise the ventricle and bioptome [42]. This allows more precise positioning of the biotome within

Table 4.2. Major complications of endomyocardial biopsy

1. Cardiac perforation, haemopericardium $\pm$ tamponade
2. Systemic (left ventricular) or pulmonary (right ventricular) embolisation of air, tissue or clot
3. Chordal rupture/papillary muscle damage
4. Aortic or tricuspid valve perforation
5. Cardiac arrhythmias
6. Pneumothorax (only with jugular/subclavian approach)

the ventricle, so that biopsies might be obtained from places where ventricular function was seen to be abnormal (such as areas of localised hypokinesia). This technique provides more precise definition of the site of biopsy than does fluoroscopy and offers the possibility of greater reproducibility of biopsy sites when serial biopsies are required. The recent development of percutaneous fibre-optic angioscopy has opened up an entirely new method for the identification of abnormal areas of endocardium and the possibility of angioscope-guided biopsy [43]. In a preliminary study angioscopy of the left ventricle was performed in 13 patients with dilated cardiomyopathy and 4 patients with acute myocarditis. Eight of these underwent endomyocardial biopsy with angioscopic guidance. Visualisation of the endocardium permitted the identification of mural thrombus and the degree of endocardial involvement by the disease process.

Special Technologies

Myocardial Tissue Enzyme Analysis

The measurement of myocardial enzyme activity using microassay techniques of tissue obtained by endomyocardial biopsy was first suggested by Peters et al. [44]. Subsequently, using less sophisticated separation techniques, similar measurements have been made [45, 46]. Wide variations in activities of several myocardial tissue enzymes including creatinine phosphokinase (CPK), lactate dehydrogenase (LDH), α-hydroxybutyric dehydrogenase (α-HBD), malic dehydrogenase (MDH) and aspartate aminotransferase (AST) were found in patients with dilated heart disease who were haemodynamically and histologically indistinguishable [45]. Analysis of the latter data demonstrated that the differences in enzyme activity levels appeared to relate to the intake of alcohol by patients, the highest levels being found in those diagnosed clinically as having alcoholic heart muscle disease.

Although the association between excessive alcohol consumption and dilated cardiomyopathy has long been known [47], the causal relationship has remained controversial [48]. Whilst endomyocardial biopsy had provided the means of obtaining myocardial tissue for histopathological evaluation of the myocardium during life, there were no histological features that appeared to be specific for alcoholic heart muscle disease [33]. Whilst a quantitative relationship between alcohol consumption and alcoholic liver disease had been established [49, 50] there were no similar studies relating alcohol intake to myocardial disease. Indeed, the clinical diagnosis of alcohol-induced heart muscle disease merely reflected the coexistence of global myocardial dysfunction in a heavy drinker in whom no other cause of myocardial disease had been demonstrated.

In view of the preliminary evidence of differing levels of enzyme activity in dilated cardiomyopathy according to alcohol consumption, this relationship was further investigated [51]. In 38 patients regularly consuming more than 40 g alcohol daily a bimodal distribution of cumulative lifetime alcohol intake was demonstrated. The patients thus fell into two groups: the first group (20 patients) were light drinkers who had cumulative lifetime intakes of <250 kg whilst the second group (18 patients) were heavy drinkers who, with one exception, had cumulative lifetime intakes in excess of 500 kg. The mean daily alcohol intake in this latter group was 114 g with a mean duration of drinking of 25 years. Fifteen of these 18 patients were predominantly beer drinkers.

Against the background of the alcohol consumption there were significant correlations between the myocardial tissue enzyme activites and both cumulative lifetime alcohol intake and maximal daily consumption. Significantly higher levels of CPK, α-HBD, LDH and MDH were found in the heavy drinkers compared with the light drinkers. Furthermore there was a strong correlation between myocardial enzyme activity and alcohol intake for the same enzymes.

Multiple regression analysis was performed in order to evaluate the possible relationship between alcohol consumption, left ventricular ejection fraction, blood pressure and myocardial enzyme activities. Levels of CPK and α-HBD correlated significantly with both ejection fraction and cumulative lifetime alcohol intake. LDH only correlated with the cumulative lifetime alcohol intake. There was no correlation of diastolic blood pressure with levels of any of the enzymes measured.

Whilst the increases in myocardial enzyme activity in the heavy drinking group may be adaptive and simply reflect chronic exposure to alcohol, increased levels of several mitochondrial enzymes such as MDH and AST have been found in patients with alcoholic fatty liver [52]. This has been attributed to reoxidation of NADH to NAD^+ which is an essential co-factor in the metabolism of alcohol. Another mechanism by which α-HBD and LDH levels might also increase is as an adaptive response to increased circulating levels of lactate derived from hepatic glycolysis. In order to investigate this, the effect of acute alcohol consumption on myocardial metabolism was studied in 12 patients using coronary sinus catheterisation. Various substrates were measured in arterial, venous and coronary sinus blood samples over a period of 1 h following the oral administration of alcohol (1 g/kg body weight). The substrates measured included lactate, pyruvate, glucose, oxygen and noradrenaline. The levels of arterial and venous lactate rose significantly, suggesting lactate release from the liver. In addition there was a significant rise in both the lactate arteriovenous difference and lactate extraction ratio. The coronary sinus lactate/pyruvate ratio rose significantly, reflecting an increase in the myocardial redox potential. These results suggest that the effect of alcohol on myocardial metabolism in patients with alcohol-induced heart muscle disease may be mediated by alcohol affecting hepatic metabolism and producing increased lactate levels. The increased myocardial redox potential resulting from this alters the oxidative capacity of the myocardium, and on a chronic basis may lead to the development of myocardial damage. The data do not preclude a direct cytotoxic effect of alcohol or its metabolites upon the myocardium.

Antioxidant Status and Alcoholic Heart Muscle Disease

It has been clearly demonstrated that skeletal myopathy can result from chronic alcohol abuse and is associated with an altered antioxidant status [53]. Metabolism of excessive alcohol induces hepatic microsomal enzyme P450-IIE1 with an increased production of reactive oxygen species. These may deplete the antioxidant pool and result in myopathy. To determine whether a similar mechanism may be responsible for the pathogenesis of alcoholic heart muscle disease, plasma α-tocopherol, β-carotene and retinol were measured using reverse phase high performance liquid chromatography in 46 patients with heart muscle disease and impaired left ventricular function. No significant difference was found between those with alcohol-induced heart muscle disease and those with dilated cardiomyopathy. Similarly there was no significant difference between patients who were drinking at the time of investigation and those who had been abstinent. This aspect will need further investigation, but at the present time there is no evidence that measurement of plasma antioxidant levels in patients with alcoholic heart muscle disease indicates any increased free radical activity.

Analysis of Myocardial Proteins

Alteration in the expression of myocardial proteins, whatever the initial mechanism for the disease process, may lead to altered function of the heart muscle. Even minor changes in protein expression may give rise to sufficient disturbance of cardiac contraction to produce a cardiomyopathic ventricle. Recent studies have demonstrated mutation in the cardiac myosin heavy chain genes with production of α/β myosin heavy chain hybrid gene [54] or a point mutation of the β myosin heavy chain gene [55]. These latter changes were detected in familial hypertrophic cardiomyopathy. However, evidence for changes in dilated cardiomyopathy comes from studies showing an abnormal distribution and expression of myosin isoforms involving both the myosin heavy [56, 57] and light chains [58–61] in the myocardium in this disease. Whilst these findings have been interpreted as being specific for dilated cardiomyopathy, it is recognised that other types of cardiac hypertrophy are known to be associated with changes in the expression of myosin and other contractile proteins [62]. It is known that persistent viral infections can interfere with normal gene expression [63]. It remains to be determined whether the persistence of enteroviral infection in dilated cardiomyopathy can result in the modification of specific cellular gene expression.

The investigation of myocardial gene expression in dilated cardiomyopathy ideally requires a technique which can simultaneously resolve several thousand proteins. Two-dimensional polyacrylamide gel electrophoresis (2D PAGE) has the resolution capacity required [64]. The proteins are separated according to their charge properties in the first dimension, and then according to their molecular size in the second dimension. The 2D protein profiles thus obtained are very complex and therefore computer systems are required to ensure accurate analysis. This enables construction a 2D protein database for the myocardial proteins which may enable detection of altered expression associated with a particular disease process. An initial study using 2D PAGE and computer analysis has enabled the identification of a group of 20 proteins which differed between patients with dilated cardiomyopathy and those with ischaemic heart disease [65].

Metabolic Applications of NMR Spectroscopy

Nuclear magnetic resonance (NMR) has been employed as an imaging technique but can also be used for in vivo biochemical analysis. A preliminary study in 7 patients with dilated cardiomyopathy and 14 controls using phosphorus-31 NMR spectroscopy has shown the feasibility of analysing energy metabolism [66]. There were no differences between dilated cardiomyopathy patients and controls in the ratio of phosphocreatine to ATP. There were, however, higher ratios of phosphodiester to phosphocreatine and phosphodiester to ATP in patients with dilated cardiomyopathy. The significance of these findings is as yet unclear but the ability to study high-energy phosphates non-invasively may provide further insights to the biochemical basis for the myocardial dysfunction in dilated cardiomyopathy.

Further research applications for NMR spectroscopy may include the measurement of RNA metabolites in the urine. These may reflect alterations in both myocardial and skeletal protein turnover and synthesis. The measurement of whole body RNA metabolism has, to date, been handicapped by the lack of suitable methodology.

References

1. International Society and Federation of Cardiology/World Health Organization (1980). Task Force on the definition and classfication of cardiomyopathies. Report. Br Heart J 44: 672–673
2. Why HJF, Cutler SJ, Wright DJM, Olsen EJG, Richardson PJ (1990) *Borrelia burgdorferi* infection: an aetiological factor in dilated cardiomyopathy (Abstr). Br Heart J 64: 48
3. Klein J, Stanek G, Bittner R, Horvat R, Holzinger C, Glogar D (1991) Lyme borreliosis as a cause of myocarditis and heart muscle disease. Eur Heart J 12 Suppl D: 73–75
4. Stanek G, Klein J, Bittner R, Glogar D (1990) Isolation of of *Borrelia burgdorferi* from the myocardium of a patient with longstanding cardiomyopathy. N Engl J Med 322: 349–352
5. de Koning J, Hoogkamp-Korstanje JAA, van der Linde MR, Crijns HJGM (1989) Demonstration of spirochetes in cardiac biopsies of patients with Lyme disease. J Infect Dis 160: 150–153
6. Jacob AJ, Boon NA (1991) HIV cardiomyopathy: a dark cloud with a silver lining. Br Heart J 66: 1–2
7. Olsen EGJ (1980) Morphologic evaluation (histologic, histochemical, and ultrastructural) of endomyocardial biopsies. In: Bolte H-D (ed) Myocardial biopsy: diagnostic significance. Springer Berlin Heidelberg New York, pp 13–18

8. Mason JW, Billingham ME, Ricci DR (1980) Treatment of acute inflammatory myocarditis assisted by endomyocardial biopsy. Am J Cardiol 45: 1037–1044
9. Nippoldt TB, Edwards W, Holmes DR, Reeder GS, Hartzler GO, Smith HC (1982) Right ventricular endomyocardial biopsy: clinicopathologic correlates in 100 consecutive patients. Mayo Clin Proc 57: 407
10. Chow LC, Dittrich HC, Shabetai R (1988) Endomyocardial biopsy in patients with unexplained congestive heart failure. Ann Intern Med 109: 535–539
11. Dec GW, Palacios IF, Fallon JT et al. (1985) Active myocarditis in the spectrum of acute dilated cardiomyopathies: clinical features, histologic correlates and clinical outcome. N Engl J Med 312: 885–890
12. Zee-Cheng CS, Tsai CC, Palmer DC, Codd JE, Pennington DG, Williams GA (1984). High incidence of myocarditis by endomyocardial biopsy in patients with idiopathic congestive cardimyopathy. J Am Coll Cardiol 3: 63
13. Levi G, Scalvini S, Volterrani M, Marangoni S, Arosio G, Quadri A (1987) Coxsackie virus heart disease: 15 years after. Eur Heart J 8 Suppl J: 1303–1307
13a. Caforio AL, Bonifacio E, Stewart JT et al. (1990) Novel organ-specific circulating cardiac autoantibodies in dilated cardiomyopathy. J Am Coll Cardiol 15: 1527–1534
14. Quigley PJ, Richardson PJ, Meaney BT, Olsen EGJ, Monaghan MJ, Jackson G, Jewitt DE (1987) Long-term follow-up of acute myocarditis: correlation of ventricular function and outcome. Eur Heart J 8 Suppl J: 39–42
15. Olsen EJG (1979) Pathology of cardiomyopathies: a critical analysis. Am Heart J 98: 385–392
16. Bowles NE, Richardson PJ, Olsen EGJ, Archard LC (1986) Detection of Coxsackie-B-virus-specific RNA sequences in myocardial biopsy samples from patients with myocarditis and dilated cardiomyopathy. Lancet: 1120–1123
17. Bowles NE, Rose ML, Taylor P et al. (1989) End-stage dilated cardiomyopathy: persistence of enterovirus RNA in myocardium at cardiac transplantation and lack of immune response. Circulation 80: 1128–1136
18. Perez JE, Barzilai B, Madaras EL et al. (1984) Applicability of ultrasonic tissue characterisation for longitudinal assessment and differentiation of calcification and fibrosis in cardiomyopathy. J Am Coll Cardiol 4: 88–95
19. Picano E, Pelosi G, Marzilli M et al. (1990) In vivo quantitative ultrasonic evaluation of myocardial fibrosis in humans. Circulation 81: 58–64
20. Alam M, Sun I (1991) Transesophageal echocardiographic evaluation of left atrial mass lesions. J Am Soc Echocardiogr 4: 323–330
21. Sunnerhagen KS, Bhargava V, Shabetai R (1990) Regional left ventricular wall motion abnormalities in idiopathic dilated cardiomyopathy. Am J Cardiol 65: 364–370
22. Ng KSK, Gibson DG (1990) Relation of filling pattern to diastolic function in severe left ventricular disease. Br Heart J 63: 209–214
23. Chandratna PAN, Bradley WG, Kortman KE, Minagoe S, Delvicario M, Rahimtoola SH (1987) Detection of acute myocarditis using nuclear magnetic resonance imaging. Am J Med 83: 1144–1146
24. Matsumori A, Kadota K, Kawai C (1980) Technetium-99m pyrophosphate uptake in experimental viral perimyocarditis: sequential study of myocardial uptake and pathologic correlates. Circulation 61: 802–807
25. O'Connell JB, Henkin RE, Robinson JA, Subramanian R, Scanlon PJ, Gunnar RM (1984) Gallium-67 imaging in patients with dilated cardiomyopathy and biopsy proven myocarditis. Circulation 70: 58–62
26. Yasuda TS, Palacios IF, Dec W et al. (1987) Indium-111 monoclonal antimyosin antibody imaging in the diagnosis of acute myocarditis. Circulation 76: 306–311
27. Rezkella S, Kloner RA, Khaw BA et al. (1989) Detection of experimental myocarditis by monoclonal antimyosin antibody, Fab fragment. Am Heart J 117: 391–395
28. Obrador D, Ballester M, Carrio I, Berna L, Pons-Llado G (1989) High prevalence of myocardial monoclonal antimyosin antibody uptake in patients with chronic idiopathic dilated cardiomyopathy. J Am Coll Cardiol 13: 1289–1293

29. Clements IP, Brown ML, Zinsmeister AR, Gibbons RJ (1991) Influence of left ventricular diastolic filling on symptoms and survival in patients with decreased left ventricular systolic function. Am J Cardiol 67: 1245–1250
30. Raftery EB, Banks DC, Oram S (1969) Occlusive disease of the coronary arteries presenting as primary congestive cardiomyopathy. Lancet 2:1147–1150
31. Sakakibara S, Konno S (1962) Endomyocardial biopsy. Jpn Heart J 3: 537–543
32. Richardson PJ (1984) Endomyocardial biopsy technique and evaluation of a new disposable forceps and catheter sheath system. In: Bolte H-D (ed.) Viral heart disease. Springer, Berlin Heidelberg New York, pp 173–176
33. Olsen EGJ (1975) Pathololological recognition of cardiomyopathy. Postgrad Med J 51: 277–281
34. Mason JW, Billingham ME, Ricci DR (1980) Treatment of acute inflammatory myocarditis assisted by endomyocardial biopsy. Am J Cardiol 45: 1037–1044
35. Daly K, Richardson PJ, Olsen EJG et al. (1984) Acute myocarditis: role of histological and virological examination in the diagnosis and assessment of immunosuppressive treatment. Br Heart J 51: 30–35
36. Caves PK, Schulz WP, Dong E Jr, Stinson EB, Schumway NE (1974) A new instrument for transvenous cardiac biopsy. Am J Cardiol 33: 264–267
37. Billingham ME (1990) Endomyocardial biopsy diagnosis of acute rejection in cardiac allografts. Prog Cardiovasc Dis 33: 11–18
38. Richardson PJ (1974) King's endomyocardial bioptome. Lancet: 660–661
39. Richardson PJ (1980) Endomyocardial biopsy technique. In: Bolte H-D (ed) Myocardial biopsy. Springer, Berlin Heidelberg New York
40. Baandrup U, Florio RA, Olsen EGJ (1982) Do endomyocardial biopsies represent the morphology of the rest of the myocardium? Eur Heart J 3: 171–178
41. Starling RC, van Fossen DB, Hammer DF, Unverferth DV (1991) Morbidity of endomyocardial biopsy in cardiomyopathy. Am J Cardiol 68: 133–136
42. Mortensen SA, Egeblad H (1983) Endomyocardial biopsy guided by cross-sectional echocardigraphy. Br Heart J 50: 246–251
43. Uchida Y, Nakamura F, Oshima T, Fujimori Y, Hirose J (1990) Percutaneous fiberoptic angioscopy of the left ventricle in patients with dilated cardiomyopathy and acute myocarditis. Am Heart J 120: 677–687
44. Peters TJ, Wells G, Oakley CM et al. (1977) Enzymic analysis of endomyocardial biopsy specimens from patients with cardiomyopathies. Br Heart J 39: 1333–1339
45. Richardson PJ, Atkinson L (1980) The measurement of enzyme activities in endomyocardial biopsy samples from patients with cardiomyopathy. In: Sekiguchi M, Olsen EGJ (eds) Cardiomyopathy: clinical, pathological and theoretical aspects. University of Tokyo Press, Tokyo, pp 149–156
46. Lehmann I, Papies B, Parsi RA et al. (1988) Enzyme pattern and lipid peroxides in endomyocardial biopsies from patients with cardiomyopathy and myocarditis. Clin Chim Acta 173: 193–200
47. Brigden W, Robinson J (1964) Alcoholic heart muscle disease. Br Med J 2: 1283–1289
48. Goodwin JF (1973) Treatment of the cardiomyopathies. Am J Cardiol 32: 341–351
49. Pequignot G, Chabert C, Eydoux H, Courcoul MA (1974) Augmentation du risque de cirrhose on fonction de la ration d'alcool. Rev Alcol 20: 191–202
50. Lelbach WK (1974) Organic pathology related to volume and patterns of alcohol use. In: Gibbons RJ, Israel Y, Kalant H, Popham RE, Schmidt W, Smart RD (eds) Research advances in alcohol and drug problems. Wiley, New York, pp 93–198
51. Richardson PJ, Wodak AD, Atkinson L, Saunders JB, Jewitt DE (1986) Relation between alcohol intake, myocardial enzyme activity and myocardial function in dilated cardiomyopathy: evidence for the concept of alcohol induced heart muscle disease. Br Heart J 56: 165–170
52. Jenkins WJ, Peters TJ (1978) Mitochondrial enzymes activities in liver biopsies in patients with alcoholic liver disease. Gut 19: 341–345
53. Ward RJ, Peters TJ (1992) The antioxidant status in patients with alcohol induced live damage or muscle damage. Alcohol Alcohol (in press)

54. Tanigawa G, Jarcho JA, Kass S, Solomon SD, Vosberg HP, Seidmann JG, Seidman CE (1990) A molecular basis for familial hypertrophic cardiomyopathy: an α/β cardiac myosin heavy chain hybrid gene. Cell 62: 991
55. Geisterfer-Lowrance AAT, Kass S, Tanigawa G, Vosberg HP, McKenna W, Seidman CE, Seidman JG (1990) A molecular basis for familial hypertrophic cardiomyopathy: a β cardiac myosin heavy chain gene missense mutation. Cell 62: 999
56. Yazaki Y, Tsuchimochi H, Kurabyashi M, Kawana M, Kimata S-I (1987) Distribution of cardiac myosin isoenzymes in cardiomyopathy: immunohistochemical and gene analysis. Jpn Circ J 51: 676
57. Bouvagnet P, Leger J, Dechesne CA, Dureau G, Ansal M, Leger JJ (1985) Local changes in myosin types in diseased human atrial myocardium: a quantitative immunofluorescent study. Circulation 72: 272
58. Hirsel HO, Tuchschmid CR, Schneider J, Krayenbuhl HP, Schaub MC (1985) Relationship between myosin isoenzyme composition, haemodynamics, and myocardial structure in various forms of human hypertrophy. Circ Res 57: 729
59. Schaub MC, Hirzel HO (1987) Atrial and ventricular isomyosin composition in patients with different forms of cardiac hypertrophy. Basic Res Cardiol 82 Suppl 2: 357
60. Kovalyov L, Naumov VG, Pulyaeva HV et al. (1990) Two dimensional electrophoresis of heart muscle proteins in human cardiomyopathies. Electrophoresis 11: 333
61. Dalla Libra L, Pauletto P, Piccolo D, Scannapieco G, Vescovo G (1991) The idiopathic dilated cardiomyopathy in man: a biochemical and molecular study on myosin. Basic Res Cardiol 86: 70
62. Swynghedauw B (1986) Developmental and functional adaptation of contractile proteins in cardiac and skeletal muscles. Physiol Rev 66: 710
63. Oldstone MBA (1989) Viral alteration of cell function. Sci Am 261: 42
64. Dunn MJ (1987) Two-dimensional polyacrylamide gel electrophoresis. In: Chambach A, Dunn MJ, Radola BJ (eds) Advances in electrophoresis, Vol l. VCH, Weinheim, p 1
65. Corbett JM, Dunn MJ, Yacoub MH (1991) Computer analysis of two-dimensional protein patterns from human heart disease. In: Dunn MJ (ed), 2-D PAGE'91. NHLI, London, p 202
66. Schaefer S, Gober JR, Schwartz GG, Tweig DB, Weiner MW, Massie B (1990) In vivo phosphorus-31 spectroscopic imaging in patients with global myocardial disease. Am J Cardiol: 1154–1161

CHAPTER 5

Prognosis and Management

E. M. Gilbert, A. Di Lenarda, and J. B. O'Connell

Introduction

Dilated cardiomyopathy is a disease of unknown etiology that principally affects the myocardium [1]. The diagnosis of dilated cardiomyopathy is established by the presence of left ventricular dilatation and systolic dysfunction in the absence of congenital, coronary, valvular, or pericardial heart disease [2]. In some patients the development of dilated cardiomyopathy is associated with clinical factors such as alcoholism, pregnancy or a family history of cardiomyopathy [1, 2]. However, dilated cardiomyopathy is distinct from specific heart muscle disease ("secondary myocardial disease"), which occurs with a specific systemic disorder that may be metabolic, collagen-vascular, infiltrative, neuromuscular, inflammatory, or neoplastic in origin [1, 2] (see Chap. 1). There are currently no specific gross anatomic, histologic, or ultrastructural morphologic features which can differentiate dilated cardiomyopathy from other causes of heart failure [3]. Since dilated cardiomyopathy is defined clinically, it is likely that several specific etiologies are responsible for this condition. It is therefore not surprising that patients with dilated cardiomyopathy have a heterogeneous clinical presentation and prognosis.

The incidence of dilated cardiomyopathy is estimated at 3–10 cases per 10000 and approximately 20000 new cases are diagnosed annually in the United States [4, 5]. Patients with dilated cardiomyopathy usually develop progressive deterioration of ventricular function resulting in death from either pump failure or arrhythmia [5–8]. Currently, the 5 year mortality is estimated at 40%–80% [5–8]. However, a subset of patients with dilated cardiomyopathy have a stable clinical course with a good long-term prognosis [6, 8].

The modern management of dilated cardiomyopathy requires an individualized approach for medical treatment of heart failure that is based on the patient's hemodynamic abnormalities. In addition, it is necessary to understand the prognostic factors that predict a poor short-term outcome so that suitable candidates can be referred for transplantation. To these ends, this chapter will review previously described predictors of prognosis in dilated cardiomyopathy and will summarize the evaluation and therapy of patients with dilated cardiomyopathy.

Survival

The poor long-term prognosis of patients with dilated cardiomyopathy has been universally reported [6–22]. Representative survival curves are shown in Figs. 5.1 and 5.2. In the majority of reports, 1-year mortality is about 35%–40% (with a range from 18% [9] to 35% [12] and 2-year mortality is about 35%–40% (with a range from 26% [6] to 48% [13, 21]. However, some authors have reported that patients who survive more than 2 or 3 years have a relatively good

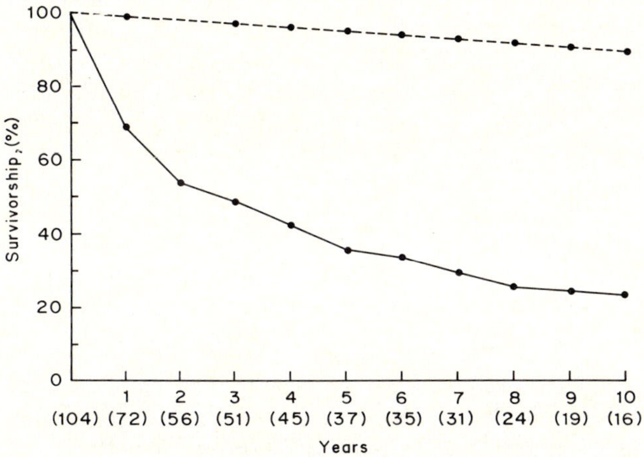

Fig. 5.1. Observed survival of 104 patients with dilated cardiomyopathy (*continuous line*) and their expected survival based on age and sex distribution according to the death rates of the Minnesota 1970 White Population Life Table (*dashed line*). The number of surviving patients under observation at each follow-up interval is indicated in parentheses. From [8]

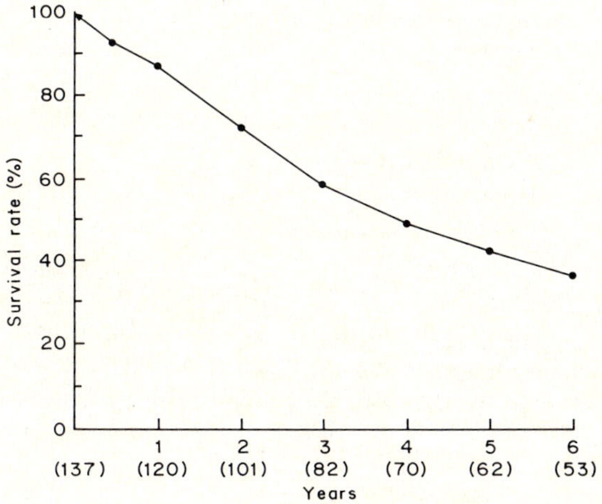

Fig. 5.2. Cumulative survival in 137 patients with dilated cardiomyopathy from the time of diagnosis to the end of the observation period. The number of surviving patients under observation at each follow-up interval is indicated in parentheses. From [6]

long-term prognosis and survival curves or such long-term survivors may even parallel survival curves of the general population [8, 10]. Stabilization and even spontaneous improvement have been observed in 20%–50% of patients [6, 8, 10, 11, 14, 21].

What accounts for the large variability in patient survival in dilated cardiomyopathy reported by these different authors? Several potential factors can be suggested including differences in underlying pathogenic mechanism for dilated cardiomyopathy, differences in duration of disease before presentation, and differences in the severity of disease, as well as differences in medical therapy after diagnosis.

Currently, patients with dilated cardiomyopathy are being identified earlier in the course of their disease due to both technologic advances in noninvasive cardiac imaging and a greater awareness of the disease among clinicians. Recent advances in medical therapy [23–25] may also produce a favorable effect on long-term outcome. Thus, the patient with dilated cardiomyopathy in the 1990s may have a better prognosis than patients reported in the literature.

Prediction of Prognosis

An understanding of factors which affect prognosis in dilated cardiomyopathy is important for proper patient management and may also improve our understanding of the pathophysiologic processes involved in the progression of disease. Several authors have analyzed the impact of multiple clinical, hemo-

Table 5.1. Predicting prognosis in dilated cardiomyopathy

	Predictive	Possibly predictive	Not predictive
Clinical factors	Symptoms	Alcoholism Peripartum presentation Family history	Age Duration of illness Preceding viral illness
Hemodynamic factors	LV ejection fraction Cardiac index	LV chamber size Atrial pressures	
Arrhythmia	LV conduction delay Complex ventricular ectopy	Atrioventricular block Atrial fibrillation	Simple ventricular ectopy
Histologic morphology		Myofibril volume	Other histologic findings
Neuroendocrine factors	Plasma noradrenaline Atrial natriuretic factor[a] Hyponatremia[a]		

LV, left ventricular
[a] Identified as prognostic factors for all causes of heart failure.

dynamic, electrocardiographic, and histologic parameters on survival in dilated cardiomyopathy. The prognostic significance of these parameters is summarized in Table 5.1. Unfortunately, most of these studies have been relatively small and only utilized univariate statistical analysis.

A variety of clinical factors including a family history of dilated cardiomyopathy, history of preceding viral illness, peripartum presentation, and excessive alcohol intake have been associated with the development of dilated cardiomyopathy (see Chap. 4). Several authors have evaluated the impact of these potential etiologic factors on survival. Unfortunately, these retrospective studies may not have had sufficient statistical power to identify any differences in outcome because of the small number of patients presenting with any of these specific factors.

Several authors have reported that the survival of patients with familial dilated cardiomyopathy does not differ from other patients with dilated cardiomyopathy [6, 10, 12, 14]. Although spontaneous improvements have been reported for patients with biopsy-proven myocarditis [23, 24], preceding viral illness does not appear to affect overall survival in patients with dilated cardiomyopathy [10, 12, 14].

The influence of peripartum presentation on survival is uncertain (see Chap. 13). Demakis et al. [25] followed 27 women with peripartum cardiomyopathy and demonstrated that the clinical course of patients with peripartum cardiomyopathy is highly variable [25]. Heart size had returned to normal within 6 months in 14 of their patients and none of these patients died of cardiac illness during an average follow-up of 10.7 years. In the remaining 13 patients, cardiomegaly persisted at 6 months and 85% died an average of 4.7 years after diagnosis. Their findings suggest that patients with peripartum cardiomyopathy have an increased probability of spontaneous improvement relative to other dilated cardiomyopathy patients. In contrast, Koide et al. [19] reported that patients with peripartum cardiomyopathy had a prognosis that was worse than other dilated cardiomyopathy patients. However, in several larger series of patients there were no differences between survival of patients with peripartum cardiomyopathy and other patients with dilated cardiomyopathy [8, 10, 12]. The differences in these reports can be reconciled by recognizing that prognosis in peripartum cardiomyopathy is good when there is early improvement in heart failure and poor when spontaneous improvement is not observed, or when relapse occurs in subsequent pregnancy (see Chaps.4 and 13). Cardiomyopathy has been associated with alcoholism [1, 2, 26, 27]. Demakis et al. [25] followed the clinical course of 57 patients with alcoholic heart muscle disease. All patients had used alcohol for more than 5 years and had a daily alcohol intake in excess of 8 ounces (0.24 l) of whiskey or gin, 1 quart (0.95 l) of wine, or 2 quarts (1.9 l) of beer. During an average follow-up period of 40.5 months, clinical status improved in 15 patients was stable in 12 patients and deteriorated in 30 patients. Twenty-four patients (42%) died after an average follow-up of 36 months. The average duration of symptoms was significantly shorter in patients with clinical improvements. Abstention from alcohol was associated with a more favourable clinical course. Eighteen of the patients abstained from alcohol: clinical status improved in 11, was stable in 3, and deteriorated in only 4 patients. Schwartz et al. [27] reported on a patient with severe alcoholic cardiomyopathy whose cardiac function was normal after 1 year's abstinence from alcohol. Koide et al. [19] found that patients with alcoholic heart muscle disease had a significantly better prognosis than other patients with dilated cardiomyopathy. All 10 of their alcoholic patients abstained and survived for at least 10 years. However, other investigators [6, 8, 10, 14] did not find any effect of alcohol abuse on prognosis in larger series of dilated cardiomyopathy patients. Fuster et al. [8] noted a trend to improved outcome with abstinence which was offset by a poor outcome if drinking was continued. The remaining reports did not include data on whether patients continued their use of alcohol or abstained after diagnosis of dilated cardiomyopathy. The borderline between alcoholic heart muscle disease and dilated cardiomyopathy complicated by alcohol indulgence may be a fine one. Definite differentiation may depend on whether improvement occurs on withdrawal of alcohol and on the amount of alcohol consumed over a long period (see Chap. 2).

The effect of age on mortality in dilated cardiomyopathy is not well defined. Fuster et al. [8] found that patients who were older than 55 had an increased mortality compared with younger patients. In contrast, Kuhn et al. [22] found that younger patients had a higher mortality. In most reports, age did not predict survival on univariate analysis [6, 10, 14, 21, 28]. Using multivariate analysis, Unverferth et al. [12], Keogh et al. [21], and Costanzo-Nordin et al. [28] found that patient age did not correlate with clinical outcome.

Although Stevenson et al. [20] only observed clinical improvement in patients with symptom duration of less than 8 months, the duration of symptoms of heart failure has not predicted survival in the majority of reports [10, 12, 13, 28]. Most investigators have found that patients with more severe functional impairment have a greater mortality risk on univariate analysis [6, 13, 15, 16, 28]. Using a stepwise discriminant analysis, Costanzo-Nordin et al. [28] found that functional class was among a group of clinical variables which predict outcome in dilated cardiomyopathy. In contrast, Unverferth et al. [12] performed multivariate analysis of 69 patients with dilated cardiomyopathy and found that heart failure symptoms did not predict 1-year mortality. Stevenson et al. [20] observed that patients referred for transplantation for dilated cardiomyopathy with a left ventricular ejection fraction ≤ 0.25 have a poor prognosis even if symptoms are mild.

Left ventricular enlargement has been reported to correlate with poor prognosis in dilated cardiomyopathy by most authors using univariate analysis [6, 8–10, 17, 18, 22]. For example, Gavazzi et al. [6] found that mortality was 77% in patients with left ventricular end-diastolic volume $> 185\ \text{ml/m}^2$ compared with 23% in patients with left ventricular end-diastolic volume $\leq 185\ \text{ml/m}^2$. Fuster et al. [8] assessed cardiac enlargement using the cardiothoracic ratio from chest roentgenogram. Mortality was 86% in patients with a cardiothoracic ratio ≥ 0.55, but only 40% in patients with a ratio < 0.55. However, left ventricular enlargement has not been shown to correlate with prognosis using multivariate analysis [9, 12, 21, 28] and may simply reflect the presence of left ventricular dysfunction.

The severity of left ventricular dysfunction appears to be a better predictor of prognosis. Left ventricular ejection fraction is significantly lower in patients who die from dilated cardiomyopathy [6, 9, 10, 12, 15, 18, 21, 28]. Left ventricular ejection fraction has been found to be an independent predictor of survival by multivariate analysis by Hofmann et al. [9] and Keogh et al. [4], but not by Unverferth et al. [12] or Costanzo-Nordin et al. [28]. In the report of Hofmann et al. [9], 84% of patients with left ventricular ejection fraction ≤ 0.35 died during the follow-up period compared with only 46% of patients with left ventricular ejection fraction >0.35. No patient with a left ventricular ejection fraction >0.40 died during an average follow-up period of 53 months. Meinertz et al. [17] prospectively followed 74 patients with dilated cardiomyopathy for an average of 11 months and also found that no deaths occurred in patients with a left ventricular ejcction fraction >0.40. Keogh et al. [21] studied 79 patients with dilated cardiomyopathy who were referred for cardiac transplantation. After 6 months of prospective follow-up there were no deaths of patients with a left ventricular ejection fraction >0.20, but an 87% mortality of patients with left ventricular ejection fraction ≤ 0.10.

Cardiac index, another measure of left ventricular function, has also been shown to correlate with clinical outcome in dilated cardiomyopathy in the majority of reports [6, 8, 9, 17, 19, 28]. Fuster et al. [8] noted that mortality during their 6–20 years of follow-up was 85% in patients with a cardiac index <3.0 l/min per m^2, but only 35% in patients with a cardiac index ≥ 3.0 l/min per m^2. However, the majority of their patients (62%) had a cardiac index <2.5 l/min per m^2, so their arbitrarily chosen division point of 3.0 l/min per m^2 would not be helpful in predicting outcome in most patients. Hofmann et al. [9] used a survival time of only 29.6 months while patients with a cardiac index >2.5 l/min per m^2 had a mean survival time of 51.9 months. Franciosa et al. [13] found that 14-months mortality of patients with a cardiac index ≤ 2.25 l/min per m^2 was 75% compared with 50% in patients with a cardiac index >2.25 l/min per m^2. Multivariate analysis of dilated cardiomyopathy patients reported by Hofmann et al. [9] and Costanzo-Nordin et al. [28] identified cardiac index as an independent prognostic factor. However, cardiac index did not predict prognosis by multivariate analysis in the patients reported by Unverferth et al. [12] or Keogh et al. [21].

The impact of left ventricular diastolic function on survival has been indirectly assessed using left ventricular end-diastolic pressure or pulmonary artery wedge pressure. Higher filling pressures have been observed in patients who died from dilated cardiomyopathy in the majority of reports [6, 8, 10, 12, 15, 17, 28]. Fuster et al. [8] reported that only 13% of patients with left ventricular end-diastolic pressure >20 mmHg survived after 6 years. Both Diaz et al. [10] and Franciosa et al. [13] noted a significant inverse correlation between left ventricular end-diastolic pressure and length of survival. Right atrial and pulmonary artery pressures have also been reported to be higher in patients who die from dilated cardiomyopathy [12, 18]. However, Keogh et al. [21] did not observe any differences in either right or left ventricular filling pressures between survivors and non-survivors.

Atrioventricular and intraventricular conduction abnormalities are frequently observed in dilated cardiomyopathy. Convert et al. [15] observed an increase in mortality in patients with atrioventricular conduction abnormalities (43% vs 23%), but others have not confirmed their findings. Intraventricular conduction abnormalities, in particular left bundle branch block, have frequently been identified as predicting a poor prognosis [6, 9, 15, 16, 22, 29], but have not been a significant factor in all reports [16, 28]. Unverferth et al. [12] found that the presence of left-sided conduction abnormalities were the most prominent factor for predicting 1-year mortality by univariate and multivariate analyses.

The impact of atrial fibrillation on survival is controversial. Many authors have reported that patients with atrial fibrillation have a worse prognosis [9, 12, 16, 18], but others have not found this association [6, 28]. Contrary to these reports, Convert et al. [15] noted that patients with sinus rhythm had a worse prognosis than patients with atrial fibrillation.

It is well recognized that ventricular arrhythmias are common in patients with dilated cardiomyopathy [17], but their significance remains controversial. It is not surprising that many authors have reported that the incidence of sudden death is increased in patients with ventricular arrhythmias [17, 20, 30]. For example, Holmes et al. [30] noted that the risk of sudden death was 11% in patients with only simple ventricular arrhythmias and 59% in patients with complex ventricular arrhythmias. Patients with both complex ventricular arrhythmias and a reduced left ventricular ejection fraction have the greatest risk for sudden death [17]. In addition to sudden death, patients with complex ventricular arrhythmias also have an increased incidence of deaths from heart failure [9, 12, 16, 18, 30]. Using multivariate analysis, Olshausen et al. [29] found that complex ventricular arrythmias were a risk factor, independent of heart failure, for death. In their study, left bundle branch block and left ventricular ejection fraction, but no form of ventricular arrhythmia, were major risk factors for sudden death.

Programmed electrical ventricular stimulation has been evaluated in dilated cardiomyopathy in an attempt to define better which patients are at risk for sudden death. Das et al. [31] studied the prognostic usefulness of programmed stimulation in 24 dilated cardiomyopathy patients without symptomatic ventricular arrhythmias. Ventricular tachycadia or ventricular fibrillation was induced in approximately 40% of their patients. Inducibility of polymorphic ventricular tachycardia or ventricular fibrillation did not correlate with clinical or hemodynamic variables or with the risk of sudden death. However, induction of unimorphic ventricular tachycardia appeared to predict the later occurrence of spontaneous unimorphic ventricular tachycardia. Poll et al. [32] studied the usefulness of programmed stimulation in 47 dilated cardiomyopathy patients presenting with clinically significant arrhythmias. Sustained, uniform ventricular tachycardia was induced in all patients presenting with this arrhythmia, but it was unusual to induce ventricular tachycardia in patients who presented with cardiac arrest or non-sustained ventricular tachycardia. Nine of 23 patients in whom no sustained ventricular arrhythmia was induced died suddenly, with 5 of the 9 receiving empiric antiarrhythmic therapy. Inducible ventricular tachycardia was suppressed with antiarrhythmic therapy in only 4 of 16 patients. These 4 patients survived a mean follow-up of 18 months, while the remaining patients with inducible venticular tachycardia which was not suppressed by antiarrhythmic therapy died suddenly.

The prognostic significance of morphologic features on endomyocardial biopsy has also been evaluated by several authors [12, 14, 21, 22, 33, 34]. Unverferth et al. [12] reported that cell diameter, endocardial thickness and percentage fibrosis were not significantly different between survivors and non-survivors. Baandrup [33] studied morphologic variations in biopsy materials from 125 patients with dilated cardiomyopathy and found that neither the severity of the disease nor the prognosis could be assessed from histologic changes. Keogh et al. [21] also found no significant histologic differences in the endomyocardial biopsy specimens of survivors and non-survivors. Kuhn et al. [22] reported severe morphologic changes in non-survivors, but their observations were not well quantified. Figulla et al. [14] evaluated the volume fraction of myofibrils using light microscopy. A relationship between hemodynamic status and the myofibril volume fraction was not found. However, a reduced myofibril volume fraction (<60%) had prognostic significance for both hemodynamic deterioration and death. Using electron microscopy, Hammond et al. [34] graded myofilament loss. Mortality at 18 months was 37% for patients with extensive myofilament loss and only 10% in patients with little or no myofilament loss. Confirmation by other investigators will be necessary before the clinical usefulness of estimates of myofibril loss on endomyocardial biopsy is established.

Neuroendocrine activation occurs in patients with left ventricular dysfunction and congestive heart failure [35–38]. Patients with heart failure who have the most marked elevation of plasma catecholamines have the most unfavourable long-term prognosis [38, 39]. Patients with heart failure who die within 6 months of evaluation have significantly higher venous plasma concentrations of angiotensin II, aldosterone, atrial natriuretic factor, norepinephrine, and epinephrine than patients who survive beyond 6 months [39]. The presence of hyponatremia is also a powerful predictor of cardiovascular mortality [40]. It is likely that hyponatremia is related to the marked elevation in plasma renin activity observed in these patients. The poor prognosis of heart failure patients with elevation of neuroendocrine hormones or hyponatremia appears to be improved with the administration of angiotensin converting enzyme inhibitors [39, 40].

Management

Importance of Diagnostic Studies

Diagnostic studies can be used to establish the diagnosis of dilated of cardiomyopathy, evaluate prognosis, and direct medical therapy. All potential dilated cardiomyopathy patients should be evaluated with a complete history and physical examination of all systems: chest radiograph, electrocardiogram and echocardiogram with Doppler studies. These studies will exclude most known causes of heart failure. Patients who are more than 30 years of age or who have a history suggestive of ischemia or a high coronary risk profile should also undergo coronary angiography to exclude coronary artery disease. Because arrhythmias have prognostic importance, a 24-h ambulatory electrocardiogram is warranted in most patients. Exercise tolerance testing is useful in selected patients for measurement of functional capacity. Endomyocardial biopsy is frequently performed in patients with unexplained heart failure since this procedure is the only accurate technique for the diagnosis of myocarditis [41] (see Chap. 4). The interest in diagnosing myocarditis is based on anecdotal reports that patients with biopsy-proven myocarditis may respond to immunosuppressive therapy [42]. But until clinical trials have established that immunosuppression is effective for the treatment of myocarditis, the role of endomyocardial biopsy in the evaluation of dilated cardiomyopathy remains undefined. A multicenter study sponsored by the National Institutes of Health is currently in progress to resolve this issue. The importance of endomyocardial biopsy lies in the detection or exclusion of specific heart muscle disease and the diagnosis of healed, healing or active myocarditis (see Chaps. 3 and 4).

Medical Therapy

Medical therapy of dilated cardiomyopathy is directed at controlling heart failure. This is accomplished by controlling salt and water retention, reducing the workload of the heart, and improving its pumping performance.

Patients should be counseled to limit their physical activities based on their functional capacity and to reduce their dietary intake of sodium. Although a "no added salt" diet (4 g Na) may be sufficient restriction for patients with well-compensated symptoms, patients with congestive symptoms will need the stricter salt restriction of a 2 g Na diet. Patients with significant hyponatremia should also restrict fluid intake.

Diuretic therapy must be individualized to account for variations in intravascular volume and renal function. Inadequate diuretic therapy will result in symptomatic pulmonary and systemic venous congestion. Over-diuresis will result in azotemia and electrolyte disorders, and will ultimately decrease cardiac output. While the physical examination is usually adequate in assessing a patient's intravascular volume, right heart catheterization is sometimes necessary to guide therapy. Patients should be instructed to follow their weights daily so that diuretic doses can be changed in response to weight changes, which usually occur prior to the development of frank symptoms. Serum electrolytes, including magnesium, should be carefully monitored with diuretic therapy.

Loop diuretics such as furosemide or bumetanide are the agents of choice when dietary measures are not adequate for controlling congestive failure [43].

Thiazide diuretics are frequently ineffective at the low glomerular filtration rates that occur with heart failure [44]. Most patients receiving diuretics will also require potassium-sparing diuretic such as amiloride to maintain serum potassium levels at >4.5 mequiv/dl. When patients are refractory to loop diuretic therapy alone, the addition of metolazone can result in marked diuresis. Metolazone is a potent long-acting diuretic, the site of action of which is primarily the cortical diluting segment, and secondarily the proximal tubule [44, 45]. It is unique among the thiazide class of diuretics because it is effective when the glomerular filtration rate is less than 25 ml/min [44]. Combined therapy with furosemide and metolazone should be initiated with caution because of the potential for excessive diuresis and electrolyte loss.

Vasodilator therapy reduces the workload of the heart and improves pumping performances. The angiotensin converting enzyme inhibitors (captopril, enalapril and lisinopril) and the combination of hydralazine and isosorbide dinitrate are the two established effective vasodilator regimens. Therapy with angiotensin converting enzyme inhibitor [46] or the combination of hydralazine and isosorbide dinitrate [47] also improves survival in heart failure. The angiotensin converting enzyme inhibitors have important metabolic effects in addition to their vasodilator activity. Treatment of heat failure with angiotensin converting enzyme inhibitors reduces circulating norepinephrine [48]. In addition, patients experience less hypokalemia and less hyponatremia on angiotensin converting enzyme inhibitor therapy [49]. Vasodilator therapy should be initiated at low dose and titrated upwards with careful observation for orthostatic hypotension. Hypotension is most frequently observed in volume-depleted patients. It is therefore, necessary to assess intravascular volume status carefully and, when necessary to correct relative hypovolemia prior to initiation of vasodilator therapy.

Digitalis is a complex drug and observed beneficial clinical responses may be related to a variety of properties, not only its positive inotropic effects. Digitalis is the undisputed drug of choice for the control of ventricular rate in atrial fibrillation or flutter. The use of digoxin in sinus rhythm has been more controversial. Two recent "blind" drug trials [50, 51] have shown that digitalis improves ejection fraction, exercise tolerance and clinical symptoms compared with a placebo. However, digitalis therapy is also associated with arrhythmias, particularly in patients with hypokalemia or hypomagnesemia. It is our practice to use digoxin in sinus rhythm when cardiomegaly and left ventricular systolic dysfunction are present and heart failure symptoms have not been controlled with diuretics and vasodilators. It is important to follow digoxin and serum electrolyte concentrations to avoid lethal arrhythmias of digitalis toxicity. Because of the risk for pulmonary and systemic emboli, it is our practice to initiate warfarin anticoagulation in patients with left ventricular mural thrombus, atrial fibrillation, left ventricular ejection fracton <20%, New York Heart Association (NYHA) class IV symptoms, or a history of systemic embolus disease. Anticoagulant therapy must be carefully monitored, with warfarin dose adjusted to maintain prothrombin time 1.5–2 times control.

Treatment of arrhythmias in dilated cardiomyopathy is a difficult problem, and the roles for antiarrhythmic drugs, electrophysiologic testing to guide therapy, and the automatic implantable defibrillator still need to be defined. The most important steps in the management of arrhythmia are to correct hypoxia, electrolyte and acid–base abnormalities and to treat heart failure. Antiarrhythmic medications have not been shown to improve survival in dilated cardiomyopathy. All antiarrhythmic drugs with the exception of amiodarone have at least some significant negative inotropic effects. In addition, many antiarrhythmic drugs are also potentially proarrhythmic, particularly in patients with severe heart failure. Because of these problems it is our practice to reserve antiarrhythmic therapy for patients with sustained ventricular tachycardia or syncope, to prevent sudden death. Therapy for these patients is guided by electrophysiologic study. Patients with spontaneous inducible ventricular tachycardia and/or sustained ventricular tachycardia that is not suppressed with antiarrhythmic therapy are given an automatic implantable defibrillator.

Beta–adrenergic Blockade

The morbidity and mortality of dilated cardiomyopathy remains very high despite the therapeutic interventions described above. Thus, alternative thera-

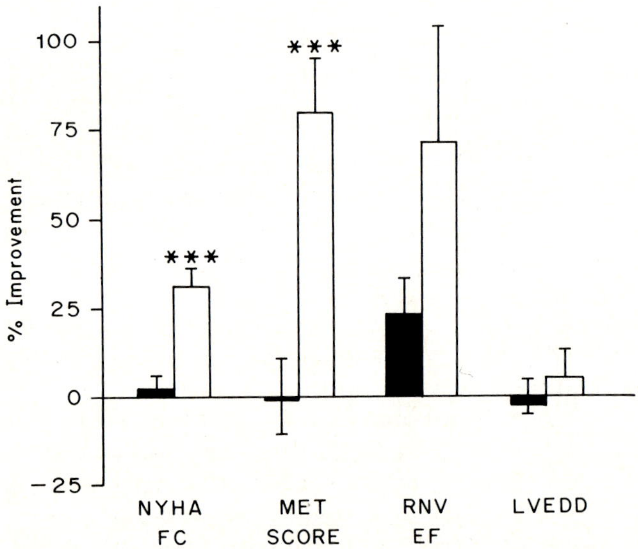

Fig. 5.3. Percentage improvement in mean NYHA functional class, treadmill exercise tolerance, left ventricular ejection fraction, and chamber size in 21 dilated cardiomyopathy patients given metoprolol (*open bars*) or a placebo (*black bars*). Results are given as mean $\pm$SEM. *NYHA FC*, NYHA functional class; *MET SCORE*, maximal oxygen consumption estimated by treadmill test; *RNV EF*, resting radionuclide left ventricular ejection fraction; *LVEDD*, left ventricular end-diastolic diameter. ***$p < 0.001$. From [54]

peutic approaches must be developed to alter favorably the natural history of the disease. One promising new approach to therapy of dilated cardiomyopathy is beta-adrenergic blockade [52]. The potential mechanisms for benefit from beta-blockade include protection from catecholamine cardiotoxicity, up-regulation of myocardial beta-adrenergic receptors, reduction in risk of sudden death, reduction in heart rate, improved ventricular diastolic function, and reduction in afterload.

Beginning with the report of Waagstein et al. [53] in 1975, several investigators have suggested that long-term beta-blockade may improve hemodynamic function, clinical symptoms, and survival in patients with dilated cardiomyopathy. Although data from controlled trials is limited and some reports have been negative, recent studies of beta-adrenergic blockade have been very encouraging. In a placebo-controlled study, Engelmeier et al. [54] administered metoprolol to 21 patients with dilated cardiomyopathy. Metoprolol-treated patients had significant improvements in exercise capacity, NYHA functional class, and left ventricular ejection fraction (Fig.5.3). These changes were not observed in control patients receiving placebo. Gilbert et al. [55] reported on a controlled study of the beta-blocker vasodilator bucindolol. Patients treated with bucindolol had significant improvements in resting hemodynamic function, and rest and exercise left ventricular ejection fraction, and a reduction in questionnaire-measured symptoms (Fig. 5.4). In addition, central venous norepinephrine level decreased

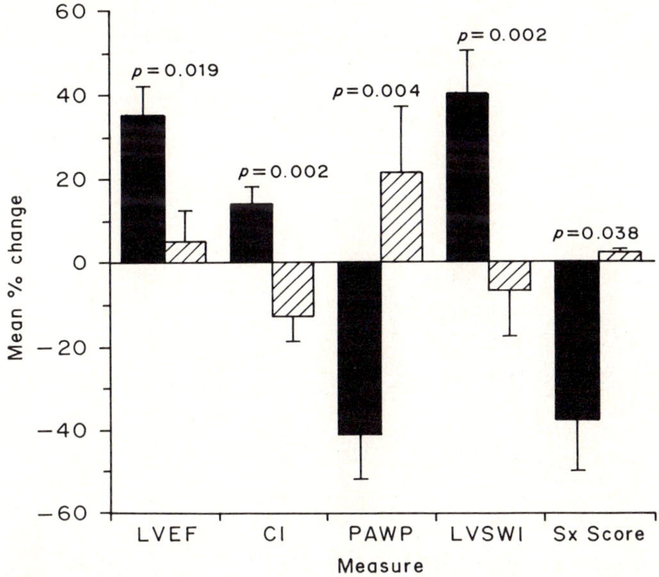

Fig. 5.4. Mean percentage change from baseline in selected functional measures in patients treated with bucindolol (*black bars*) or a placebo (*hatched bars*). *LVEF*, resting radionuclide left ventricular ejection fraction; *Cl*, cardiac index; *PAWP*, pulmonary artery wedge pressure; *LVSWI*, left ventricular stroke work index; *Sx Score*, heart failure symptom score (negative value = improvement). Values are given as mean ± SEM. From [55]

significantly in the bucindolol-treated group, but was unchanged in the placebo group.

Therapy with beta-adrenergic blockers can be successfully initiated in most patients with dilated cardiomyopathy and heart failure (95% of patients tolerated beta-blockade in the metoprolol [54] and bucindolol [55] studies cited above). Clinical experience suggest that beta-selective antagonists (such as metoprolol) or nonselective beta-antagonists with vasodilator properties (such as bucindolol or carvedilol) are better tolerated than nonselective beta-antagonists such as propranolol. Beta-blocker therapy must be initiated at very low doses and the dose must be titrated upwards very slowly. For example, the usual starting dose of metoprolol for hypertension or angina is 50 mg twice daily. For patients with dilated cardiomyopathy, we begin metoprolol at 5 mg twice daily and reach the target dose of 50 mg three times a day after 8 weeks of therapy. Using these agents we have observed a significant improvement in left ventricular ejection fraction and clinical symptoms in more than 50% of our treated patients [56]. Therapy with beta-adrenergic blocking agents must be frequently and meticulously monitored.

Clinical studies suggest that survival of patients with dilated cardiomyopathy may increase with chronic beta-blocker therapy. Swedberg et al. [57] reported that the survival of 24 dilated cardiomyopathy patients treated with beta-blockers was significantly better than that of 13 retrospective controls. Anderson et al. [58] studied 50 patients with dilated cardiomyopathy, symptomatic heart failure, and left ventricular ejection fraction <40%. Patients were randomized in pairs to receive standard therapy alone or therapy including metoprolol. A trend towards improved survival was noted for metoprolol-treated patients; however the differences were not significant (see Fig. 5.5) A large, randomized trial will be needed to determine whether these observations are correct. The

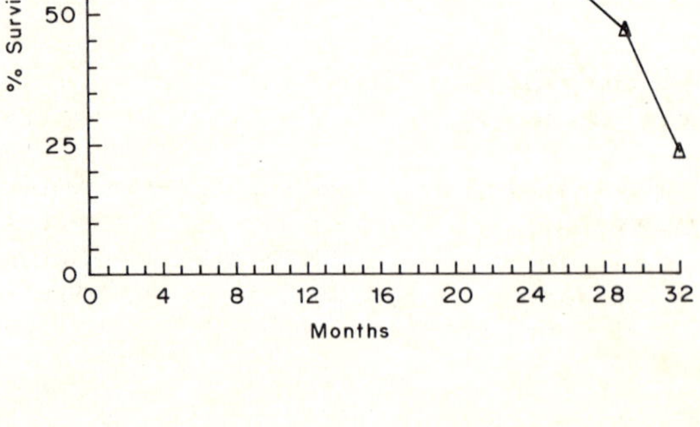

Fig. 5.5. Survival curves by actual treatment method of analysis for control (*triangles*) and β-blockade (metoprolol, *circles*) groups. The differences in curves are not significant. From [58]

Metoprolol in Dilated Cardiomyopathy study is an international trial which has been established to determine whether chronic beta-adrenergic blockade improves survival in dilated cardiomyopathy. In this double-blind, randomized trial patients receive either metoprolol or placebo along with conventional heart failure therapy for 1 year. Enrollment into the trial was completed by July 1991. It is hoped that the results of this trial will clarify the role of chronic beta-adrenergic blockade for the treatment of dilated cardiomyopathy.

Cardiac Transplantation

With improved understanding of donor and recipient selection, the establishment of an aggressive approach to the treatment of infections, the development of endomyocardial biopsy for accurate diagnosis of acute cardiac allograft rejection, and improved immunosuppression, 1-year survival for cardiac transplant recipients now exceeds 85% [59]. The survival of carefully selected transplant recipients far exceeds the survival of similar patients who are not transplanted. Patients with dilated cardiomyopathy with advanced NYHA class III or class IV symptoms refractory to medical management should be considered for transplantation. Transplantation is an important option in the management of dilated cardiomyopathy since so many patients are young adults. The indications for cardiac transplantation are reviewed in Table 5.2. Because so many patients respond to beta-adrenergic blockade, it is our practice to first try beta-adrenergic blockade before actively listing clinically stable patients for transplantation. Patients undergoing such experimental therapy are accepted as cardiac transplant recipients if suitable but placed on a "secondary" recipient list. If beta-blocker therapy fails they are then actively listed for transplantation.

Table 5.2. Indications for cardiac transplantation

1. Age ≤ 65 years
2. Heart disease:
   a) Severe functional limitation
   b) Poor prognosis
   c) Unresponsive to medical therapy or relapse after initial improvement
3. Pulmonary vascular resistance, which if elevated beyond 4–6 Wood units demonstrates reversibility
4. Lack of intrinsic disease of other organ systems which would limit long-term survival or be exacerbated by immunosuppressive therapy
5. Favorable psycho-social profile
6. Negative HIV and hepatitis B screen

Conclusion

Dilated cardiomyopathy is an important cause of morbidity and mortality in the young adult. Patients with severe clinical symptoms, marked left ventricular impairment and complex ventricular ectopy have a very poor prognosis. However, prognostication is still imprecise and much more needs to be learned about which factors predict a poor outcome. Medical management of dilated cardiomyopathy is currently directed at the treatment of heart failure. A promising new therapy is the use of beta-adrenergic blockade, but this treatment modality awaits confirmation from large, multicenter clinical trials. Cardiac transplantation should be considered for patients with severe functional impairment in whom medical therepy has failed or who have improved and then relapsed.

References

1. Shabetai R (1983) Cardiomyopathy: how far have we come in 25 years, how far yet to go? J Am Coll Cardiol 1: 252–263
2. Johnson RA, Palacios I (1982) Dilated cardiomyopathies of the adult. N Engl J Med 307: 1051–1058
3. Silver MA (1988) Anatomy of the failing heart in dilated cardiomyopathy. In: Engelmeier RS, O'Connell JB (eds) Drug therapy in dilated cardiomyopathy and myocarditis. Dekker, New York, pp 1–12
4. McKee PA, Castelli UP, McNamara PM et al. (1971). The natural history of congestive heart failure: the Framingham study. N Engl J Med 285: 1441–1446
5. Torp A (1978) Incidence of congestive cardiomyopathy. Postgrad Med J 54: 435–437
6. Gavazzi A, Lanzarini L, Cornalba C, Desperati M, Raisaro A, Angoli L, de Servi S, Specchia G (1984) Dilated (congestive) cardiomyopathy. G Ital Cardiol 14: 492–498
7. Gorlin R (1983) Incidence, etiology and prognosis of heart failure. Cardiovasc Rev Rep 4: 765
8. Fuster V, Gersh BJ, Giuliana ER, Tajik AJ, Brandenburg RO, Frye RL, (1981) The natural history of idiopathic dilated cardiomyopathy. Am J Cardiol 47: 525
9. Hofmann T, Meinertz T, Kasper W, Geibel A, Zehender M, Hohnloser S, Stienen U, Treese N, Just H (1988) Modle of death in idiopathic dilated cardiomyopathy: a multivariate analysis of prognostic determinants. Am Heart J 116: 1455
10. Diaz RA, Obasohan A, Oakley CM et al. (1987) Prediction of outcome in dilated cardiomyopathy. Br Heart J 58: 393–399
11. O'Connell JB, Costanzo-Nordin MR, Engelmeier RS, Wallis DE, Robinson JA, Scanlon PJ (1985) Prognosis and treatment of cardiomyopathy and myocarditis. Heart Vessels 1 Suppl 1: 175–179
12. Unverferth DV, Magorien RD, Mosechberger ML, Baker PB, Fetters JK, Leier CV (1984) Factors influencing the one-year mortality of dilated cardiomyopathy. Am J Cardiol 54: 147–152
13. Franciosa JA, Wilen M, Ziesche S, Cohn JN (1983) Survival in men with severe chronic left ventricular failure due to either coronary heart disease or idiopathic dilated cardiomyopathy. Am J Cardiol 51: 831–836
14. Figulla HR, Rahlf G, Nieger M, Luig H, Kreuzer H (1985). Spontaneous hemodynamic improvement or stabilization and associated biopsy findings in patients with congestive cardiomyopathy. Circulation 71: 1095–1104

15. Convert G, Delaye J, Beaune J, Biron A, Gonin A (1980). Etude pronostique des myocardiopathies primitive non obstructives. Arch Mal Coeur 27: 227–237
16. Lengyel M, Kokeny M (1981) Follow-up study in congestive (dilated) cardiomyopathy. Acta Cardiol 1: 35–48
17. Meinertz T, Hofmann T, Kasper W, Treese N, Bechtold H, Stienen U, Pop T, Leitner E-RV, Andresen D, Meyer J (1984) Significance of ventricular arrhythmias in idiopathic dilated cardiomyopathy. Am J Cardiol 53: 902–907
18. Romeo F, Pelliccia F, Cianfrocca C, Cristofani R, Reale A (1989) Predictors of sudden death in idiopathic dilated cardiomyopathy. Am J Cardiol 63: 138–140
19. Koide T, Kato A, Takabatake Y, Iizuka M, Uchida Y, Ozeki K, Morooka S, Kakihana M, Serizawa T, Tanaka S, Ohya T, Momomura S, Murao S (1980) Variable prognosis in congestive cardiomyopathy: role of left ventricular function, alcoholism, and pulmonary thrombosis. Jpn Heart J 21: 451–463
20. Stevenson LW, Fowler MB, Schroeder JS, Stevenson WG, Dracup KA, Fond V (1987) Poor survival of patients with idiopathic cardiomyopathy considered too well for transplantation. Am J Med 83: 871–876
21. Keogh AM, Freund J, Baron DW, Hickie JB (1988) Timing of cardiac transplantation in idiopathic dilated cardiomyopathy. Am J Cardiol 61: 418–422
22. Kuhn H, Becker R, Fischer J, Curtius JM, Losse B, Hort W, Loogen F (1982)Untersuchungen zur Atiologie, zum Verlauf and zur Prognose der dilatativen Kardiomyopathie (DCM). Z Kardiol 71: 497–508
23. Strain JE, Grose RM, Cho S, Factor SM (1985) Short term natural history of untreated myocarditis (Abstr). Circulation 72-III: 110
24. Quigley PJ, Richardson PJ, Meany BT, Olsen EGJ,Monaghan M, Jackson G, Jewitt DE (1987) Long term follow up in biopsy proven myocarditis: progression to dilated cardiomyopathy. Br Heart J 57: 71
25. Demakis JG, Rahimtoola SH, Sutton GC, Meadows WR, Szanto PB, Tobin JR, Gunnar RM (1971) Natural course of peripartum cardiomyopathy. Circulation 44: 1053–1061
26. DeMakis JG, Proskey A, Rahimtoola SH, Jamil M, Sutton GC, Rosen KM, Gunnar RM, Tobin JR (1974) The natural course of alcoholic cardiomyopathy. Ann Intern Med 80: 293–297
27. Schwartz L, Sample KA, Wigle ED (1975) Severe alcoholic cardiomyopathy reversed with abstention from alcohol. Am J Cardiol 36: 963–966
28. Costanzo-Nordin MR, O'Connell JB, Engelmeier RS, Moran JF, Scanlon PJ (1985) Dilated cardiomyopathy: functional status, hemodynamics, arrhythmias, and prognosis. Cathet Cardiovasc Diagn 11: 445–453
29. Olshausen AV, Stienen U, Schwarz F, Kubler W, Meyer J (1988) Long-term prognostic significance of ventricular arrhythmias in idiopathic dilated cardiomyopathy. Am J Cardiol 61: 146–151
30. Holmes J, Kubo SH, Cody RJ, Kligfield P (1985) Arrhythmias in ischemic and nonischemic dilated cardiomyopathy: prediction of mortality by ambulatory electrocardiography. Am J Cardiol 55: 146–151
31. Das SK, Mordy F, DiCarlo L, Baerman J, Krol R, de Buitleir M, Crevey B (1986) Prognostic usefulness of programmed ventricular stimulation in idiopathic dilated cardiomyopathy without symptomatic ventricular arrhythmias. Am J Cardiol 58: 998–1000
32. Poll DS, Marchlinski FE, Buxton AE, Josephson ME (1986) Usefulness of programmed stimulation in idiopathic dilated cardiomyopathy. Am J Cardiol 58: 992–997
33. Baandrup U, Florio RA, Rehahn M, Richardson PJ, Olsen EGJ (1981) Critical analysis of endomyocardial biopsies from patients suspected of having cardiomyopathy. Br Heart J 45: 487–493
34. Hammond EH, Menlove RL, Anderson JL (1987) Predictive value of immunofluorescence and electron microscopic evaluation of endomyocardial biopsies in the diagnosis and prognosis of myocarditis and idiopathic dilated cardiomyopathy. Am Heart J 114: 1055
35. Levine TB, Francis GS, Goldsmith SR, Simon AB, Cohn JN (1982) Activity of the sympathetic

nervous system and renin–angiotensin system assessed by plasma hormone levels and their relation to hemodynamic abnormalities in congestive heart failure. Am J Cardiol 49: 1659
36. Francis GS, Benedict C, Johnstone DE, Kirlin PC, Nicklas J, Liang C-S, Kubo SH, Rudin-Toretsky E, Yusuf S (1990) Comparison of neuroendocrine activation in patients with left ventricular dysfunction with and without congestive heart failure. Circulation 82: 1724–1729
37. Maisel AS, Scott NA, Motulsky HJ, Michel MC, Boublik JH, Rivier JE, Ziegler M, Allen RS, Brown MR (1989) Elevation of plasma neuropeptide Y levels in congestive heart failure. Am J Med 86: 43
38. Cohn JN, Levine TB, Olivari MT, Garberg V, Lura D, Francis GS, Simon AB, Rector T (1984) Plasma norepinephrine as a guide to prognosis in patients with chronic congestive heart failure. N Engl J Med 311: 819–823
39. Swedberg K, Eneroth P, Kjekshus J, Wilhelmsen L (1990) Hormones regulating cardiovascular function in patients with severe congestive heart failure and their relation to mortality. Circulation 82: 1730–1736
40. Lee WH, Packer M (1986) Prognostic importance of serum sodium concentration and its modification by converting-enzyme inhibition in patients with severe chronic heart failure. Circulation 73: 257–267
41. Mason JW, Billinggham ME, Ricci DR (1980) Treatment of acute inflammatory myocarditis assisted by endomyocardial biopsy. Am J Cardiol 45: 1037–1044
42. Gilbert EM, Mason JW Immunosuppressive therapy of myocarditis. In: Engelmeier RS, O'Connell JB (eds) Drug therapy in dilated cardiomyopathy and myocarditis. Dekker, New York, pp 233–263
43. Doherty JE (1988) Use of digitalis and diuretics in the treatment of heart failure. In: Cohn JN (ed) Drug treatment of heart failure. Advanced Therapeutics Communications International, Secaucus, pp147–178
44. Renlin FC The actions and use of diuretics in renal disease. In: Freidkey CK (ed) Heart, kidney and electrolytes. Grune and Stratton, New York, pp 169–193
45. Craswell PW, Ezzati E, Kopstein J et al. (1973) Use of metolazone, a new diuretic, in patients with renal disease. Nephron 12: 63–73
46. CONSENSUS Trial Study Group (1987) Effects of enalapril on mortality in severe congestive heart failure: results of the Cooperative North Scandinavian Enalapril Survival Study (CONSENSUS). N Engl J Med 316: 1429–1435
47. Cohn JN, Archibald DG, Ziesche S, Franciosa JA, Harston WE, Tristani FE, Dunkman WB, Jacobs W, Francis GS, Flohr KH, Goldman S, Cobb FR, Shah PM, Saunders R, Fletcher RD, Loeb HS, Hughes VC, Baker B (1986) Effect of vasodilator therapy on mortality in chronic congestive heart failure. N. Engl J Med 314: 1547–1552
48. Cody RJ, Franklin KW, Kluger J, Laugh LH (1982) Sympathetic responsiveness and plasma norepinephrine during therapy of chronic congestive heart failure with captopril. Am J Med 72: 791–797
49. Cleland JGF, Dangic H, Horsman GP et al. (1984) Captopril in heart failure, a double blind controlled trial. Br Heart J 52: 530–535
50. Captopril-Digoxin Multicenter Research Group (1988) Comparative effects of therapy with captopril and digoxin in patients with mild to moderate heart failure. JAMA 259: 539–554
51. DiBianco R, Shabetai R, Kostuk W et al. (1989) A comparison of oral milrinone, digoxin and their combination in the treatment of patients with chronic heart failure. N Engl J Med 320: 677–683
52. Gilbert EM, O'Connell JB, Bristow MR, (1992) Therapy of idiopathic dilated cardiomyopathy with chronic beta-adrenergic blockade. Heart Vessels (in press)
53. Waagstein F, Hjalmmarson A, Varnauskas E, Wallentin I (1975) Effect of chronic beta-adrenergic receptor blockade in congestive cardiomyopathy. Br Heart J 37: 1022–1036
54. Engelmeier RS, O'Connell JB, Walsh R, Rad N, Scanlon PJ, Gunnar RM (1985) Improvement in symptoms and exercise tolerance by metoprolol in patients with dilated cardiomyopathy: a double blind, randomized, placebo-controlled trial. Circulation 72: 526–546

55. Gilbert EM, Anderson JL, Deitchman D, Yanowitz FG, O'Connell JB, Renlund DG, Bartholomew M, Mealey PC, Larrabee P, Bristow MR (1990) Long-term beta-blocker vasodilator therapy improves cardiac function in idiopathic dilated cardiomyopathy: a double-blind, randomized study of bucindolol versus placebo. Am J Med 88: 223–229
56. Gilbert EM, Mestroni L, Anderson JL, Woodley SL, Bristow MR (1989) Can response to beta-blocker therapy in idiopathic dilated cardiomyopathy be predicted by baseline parameters? Circulation 80: II-428
57. Swedberg K, Waagstein F, Hjalmarson S, Wallentin I (1979) Prolongation of survival in congestive cardiomyopathy by a beta receptor blockade. Lancet 1: 1374–1376
58. Anderson JL, Lutz JR, Gilbert EM, Sorenson SG, Yanowitz FG, Menlove RL, Batholomew M (1985) A randomized trial of low dose beta-blockade therapy for idiopathic dilated cardiomyopathy. Am J Cardiol 55: 471–475
59. O'Connell JB, Renlund DG, Bristow MR (1989) Cardiac transplantation: emerging role of the internist/cardiologist. J Intern Med 225: 147–156

Part III
Hypertrophic Cardiomyopathy

CHAPTER 6

Clinical Aspects

J. F. Goodwin

Although it has recently been suggested again that hypertrophic cardiomyopathy may be not one disease but many [1, 2], the undoubted existence of the disease in the absence of any identifiable cause for ventricular hypertrophy—that is other heart or cardiovascular disease, such as aortic stenosis or hypertension—suggests that it certainly is a definite entity [3]. But there is no doubt that the manifestations of the disorder are protean and that their wide spectrum influences the clinical picture, diagnosis and prognosis. One of the difficulties of supporting a unitarian hypothesis is the lack of a single specific pathological feature, for even the characteristic myofibrillar disarray is not pathognomonic [2, 3], because such areas can be found in normal fetal hearts at certain stages of development, in normal hearts and in other forms of heart disease. However a definitive diagnosis of hypertrophic cardiomyopathy can be made on the basis of the association of essential clinical and investigative diagnostic features in a given patient. The diagnosis can, in typical cases, be determined at the bedside. Conversely, there may be no abnormal physical signs and even sophisticated investigations may fail to give a definite answer, though this is now unusual. But it is probable that there are cases in which a confident diagnosis cannot be made on one examination though time may sometimes reveal the disease. Accurate diagnosis in such cases will depend on identification of the gene responsible. Already a site on chromosome 14 has been identified in three families [4].

Causation and Geographical Distribution

Hypertrophic cardiomyopathy is found world-wide, with no especial climatic or geographical bias. The finding of well-developed hypertrophic cardiomyopathy in the hearts of newborn infants suggests that it may be a disorder of the growth of developing myocardium in utero. The myofibrillar disarray found in hypertrophic cardiomyopathy is similar to that seen in primitive hearts such as that of the salamander. Ferrans et al. [5] and Manasek [6] have noted that mechanical forces of contraction determine the pattern of orientation of muscle fibres, and derangement of the orientation of myofibres into parallel lines during intrauterine development may be caused by abnormally orientated forces. The myofibrillar disarrangement in hypertrophic cardiomyopathy suggests a cell type less well differentiated than in the fully developed heart.

Goodwin [7] in 1974 suggested that abnormal orientation of myofibrils in hypertrophic cardiomyopathy might be a genetically determined aberration of catecholamine function in the embryo heart, because clinically there are a number of conditions that have been described in connection with hypertrophic cardiomyopathy which have a basis in abnormal catecholamine function. These are: systemic hypertension, phaeochromocytoma, neurofibromatosis and Friedreich's ataxia [8–12]. The association of hypertrophic cardiomyopathy with multiple symmetrical lentigens suggests that hypertrophic cardiomyopathy might be related to some defect in neural crest function [12].

Beta-adrenergic stimulation has been shown to increase the abnormalities of function in hypertrophic cardiomyopathy and beta-adrenergic blockade to suppress them [13]. Animal studies by Blaufuss et al. [14] showed that chronic subhypertensive infusions of noradrenaline produced ventricular hypertrophy in dogs with haemodynamic and angiographic changes reminiscent of those in hypertrophic cardiomyopathy. These workers thought that noradrenaline might be regarded as a "myocardial cell hypertrophy hormone". Witzke and Kaye [15] found that "nerve growth factor" (a naturally occurring glycoprotein which stimulates sympathetic nerve growth and cardiac adrenergic innervation) produced left ventricular pressure gradients and increased septal thickness and myocardial fibrillar disarray in newborn puppies in which increased catecholamines were found in the base of the heart abnormal receptors were postulated. Further experimental studies by Pearce et al. [16] support a genetic component in showing that the administration of thyroid precursor (triiodothyroacetic acid) to pregnant rats produced myofibrillar disarray in the offspring. The effect of triiodothyroacetic acid could be blocked by low doses of calcium antagonist therapy with verapamil. Wagner et al. [17] showed an increase in the number of calcium antagonist receptors in the atrial myocardium, which would reflect an increased voltage sensitivity of the calcium channel. The same authors also noted a normal density of beta-adrenergic receptors. Dargie and Goodwin [17a] reported an increase in plasma noradrenaline levels in hypertrophic cardiomyopathy at rest on standing and during the cold pressor test as compared with controls. Perloff [18] suggested that there might be faulty interaction between noradrenaline and myocardial receptor sites leading to failure of normal regression of the disproportionate septal thickness and myocardial fibre disarray found in the developing fetal heart. The findings of Wagner et al. [17] do not support the theory that the inherited abnormalities in hypertrophic cardiomyopathy are due to abnormal handling of catecholamines by the developing myocardium, but neither do they exclude it. Whatever mechanism operates it encourages persistence of abnormal myofibrillar disarray, causes disarray later, stimulates hypertrophy and impairs both contraction and relaxation. Powerful contraction of the left ventricle may be due to excess of catecholamine action, and the impaired relaxation to the "criss-cross" basket-weave arrangement of the myofibrils and abnormal calcium fluxes. Although Matsumori et al. [19] thought that the HLA system might play some role in the pathogenesis of hypertrophic cardiomyopathy with familial occurrence, at the present time there seems little evidence of a disorder of cellular immunity. The reversible echocardiographic, angiographic and haemodynamic features suggesting hypertrophic cardiomyopathy that occur in infants or diabetic mothers suggest that other hormones might be involved in causation also [20].

Structural and Functional Disorders that Determine the Pattern of the Disease

There are seven Structural and functional abnormalities that determine the pattern of the disease:

1. Massive hypertrophy of the ventricular septum that may involve its entire length, the apical or basal portions. The hypertrophy often extends to the free wall of the left ventricle, sometimes to the right ventricle.
2. Powerful rapid contraction of the left ventricle which over-empties.
3. Systolic pressure difference (gradient) between the body of the left ventricle and the aorta.
4. Delayed relaxation, increased stiffness and reduced compliance of the left ventricle that can be general or regional.
5. Occlusive changes in small intramural coronary arteries and arterioles.
6. Myofibrillar disarray and fibrosis.
7. Tendency to sudden death.

While it is commonly supposed (and is usually the case) that the degree of hypertrophy matches the extent of the myofibrillar disarray, recent reports indicate that extensive disarray may exist without comparable hypertrophy, and that hypertrophy can be extreme with little if any myofibrillar disarray [21, 22]. The lack of hypertrophy in patients who die suddenly with extensive myofibrillar disarray calls into question the validity of the terminology of the disease, but in view of the limitations of our knowledge, it is impossible to avoid a descriptive term. Since myofibrillar disarray is not pathognomonic for the disease perhaps cases with extreme disarray but not hypertrophy are examples of hypertrophic cardiomyopathy in which hypertrophy has not (yet) developed.

The Clinical Picture

For symptoms see also Chap. 9.

Dyspnoea

Dyspnoea is common, but variable in degree. It may occur on effort or occasionally spontaneously. It is due to the high left atrial pressure and pulmonary venous pressure produced by the stiffness and diastolic faults of the left ventricle. It is worsened by tachycardia, which limits the time available for filling the left ventricle and raises the left atrial pressure further. Although patients with hypertrophic cordiomyopathy are commonly physically well developed and active, they show considerable impairment of respiratory function on effort. Often they do not appear to realise that they are dyspnoeic, which is not surprising since the sensation of dyspnoea is a complex one involving central and peripheral influences as well as pulmonary causes. While dyspnoea is undoubtedly associated with raisd left atrial and pulmonary venous pressure due to abnormal left ventricular diastolic function [23], while impaired filling of the left ventricle impedes exercise capacity, doubts have been expressed about this simplistic explanation. Maximum oxygen consumption and anaerobic threshold have been related to peak cardiac index on effort, but not to cardiac index at rest nor to the rise of pulmonary venous pressure on effort, suggesting that other mechanisms may be at work [24]. Furthermore, the status of atrial natriuretic protein at rest and on effort in hypertrophic cardiomyopathy has not been studied. Spontaneous episodes of dyspnoea are rare. Sometimes they are due to transient atrial fibrillation which impairs systolic and diastolic function, to acute left ventricular failure or to sudden myocardial ischaemia.

Ischaemic Cardiac Pain

Ischaemic cardiac pain is frequent, usually occurring as typical angina of effort [25]. However, severe persistent pain resembling coronary thrombosis can occur and myocardial infarction has been described with normal major coronary arteries in hypertrophic cardiomyopathy [26]. The reasons for ischaemic pain are not entirely clear. Several mechanisms may operate: excess of demand over supply to the greatly hypertrophied myocardium, compression of septal perforating arteries, small vessel disease, impaired diastolic relaxation, abnormal wall stress and increased oxygen demand. Possibly all these factors participate, but the most important link may be the impairment of diastolic function. Whatever the cause of the pain, metabolic abnormalities consistent with ischaemia are present [27] and coronary vasodilator reserve is impaired [28]. Furthermore there is ST segment depression at rest and on effort during electrocardiographic ambulatory monitoring in many, if not most, cases.

Disturbance of Consciousness

Dizziness, feelings of faintness and syncope are all common symptoms tending to occur on or after effort, tachycardia or emotional disturbance. A rapid fall in blood volume or pressure with vasodilatation precipitates syncope due to reduction in volume of the left ventricle. Syncopal attacks can be fatal and sudden death is the single commonest mode of termination. Episodes of impaired consciousness can occur without any obvious precipitating factor.

There are a number of reasons for disturbance of consciousness and for sudden death, notably serious arrhythmia, haemodynamic faults and possibly ischaemic episodes.

Arrhythmic Causes

Repetitive non-sustained ventricular tachycardia is common, and most patients show evidence of ventricular irritability in one form or another varying from isolated unifocal ventricular contractions to multifocal multiple ectopic beats. Serious ventricular arrhythmia has been reported in 50% of cases [29]. While ectopic beats alone are not likely to impair consciousness, runs of ventricular tachycardia may well do so. Paroxysmal atrial fibrillation, especially when the ventricular rate is rapid, may cause syncope. Patients who have Pre-excitation [30] (which is rare) may have attacks of atrial fibrillation and die suddenly. Heart block is rare in hypertrophic cardiomyopathy but Adams–Stokes attacks can occur. The tachycardia–bradycardia syndrome may accompany hypertrophic cardiomyopathy and cause symptoms also. (see Chap. 9).

Haemodynamic Causes

The combination of impaired relaxation and delayed filling with excessive emptying of the left ventricle may induce a state of "no flow" through the heart and is a major cause of disturbance of consciousness or sudden death. The importance of these haemodynamic factors is emphasised by the fact that sudden death in children is apparently not related to arrhythmia—in contrast to adults in whom severe ventricular arrhythmia is an important marker for sudden death [31]. A case report [32] testifies to the haemodynamic mechanism: a woman with hypertrophic cardiomyopathy collapsed pulseless while walking equipped with an electrocardiographic monitor which continued to record while she was unconscious. The monitor did not reveal any ventricular arrhythmia, but showed ischaemia on her recovery. It is likely that both haemodynamic and arrhythmic causes may operate together to cause syncope or sudden death [11]. Outflow tract "obstruction" is probably a less important influence than previously thought [11]. Syncope, during or after effort, can be due to tachycardia limiting diastolic filling and reducing ventricular volume. Recent work [33] has identified patients with hypertrophic cardiomyopathy who develop hypotension due to vasodilatation in non-excercising muscles on effort. These patients have an adverse prognosis (see Chaps. 8 and 9). Further work is necessary to determine whether a peripheral reflex is triggered by the hypertrophied heart in some way.

Ischaemic Causes

It is likely that transient ischaemia could cause disturbance of consciousness, but it is worth noting that anginal pain is rare during episodes of dizziness or near-syncope.

Palpitations

Palpitations are usually due to arrhythmia, but are sometimes a symptom of the powerful, rapidly contracting heart. However, attacks of regular or irregular rapid heart beat which start and stop suddenly strongly suggest paroxysmal atrial fibrillation or flutter. Although episodes of ventricular tachycardia may give rise to a sensation of palpitations and other symptoms, it is remarkable that many such episodes go completely unrecognised by the patient, presumably because they are often of short duration. By contrast, atrial fibrillation tends usually to produce symptoms.

Fatigue

Fatigue is a well-recognised though not a frequent symptom. It occurs more often in older age groups and is difficult to evaluate because of its vague subjective character. It is, however, a real component of the disease. The cause is uncertain, but it probably reflects impairment of cardiac output possibly related to diminished coronary reserve. It may be the equivalent of "silent angina". Fatigue is not related to any particular event, action or time and may occur on effort or at rest; sometimes patients complain of overwhelming tiredness for no apparent reason.

Symptoms Due to Complications

Infective Endocarditis

Infective endocarditis causes fever, shivering and general malaise, but in elderly people symptoms may be much more subtle: fatigue, anorexia, vague muscle pains, dyspnoea. At any age neuropsychiatric symptoms can predominate and disturbance of mood, such as depression, can be the first symptom. A history of dental work not covered by antibiotics should arouse suspicion. The mitral valve is the commonest site for infection, followed by the aortic valve. The incidence has been reported as 5%–9% of cases of hypertrophic cardiomyopathy [34].

Valvar Disease

Calcification of the mitral valve can occur in older patients [35]. It may be associated with severe or extreme mitral regurgitation which can also occur after infective endocarditis or as a result of progressive damage due to the turbulent blood flow in the left ventricle. The impact of the anterior mitral valve leaflet on the ventricular septum can cause damage and mitral prolapse. Severe mitral regurgitation produces extreme dyspnoea, even pulmonary oedema, and may precipitate right heart failure due to severe pulmonary hypertension.

Aortic regurgitation

Aortic regurgitation is more common than previously realised and is presumably due either to minor associated congenital abnormality of the aortic valve or to previous endocarditis. Murmurs of aortic reflux were recorded in 3 of a series of 87 patients, but Doppler echocardiography showed the regurgitant signal in 23% [36]. However, Doppler techniques tend to overestimate valvar reflux and a positive signal does not necessarily indicate a defective valve. There are no symptoms unless the aortic reflux is clinically appreciable.

Systemic Embolism

Systemic embolism is a serious hazard if atrial fibrillation has developed or infective endocarditis has occured. Symptoms depend upon the location of the embolism, common sites being the brain, limbs, gut or kidney. Occasionally coronary embolism producing myocardial infarction may occur.

Symptomps Due to Associated Conditions

Atherosclerotic Coronary Artery Disease in the Major Coronary Arteries

Atherosclerois may occur in up to 15%–20% of patients with hypertrophic cardiomyopathy. Many of the symptoms overlap those of hypertrophic cardiomyopathy, though symptoms alone do not make the diagnosis. Neither the resting cardiogram nor effort test will diagnose associated coronary heart disease, so coronary arteriography may be required (see Chap. 8 for indications). In coronary heart disease the volume of the left ventricle may increase and the force of contraction diminish, temporarily improving the symptoms of the hypertrophic cardiomyopathy and reducing signs of any intraventricular pressure gradient [37].

Pregnancy

Pregnancy is well tolerated in hypertrophic cardiomyopathy [38] though angina may increase somewhat. Because of the circulatory hormonal and fluid balance changes of pregnancy, mild congestive heart failure may develop in the last trimester. Intrauterine life is usually uneventful and the risk to the fetus small. Although the fetus may inherit the disease, this does not necessarily mean that overt disease will be present at or after birth.

Hypertension

Hypertension is commonly associated with hypertrophic cardiomyopathy. Indeed, this differential diagnosis between hypertrophic cardiomyopathy and hypertension on the one hand and hypertensive heart disease on the other can be extremely difficult or occasionally impossible. It is likely that the association of hypertrophic cardiomyopathy with hypertension is part of the diverse spectrum of the former [39]. It is of interest that a recent editorial discussing the relationship of hypertension to complications of left ventricular hypertrophy considered that hypertrophy might cause or aggravate hypertension [40]. If so, this could explain hypertension in hypertrophic cardiomyopathy, though would not make clear why only some patients with the disease are hypertensive. Perhaps differences in the geometry of the left ventricle are relevant factors. As might be expected, hypertension is more common in older patients than in younger ones.

Hypertrophic Cardiomyopathy in the Elderly

In older patients, symptoms tend to be less severe and sudden death less common [41]. Mitral valve calcification is well recognised.

Natural History

Hypertrophic cardiomyopathy is remarkable in having an immensely variable prognosis. Infants born with serious disease usually develop heart failure shortly after birth and may die in a few weeks or months. At the other end of the spectrum, patients may be diagnosed accidentally in their seventies with few if any symptoms. A recent study documented a good prognosis in a group of asymptomatic out-patients [42]. Children and adolescents with a family history of sudden death and definite symptoms including syncope and arrhythmia have a poor outlook: sudden death can be the presenting symptom of the disease.

A recent report [43] suggested a direct relation between the extent of severity of left ventricular hypertrophy and the occurence of unexplained sudden death. Sudden death was uncommon in asymptomatic or mildly symptomatic in patients with relatively slight left ventricular hypertrophy. It seems likely that this is a reasonable generalisation, but clearly not always the case, especially if there is a strong family history of the disease. Middle-aged adults with moderate hypertrophy, no family history of sudden death and limited physical signs tend to have few or any symptoms for many years, and the risk of sudden death is small, though unexpected death can be a threat to any patient at any time. Mention has already been made of the occurrence of sudden death in patients with little or no hypertrophy but with massive myofibrillar disarray, and by contrast in those with massive hypertrophy but little disarray. The combination of widespread disarray and massive hypertrophy carries a poor prognosis. It is likely that the disease is mild in many patients who remain undetected for long periods or who, if detected, do not require treatment. Progressive T wave changes do not necessary indicate clinical deterioration, though reduction in R voltage may do so (Fig. 6.1).

The natural history of the disease is influenced by associated disorders, by the progress of the disease and by its complications. Heart failure occurs when

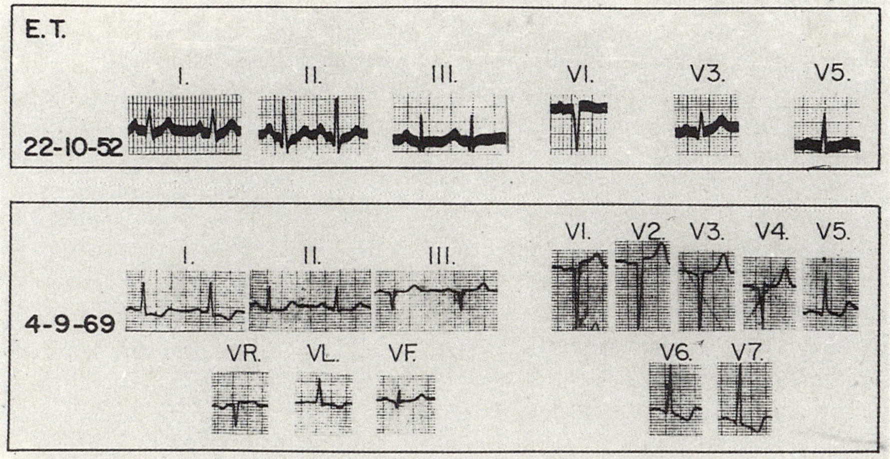

Fig. 6.1. Serial electrocardiograms in hypertrophic cardiomyopathy. *Upper panel:* Normal appearance. *Lower Panel*: 17 years later T wave inversiom has developed in leads I, V_L, V_6 and V_7. Q waves are present in III, V_F, and V_1 to V_4.

systolic failure is added to diastolic faults. Other factors in producing or exaggerating heart failure are atrial fibrillation myocardial infarction, severe mitral regurgitation and infective endocarditis.

Until recently, it was thought that atrial fibrillation was almost invariably a serious stage in the downward progress of the disease resulting in considerable increase in symptoms. While this is often true, a recent study suggests that some patients tolerate periods of atrial fibrillation very well. In a series of 52 consecutive patients with atrial fibrillation, 19 deaths were related to the disease—figures that were similar to those in a concurrent group of 122 patients who remained in sinus rhythm. Good results were dependent on restoration of sinus rhythm, which was assisted by the use of amiodarone. Despite these encouraging results, the acute onset of arrhythmia was associated with change of symptoms in 89%, but over 90% returned to their original symptoms after sinus rhythm had been restored [44].

It is not true that hypertrophic cardiomyopathy can turn into or become dilated cardiomyopathy; dilatation of the ventricles is a late stage of hypertrophic cardiomyopathy but differentiation clinically from dilated cardiomyopathy may be extremely difficult, especially if atrial fibrillation is present.

Clinical Signs

Cardiac radiography and electrocardiography will be included in the clinical assessment.

General Appearance

Most patients with hypertrophic cardiomyopathy have excellent physique, and many are competitive athletes. Their psychological make-up also appears to be stable; neurotic trends are unusual. Chest deformity, and spinal abnormalities such as kyphoscoliosis, are also unusual.

Classical Cardiovascular Signs

The signs in the cardiovascular system are clear-cut in severe cases, but there may be few if any signs in mild ones. The classical signs are: the characteristic arterial pulse, the cardiac impulse and the auscultatory features as noted below. The three significant assessments, if associated with a compatible history, can permit a confident diagnosis at the bedside without further tests.

Arterial Pulse

The character of the arterial pulse is due to the rapid powerful contraction and emptying of the left ventricle. The sharp collapse of the pulse reflects the over-emptying of the left ventricle and, in some cases, the development of an outflow tract gradient (Fig. 6.2).

Cardiac Impulse

The cardiac impulse is left ventricular in type—a localised powerful thrust that may be felt outside the left mid-clavicular line. Like the arterial pulse, it is ill-sustained. It is due to the powerful thrust of the hypertrophied left ventricle. The complete emptying of the ventricle acts as a "run-off" and accounts for the rapid decline of the beat. The left ventricular thrust is preceded by a lesser pulsation, the left atrial beat, which is due to the powerful contraction of the left atrium needed to fill the stiff left ventricle. It may be necessary to turn the patient on to the left side to feel the atrial beat (Fig. 6.2).

Ausculation

Left-Sided Events. The characteristic number is systolic in time, diamond in shape and begins after the third sound. It may give rise to a thrill. The murmur is characteristically of late onset, there being a silent period immediately after the third heart sound before the murmur begins. This murmur may be associated with mitral regurgitation or turbulence in the ventricle. Sometimes mitral valve prolapse may be associated, contributing to the systolic murmur, and occasionally producing a systolic click. When the proximal portion of the ventricular septum is greatly hypertrophied there may be a soft diastolic rumble due to relative submitral valve obstruction. The third heart sound is due to tensing of the

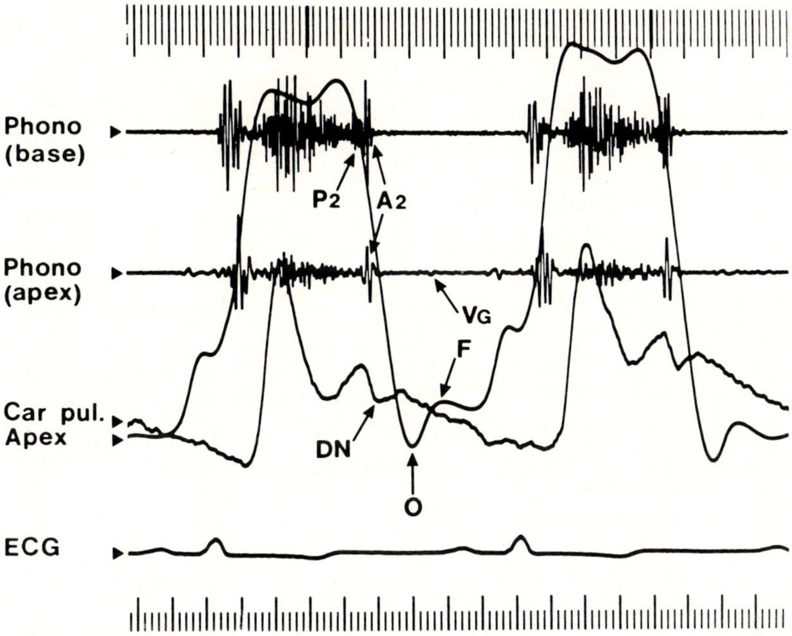

Fig. 6.2. Composite phonocardiogram, apex cardiogram, arterial pulse tracing and electrocardiogram in an adult patient with fully developed hypertrophic cardiomyopathy. The phonocardiogram shows the diamond-shaped systolic murmur of late onset heart at the base and apex. The split of the second heart sound is reversed due to late closure of the aortic valve. The apex cardiogram shows a notch on the upstroke indicating the atrial beat. The arterial pulse tracing shows the rapid upstroke, rapid decline and dicrotic notch (DN). (Courtesy of Dr. R. Alvares)

papillary muscles. It is likely to be present when there is dilataion of the left ventricle or when initial filling of the left ventricle is rapid. A further sound due to atrial contraction is to be expected but is often not heard because of its low frequency (Fig. 6.2).

Right-Sided Events. When the massive septum bulges into the right ventricle and outflow tract, there may be a right atrial systolic murmur due to relative tricuspid stenosis, and a systolic murmur due to a right ventricular/pulmonary artery gradient in systole.

Physical Signs When No Gradient Is Present

There may be no murmur or only a very soft short one, but the arterial pulse is commonly ill-sustained, the left ventricular thrust notable and the atrial beat palpable. Gallop sounds may be audible, but in mild cases there may be no abnormal physical signs.

Physical Signs Modified by Progress in the Disease, Complications or Associated Conditions

Atrial Fibrillation

The development of atrial fibrillation removes two important physical signs: the atrial beat disappears and the characteristic features of the arterial pulse tend to disappear.

Congestive Heart Failure

Congestive heart failure may occur with or without a systolic murmur. When ventricular dilatation is considerable the systolic murmur tends to diminish or disappear as the dilatation of the ventricle reduces the gradient. In congestive heart failure the murmur can be due to mitral regurgitation. The left ventricular impulse becomes less forceful and the signs of hypertrophic cardiomyopathy tend to be obscured. A clue to the underlying diagnosis may be a slow "y" descent in the jugular venous pulse due to increased resistance to filling of the right ventricle. Atrial fibrillation is often present. The electrocardiogram and echocardiogram show massive left ventricular hypertrophy.

Infective Endocarditis

Infective Endocarditis will usually cause fever, fatigue, malaise and signs of valvar regurgitation. Congestive heart failure may be precipitated. Signs of infection include anaemia, clubbing of the fingers and splinter haemorrhages. Signs of embolism may develop, such as absence of an arterial pulse and central retinal artery occlusion, but can produce a wide range of symptoms according to the organs involved and the size of the embolism. Mycotic aneurysms, as a result of infected emboli, can develop on any artery, but are most common in the brain.

Hypertension

Hypertention does not usually alter the clinical picture of hypertrophic cardiomyopathy but may produce evidence of hypertensive disease in other organs.

Electrocardiography in Diagnosis

The electrocardiogram is usually abnormal but can be completely normal, though seldom in older age groups. In screening family members for evidence of hypertrophic cardiomyopathy electrocardiographic abnormalities are an important clue. The most significant features are signs of left ventricular hypertrophy, which may be extreme with high-voltage R and S waves and deeply inverted T waves in left precordial leads. A well-recognised, though not common pattern

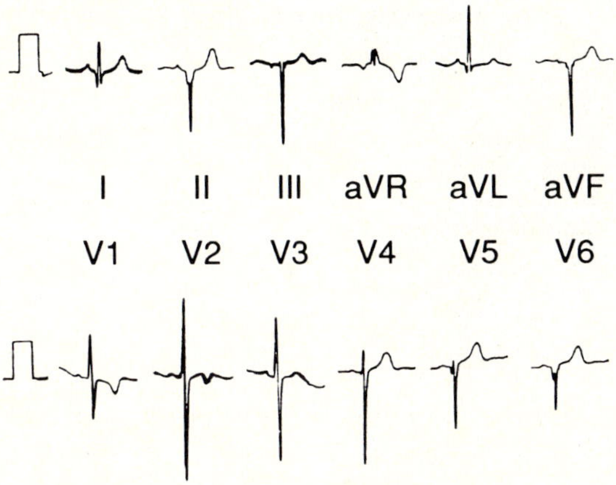

Fig. 6.3. Electrocardiogram of a 14-year-old boy with hypertrophic cardiomyopathy. Abnormal waves are present in leads I, II, aV_F, V_5 and V_6. The PR interval is 0.08/s

is the presence of Q waves in central and lateral precordial leads suggesting myocardial infarction (Fig.6.3). The frontal plane axis may be normal, but left anterior hemiblock can be found. The PR interval is usually on the short side of normal, but delta waves are uncommon and true pre-excitation unusual,though accessory atrioventricular pathways have been described by Krikler et al. [30]. There is commonly evidence of marked left atrial and sometimes right atrial enlargement. In patients with the apical type of hypertrophic cardiomyopathy extreme T wave inversion with ST segment depression may be seen in left precordial leads and can be a useful diagnostic pointer [45].

Serial electrocardiographic studies show increasing T wave inversion in some patients. This does not appear to indicate deterioration, though reduction of R wave voltage may do so.

In a personal study by McKenna et al. of 216 patients, the T wave was normal in 49%, there was left atrial hypertrophy in 8%, a normal frontal plane axis in 70%, left axis deviation in 20%, right axis deviation in 4% and bundle branch block in 2%. Sixty-eight percent of patients had no conduction defects. Various combinations of bizarre electrocardiographic appearances usually suggesting gross left ventricular hypertrophy, bi-ventricular hypertrophy, myocardial ischaemia or infarction should indicate the possibility of hypertrophic cardiomyopathy (Fig. 6.3).

Rhythm is usually sinus, but paroxysmal or established atrial fibrillation is common. Premature ventricular contractions and non-sustained ventricular tachycardia, although common on ambulatory monitoring, are uncommon on resting tracings. Complete heart block is unusual (See Chaps. 8 and 9).

Chest Radiography

Chest radiography is often unhelpful because the heart is not dilated; its size will be normal unless there is very gross hypertrophy. If the left ventricular end-

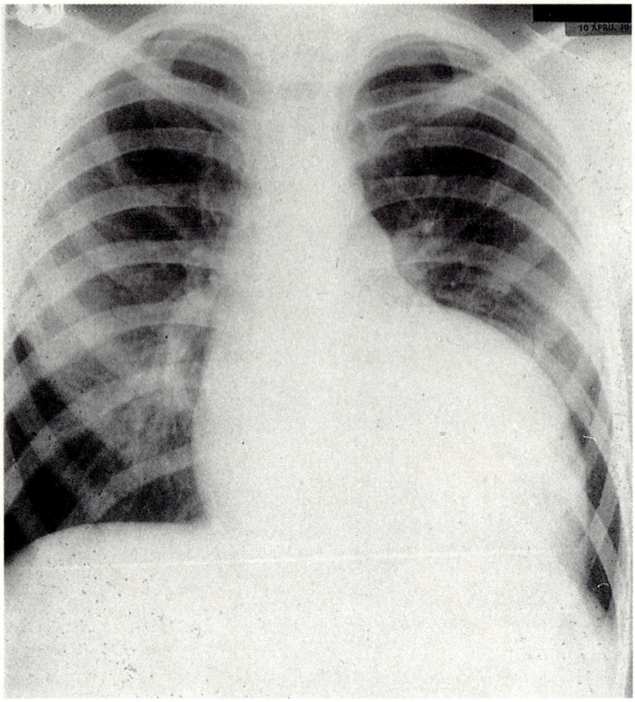

Fig. 6.4. Six-foot postero-anterior chest radiograph of a boy with hypertrophic cardiomyopathy. There is considerable cardiomegaly with a pronounced "shelf" on the left border due to massive hypertrophy of the free wall of the left ventricle. The left atrium is slightly enlarged. The lung vessels suggest some increase in left atrial pressure.

diastolic and pulmonary venous pressures are high, there may be signs of pulmonary venous hypertension, but the lung vasculature often appears normal. A characteristic but rare finding is a bulge on the left border of the heart in the postero-anterior view situated lower down the left heart border than the appendage of the left atrium (Fig. 6.4).

Differential Diagnosis

Coronary Heart Disease

Differentiation of hypertrophic cardiomyopathy from coronary heart disease may be extremely difficult in patients with angina on effort, no obvious physical signs of hypertrophic cardiomyopathy and changes on the electrocardiogram suggesting ischaemia. The correct diagnosis then will not be made without further investigation—notably coronary arteriography and left ventricular angio-

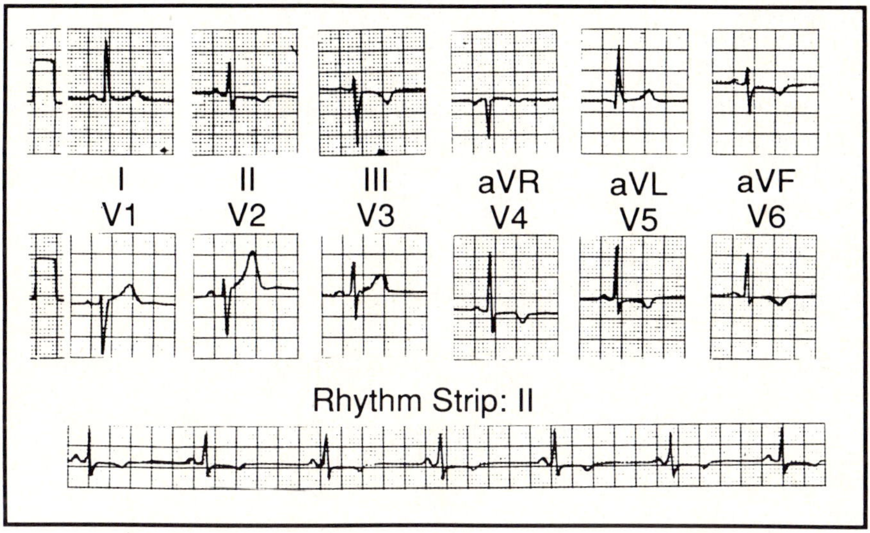

Fig. 6.5. Electrocardiogram of a man who presented with angina. The only abnormal physical sign was a presystolic gallop. There is T wave inversion in leads 2, 3, V_F, and V_4 to V_6. The PR interval is 0.1/s with no delta wave. Echocardiography and angiocardiography confirmed the diagnosis of hypertrophic cardiomyopathy: the major coronary arteries were increased in diameter with widely patent smooth lumina

graphy. Since hypertrophic cardiomyopathy and coronary heart disease can coexist, the diagnosis of one does not necessarily exclude the other. Sometimes the diagnosis of hypertrophic cardiomyopathy may be suspected when there is an unexpected gallop rhythm or left ventricular hypertrophy on the electrocardiogram, when the arterial pulse is ill-sustained or when there is an atrial beat (Fig. 6.5).

Differential Diagnosis of the Systolic Murmur

When there is a loud systolic murmur, the following conditions should be considered:supravalvar, valvar or subvalvar aortic stenosis, pulmonary stenosis, ventricular septal defect, mitral regurgitation and mitral prolapse. In all these conditions except mitral prolapse, the murmur usually starts immediately after the first sound and there is no silent gap. The murmur of mitral prolapse, can closely resemble that of hypertrophic cardiomyopathy but the presence of a systolic click strongly suggests mitral prolapse—though hypertrophic cardiomyopathy and mitral prolapse can coexist. When mitral regurgitation is appreciable and atrial fibrillation is present, the physical signs may closely resemble those of rheumatic heart disease, particularly when there is a mitral diastolic rumble and when the mitral valve is calcified.

Hypertension

The differential diagnosis between hypertensive heart disease and hypertension with hypertrophic cardiomyopathy may be virtually impossible. Evidence of hypertensive disease elsewhere, such as the retina or kidneys, may be of value in diagnosis. Mid-systolic closure of the aortic valve and SAM–septal contact does not usually occur in hypertensive heart disease (see Chapter 8).

Physiological Cardiac Hypertrophy in Athletes

Hypertrophic cardiomyopathy may be suggested in athletes who have, because of their training, a physiological bradycardia and high stroke volume. The high stroke volume at a slow heart rate may give the arterial pulse a high-volume ill-sustained quality reminiscent hypertrophic cardiomyopathy. It is now realised that exercise training and extreme physical fitness can give rise to physiological left ventricular hypertrophy; thus in young people with a thin chest wall, the left ventricular impulse may suggest left hypertrophy but there is no left atrial beat. The high stroke volume tends to cause an ejection type of systolic murmur. The electrocardiogram, especially when the chest wall is thin, may show increased R wave voltage over the left precordium, but T wave abnormalities are absent and stress testing is negative. A recent paper suggests that a thickness of the left ventricular wall greater than 16 mm in the absence of ventricular dilatation indicates a primary form of pathological hypertrophy such as hypertrophic cardiomyopathy [45].

References

1. Bulkley BH (1977) Idiopathic hypertrophic subaortic stenosis afflicted idols of the cave and marketplace. Am J Cardiol 40: 476–479
2. Davies MJ (1990) Hypertrophic cardiomyopathy: one disease or several? (Editorial). Br Heart J 63: 263–264
3. Goodwin JF (1980) Hypertrophic cardiomyopathy: a disease in search of its own identity. Am J Cardiol 45: 177–179
4. Jarcho JA, McKenna W, Pare JAP et al. (1989) Mapping a gene for familial hypertrophic cardiomyopathy to chromosome 14ql. N Engl J Med 321: 1372–1377
5. Ferrans DJ, Morrow AG, Roberts WC (1972) Myocardial ultrastructure in idiopathic hypertrophic subaortic stenosis. Circulation 45: 769.
6. Manasek FG (1970) Histogenesis of the embryonic myocardium. Am J Cardiol 25: 149.
7. Goodwin JF (1974) Prospects and predictions for the cardiomyopathies. Circulation 50: 201
8. Thoren C (1964) Cardiomyopathy in Friedreich's ataxia. Paediatrics 54: 153
9. Fitzpatrick AP, Emmanuel RW (1988) Familial neurofibromatosis and hypertrophic cardiomyopathy. Br Heart J 60: 247–251
10. Symons C, Fortune F, Greenbaum RA, Dandone P (1985) Cardiac hypertrophy, hypertrophic cardiomyopathy and hyperparathyroidism: an association. Br Heart J 54: 539–542
11. Goodwin JF (1982) The frontiers of cardiomyopathy. Br Heart J 48: 1–18

12. Goodwin JF (1978) cardiomyopathy: an interface between fundamental and clinical cardiology. In : Hayase S., Murao S. (eds) proceedings of the 8th World Congress of cardiology 1978. Excerpta Medica, Amsterdam, pp 103–116
13. Web-people MM, Oakley CM,Croxon RS, Goodwin JF (1971) Cardioselective beta-adrenergic blockade in hypertrophic obstructive cardiomyopathy. Postgrad Med J 47 [Suppl 93]
14. Blaufuss AH,Laks MM, Garner D, Ishimoto DM, Criley JM (1975) Production of ventricular hypertrophy simulating idiopathic hypertrophic subaortic stenosis (IHSS) by sub-hypertensive infusions of norepinephrine in the conscious dog. Clin Res 23: 77a
15. Witzke DJ, Kaye MP (1976) Myocardial ultrastructural changes induced by nerve growth factor. Surg Forum 27: 295
16. Pearce TC, Hawkey C, Symons C, Olsen EGJ (1985) Role of calcium in the induction of cardiac hypertrophy and myofibrillar disarray. Experimental studies of a possible cause of hypertrophic cardiomyopathy. Br Heart J 54: 420
17. Wagner JA, Sax FL, Weissman HF, Porterfield J, McIntosh C, Weisfeldt ML, Snyder SH, Epstein SE (1989) Calcium antagonist receptors in atrial tissues of patients with hypertrophic cardio-myopathy. N Engl J Med 320: 755
17a. Dargie HJ, Goodwin JF (1982) Catecholamine, cardiomyopathy and cardiac functions. In: Yu PN, Goodwin JF (eds) Progress in cardiology 1982, vol. 2. Lea and Febiger, Philadelphia, p 93
18. Perloff JK (1981) Pathogenesis of hypertrophic cardiomyopathy:hypotheses and speculations. Am Heart J 101: 219
19. Matsumori A, Hirose K, Wakabayshi A, Kawai C, Nakeya M, Sakurami T, Tsuji K (1979) HLA and hypertrophic cardiomyopathy. Am Heart J 97: 428
20. Gutgesell HP, Spear ME, Rosenberg HF (1980) Characterisation of the cardiomyopathy in infants of diabetic mothers. Circulation 61: 441
21. Maron BJ, Kragel AH, Roberts WC (1990) Sudden death in hypertrophic cardiomyopathy with normal left ventricular mass. Br Heart J 63: 308–310
22. McKenna WJ, Stewart JI, Nihoyannopoulos P, McGinty F, Davies MJ (1990) Hypertrophic cardiomyopathy without hypertrophy: two families with myocardial disarray in the absence of increased myocardial mass. Br Heart J 63: 287–290
23. Iida K, Yukisoda K, Sugishita Y, Matsuda M, Kosekis I (1987) Impaired left ventricular rapid filling during exercise in patients with hypertrophic cardiomyopathy. Clin Cardiol 10: 147–152
24. Frenneaux MP, Porter A, Caforio APL, Odawara H, Counihan P, McKenna W (1989) Determinants of exercise capacity in hypertrophic cardiomyopathy. J Am Coll Cardiol 13: 1521–1526
25. Goodwin JF (1987) Review of hypertrophic cardiomyopathy. Ergeb Inn Med Kinderheilk 55: 42–79
26. Maron BJ, Epstein JE, Roberts WC (1979) Hypertrophic cardiomyopathy and transmural myocardial infarction without significant atherosclerosis of the extramural coronary arteries. Am J Cardiol 43: 1086
27. Thompson DS, Naquie N, Juul SM, Swanton RH, Coltart DJ, Jenkins BS (1980) The effects of propranolol on myocardial oxygen consumption, substrate extraction and haemodynamics in hypertrophic cardiomyopathy. Br Heart J 44: 88
28. Canon RO III (1990) Ischaemia, coronary blood flow and coronary reserve in hypertrophic cardiomyopathy In: Baroldi G, Camerini F, Goodwin JF (eds) Advances in cardiomyopathies. Springer, Berlin Heidelberg New York, pp 44–57
29. McKenna WJ, Chetty S, Oakley CM, Goodwin JF (1980) Arrhythmia in hypertrophic cardiomyopathy: exercise and 48 hour ambulatory electrocardiographic assessment with and without beta blockade. Am J Cardiol 45: 1–5
30. Krikler DM, Davies JM, Rowland E, Goodwin JF, Evans RC, Shaw DB (1980) Sudden death in hypertrophic cardiomyopathy: associated accessory atrio-ventricular pathways. Br Heart J 43: 245–251
31. McKenna WJ, Franklin RCG, Nihoyannopoulos P, Robinson KR, Deanfield J (1988) Arrhythmia and prognosis in infants, children, and adolescents in hypertrophic cardiomyopathy. J Am Coll Cardiol 11: 147–153

32. McKenna WJ, Harris L, Deanfield J (1982) Syncope in hypertrophic cardiomyopathy. Br Heart J 47: 177–179
33. Frenneaux MP, Counihan P, Webb D, McKenna WJ (1989) Evidence for an abnormal vasodilator response in hypertrophic cardiomyopathy. J Am Coll Cardiol 13: 117a
34. Alessandri N, Pennarale G, del Morte F, Moretti F, Marino B, Reale A (1990) Hypertrophic obstructive cardiomyopathy and infective endocarditis: a report of 7 cases and a review of the literature. Eur Heart J 11: 1041
35. Nair CK, Kudesian V, Hansen D, Thomson W, Ragano T, Ryschon V, Sketch MH (1987) Echocardiographic and electro-cardiographic characteristics of patients with hypertrophic cardiomyopathy with and wihout mitral annular calcification. Am J Cardiol 59: 1428–1430
36. Takahiro S, Sakimoto T, Takenaka K, Amano K, Hada Y, Hasegawa I, Suzuki JI, Takshashi, Sugimoto T (1989) Aortic regurgitation associated with hypertrophic cardiomyopathy: a colour Doppler echocardiographic study. Br Heart J 62: 171–176
37. Caplan J, Boltwood CM, Tei C, Shah PM (1985) Clinical improvement in hypertrophic cardiomyopathy after inferior myocardial infarction. J Am Coll Cardiol 5: 797–802
38. Oakley CM, McGarry K, Limb DG (1979) Management of pregnancy in patients with hypertrophic cardiomyopathy. Br Med J 1: 1749
39. Kavan R, Lever HM, Healey BP (1989) Hypertensive hypertrophic cardiomyopathy or hypertrophic cardiomyopathy with hypertension: a study of 78 patients. J Am Coll Cardiol 13: 580–584
40. Devereux RB (1990) Does increased blood pressure cause left ventricular hypertrophy or vice versa? Ann Intern Med 112: 157–158
41. Topol EJ, Traill TA, Fortuin NJ (1985) Hypertensive hypertrophic cardiomyopathy in the elderly. N Engl J Med 312: 277–283
42. Spirito P, Chiarella F, Carratiro I, Berisso MZ, Bellotti P, Vecchuo C (1989) Clinical course and prognosis of hypertrophic cardiomyopathy in an outpatient population. N Engl J Med 320: 749·
43. Spirito P, Maron BJ (1990) Relation between extent of left ventricular hypertrophy and occurrence of sudden death in hypertrophic cardiomyopathy. J Am Coll Cardiol 15: 1521–1526
44. Robinson K, Frennaux NP, Spockins B, Karatasakis G, Poloniecki JG, McKenna WJ (1990) Atrial fibrillation in hypertrophic cardiomyopathy: a longitudinal study. J Am Coll Cardiol 15: 1279
45. Pellicia A, Maron BJ, Sataro A, Proscan MA, Spirito A (1990) The upper limit of physiologic cardiac hypertrophy in highly trained elite athletes. N Engl J Med 324: 295

CHAPTER 7

Pathology

E. G. J. Olsen and S. E. Trotter

The WHO/ISFC Task Force [1] recommendation on nomenclature of cardiomyopathy has suggested omission of the terms "with" and "without" obstruction. From a morphological point of view the concept of a difference in distribution of abnormal myocytes and their arrangement [2] has also not been substantiated (see Chaps. 1 and 9).

Macroscopy (Fig. 7.1)

The hearts are enlarged and globular in shape and firm to the touch. They are often severely overweight, and not infrequently twice the normal weight [3]. The epicardium is unremarkable.

The left (and not infrequently the right) ventricular cavity is reduced in size [4] due to muscular encroachment of the frequently asymmetric thickening of the interventricular septum, hypertrophy of the papillary muscles and rigor mortis, the heart being in end-systole at the time of death [5–9]. Asymmetric hypertrophy of the interventricular septum, once considered to be a pathognomonic feature, can be striking. The maximal bulge may be diffuse or confined to the apex, the mid-region of the septum, or beneath the aortic valve [10].

This thickening may involve the anterior or posterior left ventricular walls and even the free wall. The septal bulge leads to displacement of the anterior papillary muscles, interfering with the normal closure of the mitral valve and resulting in endocardial thickening of the left ventricular outflow tract [11] forming a "mirror image" of the anterior mitral valve leaflet. The valvar leaflets may be thicker than normal due to insufficiency during life. Mitral valve ring calcification may be striking [12]. The mitral valve leaflet is usually normal in position, but abnormal location has been described; instead of the anterior leaflet being related to the base of the right aortic valve leaflet, the anterior leaflet is inserted below the posterior aortic valve leaflet [13]. Mitral insufficiency is attributable to poor left ventricular compliance resulting in enlargement of the left atrium, turbulence and local trauma due to strong SAM–septal impact. Rarely infective endocarditis may be a cause. The myocardium is frequently arranged in whorls, particularly when seen on cross sections of the ventricles [14]. Fibrous tissue also abounds, particularly in the areas of the maximal bulge

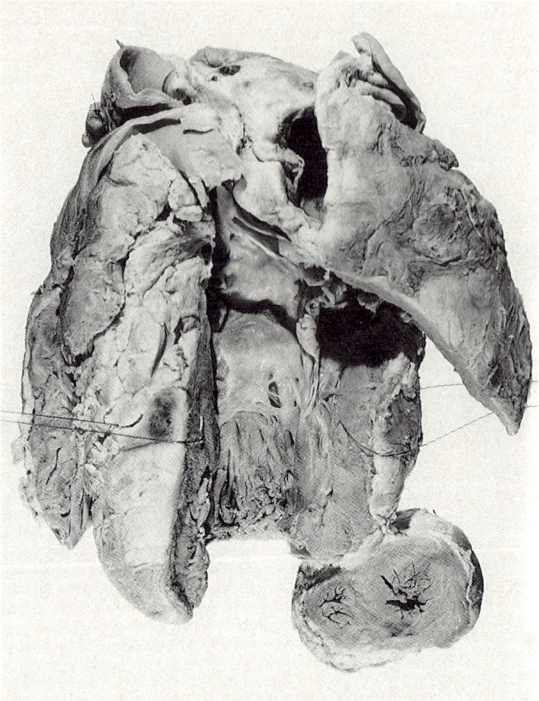

Fig. 7.1. Macroscopic view of a heart with hypertrophic cardiomyopathy. A characteristic feature that some pathologists regard as diagnostic is the distinctive endocardial impression of the anterior mitral valve leaflet overlying the septal bulge

of the septum. Infarct-like lesions have been described, but are rare [15]. Nonspecific endocardial thickening may be haphazardly distributed. Thrombus superimposition is rare. Very occasionally, vegetations on the mitral valve leaflets due to infective endocarditis are seen [16].

The extramural coronary arteries are large, smooth and usually free from atheroma. Associated atherosclerotic coronary disease is present in 15% of patients [15, 17] (See Chap. 6). If the interventricular septal bulge is twice the normal thickness of the already hypertrophied left ventricular free wall, this constitutes a pathognomonic feature [8]. If such discrepancy is not evident, caution should be exercised in formulating a diagnosis on macroscopic findings alone. Although an increase in measurement of the junction of the posterior septum with the posterior left ventricular free wall of more than 1.3 (normal 1.03) on echocardiographic examination is suggestive [18], such measurements may occur in hypertensive heart and congenital heart disease particularly when the right side of the heart is involved. Furthermore, in the newborn asymmetry of the interventricular septum is, not infrequently, present [19].

Symmetric forms affecting the left ventricle are now well recognised and echocardiographic examination has found this form of hypertrophic cardiomyopathy to occur in 31% of patients [20]. A rare form confined to the free left ventricular wall has also been described [21].

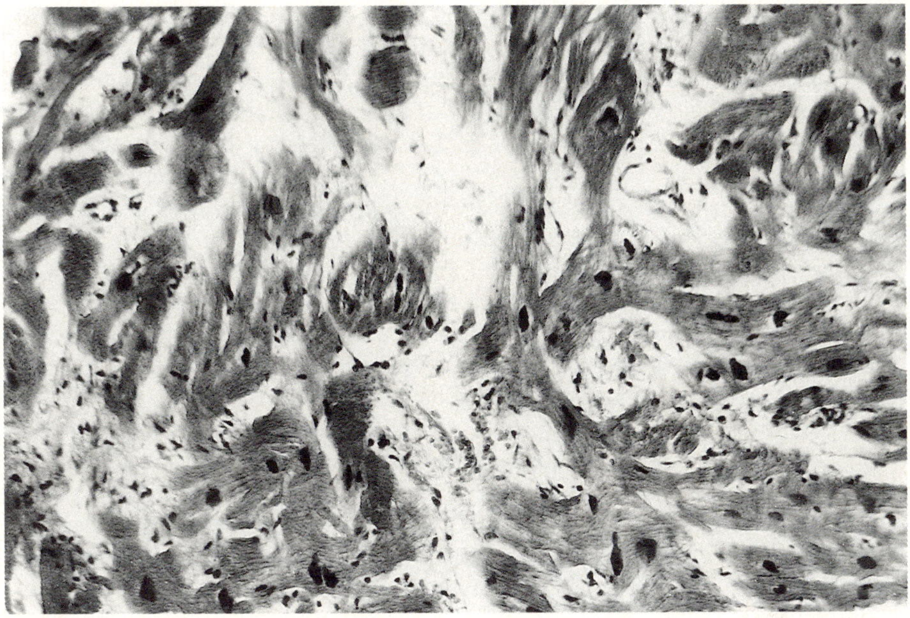

Fig. 7.2. Photomicrograph of the myocardium in hypertrophic cardiomyopathy. There is considerable hypertrophy, and disarray, including whorling of the fibres, is evident. Lymphocytes are occasionally seen in the interstitium and must not be considered to represent a myocarditic process. (Haematoxylin and Eosin × 400)

In those patients who have died suddenly no reliable morphological discriminating factors have been established [22].

Disarray of myocardial fibres together with severe hypertrophy of the myocytes are typical histological changes [6–8] (Fig. 7.2). Whereas in hypertrophy due to known cause or associations myocytes may reach a diameter of 25–30 μm, in hypertrophic cardiomyopathy individual measurements may be as high as 100 μm [23]. Bizarre-shaped nuclei, either pyknotic or vesicular, with irregular outline are typical, often surrounded with a clear zone, the so-called perinuclear halo [24]. The myocytes display a whorled arrangement, akin to a cartwheel. Frequently, the myocytes are intertwined with a side-to-side junction in addition to the end-to-end connections. The interstitium is widened and is composed of loosely arranged connective tissue, often rich in mononuclear cells. Contributing to the cellularity of the interstitium are intercellular clefts, lined by endothelial cells and often covered by sparse elastic fibres, adding also to the increased cellularity of the intercellular spaces [4]. A focal or a more widespread increase of interstitial fibrous tissue is typical, not infrequently replacing areas of myocytes. The intramural vessels may show medial hypertrophy, accompanied by intimal thickening of fibroelastic tissue, narrowing the interventricular lumina to usually less than 50%. More significant vascular changes have been described [25, 26] and it has been suggested that these may be primary [27]. However it may well be that these vascular changes are secondary as they are found most frequently in the areas of fibrosis, particularly in the interventricular septum and in patients when heart failure has supervened [28] (see Chap. 9).

Controversy as to the significance of disarray of myocytes exists. It has been found that 55%, or more, usually 30%–50% of ventricular myocytes show disarray in cases of hypertrophic cardiomyopathy [29]. It must be remembered, however, that disarray may occur normallly in the septal/free wall junction and may accompany hypertrophy from any cause, such as hypertension of aortic stenosis. It is, therefore, not the presence but the extent of disarray that would appear significant. Furthermore, during processing of tissue selected for microscopic examination, the angle of cutting of tissue may alter the parallel alignment [30]. The problem of disarray in the context of hypertrophic cardiomyopathy has been reviewed [31, 32] and it may be concluded that no histological feature alone is pathognomonic. It is the combination of disorganisation and the severe hypertrophy of myocytes together with bizarre-shaped nuclei, the peri-nuclear halo, a whorled arrangement and cellular interstitial widening which permit a confident histological assessment of hypertrophic cardiomyopathy. Cases have been described with severe hypertrophy and little disarray, and conversely with marked disarray and little hypertrophy (see Chaps. 6 and 9).

Histochemistry

Accumulation of glycogen, especially in the perinuclear region, results frequently in "pooling". A dramatic increase in succinic dehydrogenase in these areas is also of diagnostic significance [33]. A panel of histochemical parameters including neutral fat, lipofuscin dehydrogenases, succinate dehydrogenases, oxidases, monoamine oxidase, non-specific esterases, acid phosphatases, alkaline phosphatase and phosphorylase may be raised, but may reflect the severe hypertrophy. Nicotinamide adenine dinucleotide dehydrogenase and nicotinamide adenine dinucleotide phosphate dehydrogenase are also substances routinely investigated histochemically and in hypertrophic cardiomyopathy reduced levels of both are found. An increase in dehydrogenase and lysosomal markers, such as acid phosphatase and non-specific esterases, is also found. An even distribution of myosin ATPase is noted and cholinesterases are usually absent, except in nerve tissue included in the sections [33].

The finding of an increase in catecholamines—originally described by Pearse [34] but discredited because the techniques employed made a distinction from connective tissue difficult [23]—has now again gained importance, not so much diagnostically, but pathogenetically.

Ultrastructural Examination

The changes observed histologically can also be seen at the ultrastructural level of examination. The myocardial fibrils are disorganised [23] with frequent inter-

and intrafibrillar connections [35], often having a whorled appearance within the myofilaments [36]. Diffusion of Z-band material is typical. The entire arrangement of the myofibrils can be likened to basket- weave and it is tempting to speculate that this arrangement may be the cause of the haemodynamic fault, namely poor left ventricular compliance. Unfortunately, however, these changes may sometimes be focal in distribution and can be observed in hypertrophy due to known causes. There is focal accumulation of mitochondria, frequently showing cristolysis [23]. In the interstitium varying degrees of an increase in collagen fibrils are encountered. Degenerative changes are shown, not only affecting the contractile elements but also apparent by the presence of myelin bodies and membrane-bound vesicles [23, 36, 37]. The nuclei show severe infolding of their membranes. All these changes are focal in distribution and may be mild.

Semi-quantitative Examination

Van Noorden et al. compared surgically obtained tissue from the left ventricular outflow tract in cases of hypertrophic cardiomyopathy with similarly derived tissue from patients with aortic valve stenosis. The parameters used were fibrosis, short interrupted fibres, large bizarre-shaped nuclei, haloes around the nuclei, disappearing myofibrils, whorls and average fibre diameter. The results indicated considerable overlap on assessment using a "plus" system (○, +, + +, + + +, according to the severity) applied to these parameters. These semi-quantitative assessments were not only applied at histological level, but also histochemically and ultrastructurally. With a points system (maximum points of three for each of five histological changes omitting average fibre diameter), four histochemical and seven ultrastructural features were examined. The maximum number for histological features was fifteen for histochemical, twelve and seven ultrastructural features, twenty-one. Each of these figures in the three categories were expressed as 100% and according to the number obtained, the index was calculated. A result of over 50% permitted a firm diagnosis of hypertrophic cardiomyopathy on histological assessment. Between 30%–50% the changes were suggestive and below 30% no evidence of this form of cardiomyopathy could be sustained [23].

These results also showed overlap between hypertrophic cardiomyopathy and "ordinary hypertrophy" of individual parameters. Apart from glycogen accumulation, considerable overlap between the two groups existed and total overlap at ultrastructural level.

Endomyocardial Biopsy

By comparison with a large number of (nearly 2000) patients suspected of having dilated cardiomyopathy only 10% had endomyocardial tissue obtained by bioptome sent for morphological assessment. The reason for this is largely due to the fact that clinical examination, together with new sophisticated non-invasive techniques of investigation, makes endomyocardial biopsies unnecessary. Of the 200 cases thus investigated, only just over 50% showed typical changes. This low figure can, in part, be attributed to the diagnostic changes being beyond the reach of the bioptome and to the focal distribution of affected myocytes [37]. In some cases amyloid has been found [38], indicating that in rare instances amyloid may mimic or be associated with hypertrophic cardiomyopathy (see Chaps. 10 and 11). Endomyocardial biopsy [39] permits additional factors such as biochemical and enzymatic changes to be assessed [40–42], and morphometric studies to be undertaken [43, 44]. However, due to the abnormal geometry of the ventricle, biopsy is not without hazard and, since the disorder is patchy, may be unhelpful.

Associated Conditions

Hypertrophic cardiomyopathy can occur in conjunction with various types of congenital heart disease and with a number of other disease entities, such as acromegaly, hyperparathyroidism [45], in infants of diabetic mothers [46], lentiginosis [47], Friedreich's ataxia [48, 49] and hyperthyroidism [50, 51]. Clinical observations and experimental studies have shown an increase in triiodothyroacetic acid in the circulation in covert and overt hyperthyroidism. The site of action is at the cell membrane, which permits influx of calcium, resulting in extra systolic contractions [52, 53].

In individuals engaging in active competitive sport hypertrophic cardiomyopathy may be present, but unless the clinician is aware of this the clinical symptomatology may be wrongfully ascribed to athletic activity. A study on a large number of cases of hypertrophic cardiomyopathy in athletes has been analysed [54]. The incidence is high and may be due to the referral of cases to the investigators especially interested in this condition. It nevertheless emphasises the necessity for constant vigilance on the part of the examining physician. Familial recurrence of this form of cardiomyopathy is well recognised and, depending on the parameters used for diagnosis, may be as high as 60% [55]. From a morphological point of view no differences exist between familial and sporadic cases.

By definition the aetiology is unknown and the various suggestions previously made, including embryonic growth disturbances, haematoma, increased noradrenaline, primary disorders of myocardial muscle metabolism, a myopathic disorder accompanying skeletal muscle changes and hypertension, as well as endogenous changes such as an increase in circulating triiodothyroacetic acid may all, in part, be contributory [56]. The underlying cause is likely to be genetic. These new and exciting developments in this field are described in detail elsehere in the book (see Chaps. 9 and 17).

References

1. WHO/ISFC (1980) Task Force report on the definition and classification of cardiomyopathies. Br Heart J 44: 672–673
2. Edwards WD, Zakheim R, and Mattioli L (1977) Asymmetric septal hypertrophy in childhood: unreliability of histologic criteria for differentiation of obstructive and nonobstructive forms. Hum Pathol 8: 277–284
3. Gould SE (ed) (1968) Pathology of the heart and blood vessels, 3rd edn. Thomas, Springfield, p 1139
4. Adelman AG, McLoughlin MJ, Marquis Y, Auger P, Wigle ED (1969) Left ventricular cineangiographic observations in muscular subaortic stenosis. Am J Cardiol 24: 689–697
5. Teare D (1958) Asymmetrical hypertrophy of the heart in young adults. Br Heart J 20: 1–8
6. Olsen EGJ (1971) Morbid anatomy and histology in hypertrophic obstructive cardiomyopathy. Ciba Found Study Group 37: 183–191
7. Roberts WC (1973) Valvular, subvalvular and supravalvular aortic stenosis: morphologic features. Cardiovasc Clin 5: 104–126
8. Menges JH, Brandenburg RD, Brown AL Jr (1961) The clinical, haemodynamic and pathologic diagnosis of muscular subvalvular aortic stenosis. Circulation 24: 1126–1136
9. Maron BJ, Henry WL, Roberts WC, Epstein SE (1977) Comparison of echocardiographic and necropsy measurements of ventricular wall thicknesses in patients with and without disproportionate septal thickening. Circulation 55: 341–346
10. Sakamoto T, Tei C, Masahiro M, Ischiyasu M, Hada Y, Hayashi T, Amano K (1976) Giant T wave inversion as a manifestation of asymmetrical apical hypertrophy (AAH) of the left ventricle: echocardiographic and ultrasonocardiotomographic study, Jpn Heart J 17: 611–629
11. Davies MJ, Pomerance A, Teare RD (1974) Pathological features of hypertrophic obstructive cardiomyopathy. J Clin Pathol 27: 529–535
12. Motamed HE, Roberts WC (1984) Frequency and significance of mitral annular calcium in hypertrophic cardiomyopathy:analysis of 200 necropsy patients. Am J Cardiol 60: 877–884
13. Bjork VO, Hultquist G, Lodin H (1961) Subaortic stenosis produced by an abnormally placed anterior mitral leaflet. J Thorac Cardiovasc Surg 41: 659–669
14. Olsen EGJ (1980) The pathology of the heart, 2nd edn. Macmillan, London, p 318
15. Maron BJ, Epstein SE, Roberts WC (1979) Hypertrophic cardiomyopathy and transmural myocardial infarction without significant atherosclerosis of the extramural coronary arteries. Am J Cardiol 43: 1086–1102
16. Vecht RJ, Oakley CM (1968) Infective endocarditis in three patients with hypertrophic obstructive cardiomyopathy. Br Med J 2: 455–459
17. Lie JT (1980) Hypertrophic cardiomyopathy and coronary heart diesease (Editorial). Mayo Clin Proc 55: 54–55
18. Henry WL, Clark CE, Epstein SE (1973) Asymmetric septal hypertrophy (ASH): echocardiographic identification of the pathognomonic abnormality of IHSS. Circulaton 47: 225–233
19. Bulkley BH, Weisfeldt ML, Hutchins GM (1977) Asymmetric septal hypertrophy and myocardial fibre disarray:features of normal, developing and malformed hearts. Circulation 56: 292–298
20. Shapiro LM, McKenna WJ (1983) Distribution of left ventricular hypertrophy in hypertrophic cardiomyopathy: a two- dimensional echocardiographic study. J Am Coll Cardiol 2: 437–444
21. Edwards WD (1991) Cardiomyopathies. In: Virmanie R, Atkinson JB, Fenoglio JJ (eds) Cardiovascular pathology. Saunders, Philadelphia, p 274 (Major problems in pathology vol 23)
22. Maron BJ, Roberts WC, Epstein SE (1982) Sudden death in hypertrophic cardiomyopathy: a profile of 78 patients. Circulation 65: 1388–1394
23. Van Noorden S, Olsen EGJ, Pearse AGE (1971) Hypertrophic obstructive cardiomyopathy: a histological, histochemical and ultrastructural study of biopsy material. Cardiovasc Res 5: 118–131
24. James TN, Marshall TK (1975) De subitaneis mortibus. XII Asymmetrical hypertrophy of the heart. Circulation 51: 1149–1166

25. McReynolds RA, Roberts WC (1975) The intramural coronary arteries in hypertrophic cardiomyopathy (Abstr). Am J Cardiol 35: 154
26. Maron BJ, Wolfson JK, Epstein SE, Roberts WC (1986) Intramural ("small vessel") coronary artery disease in hypertrophic cardiomyopathy, J Am Coll Cardiol 8: 545–557
27. Maron BJ, Wolfson JK, Epstein SE, Roberts WC (1987) Morphologic evidence for "small vessel disease" in patients with hypertrophic cardiomyopathy. Z Kardiol 76 Suppl 3: 91–100
28. Fujiwara H, Kawai C (1988) Intramural coronary artery disease in hypertrophic cardiomyopathy. In: Toshima H, Maron BJ (eds) Hypertrophic cardiomyopathy. University of Tokyo Press, Tokyo, pp 47–58 (Cardiomyopathy update 2)
29. Maron BJ, Roberts WC (1979) Quantitative analysis of cardiac muscle cell disorganisation in the ventricular septum of patients with hypertrophic cardiomyopathy. Circulation 59: 689–706
30. Becker AE, Caruso G (1982) Myocardial disarray: a critical review. Br Heart J 47: 527–538
31. Olsen EGJ (1982) Myocardial disarray revisited (Leader). Br Med J 285: 991–992
32. Maron BJ (1982) Myocardial disorganisation in hypertrophic cardiomyopathy. Br Heart J 47: 1–8
33. Van Noorden S, Pearse AGE (1971) Histochemistry and electron microscopy of the heart in hypertrophic obstructive cardiomyopathy. Ciba Found Study Group 37: 192–210
34. Pearse AGE (1964) Ciba Found Symp 132–164
35. Ferrans VJ (1988) Light and electron microscopic features of hypertrophic cardiomyopathy. In: Toshmia H, Maron B (eds) Hypertrophic cardiomyopathy. University of Tokyo Press Tokyo, pp 27–45 (Cardiomyopathy update 2)
36. Hamjanz D, Reale E (1981) Overcontraction and excess actin filaments: basic elements of hypertrophic cardiomyopathy. Br Heart J 45: 494–499
37. Tazelaar HD, Billingham ME (1987) The surgical pathology of hypertrophic cardiomyopathy. Arch Pathol Lab Med 3: 257–260
38. Sedlis SP, Saffitz JE, Schwob VS, Jaffe AL (1984) Cardiac amyloidosis simulating hypertrophic cardiomyopathy. Am J Cardiol 53: 969–970
39. Olsen EGJ (1978) Endomyocardial biopsy (Editorial). Br Heart J 40: 95–98
40. Peters TJ, Wells G, Oakley CM, Broksby IAB, Jenkins BS, Webb-Peploe MM, Coltart DJ (1977) Enzymic analysis of endomyocardial biopsy specimens from patients with cardiomyopathies. Br Heart J 39: 1333–1339
41. Richardson PJ, Atkinson L (1980) Enzyme activities in endomyocardial biopsy samples from patients with cardiomyopathy. In:Bolte HD (ed) Myocardial biopsy: diagnostic significance. Springer, Berlin Heidelberg New York, pp 97–101
42. Schultheiss HP, Bolte HD, Cyran J (1980) Lactate dehydrogenase isoenzyme pattern in myocardial biopsies of patients with congestive cardiomyopathy and with alcoholic cardiomyopathy: clinical and experimental results. In: Bolte HD (ed) Myocardial biopsy: diagnostic significance. Springer, Berlin Heidelberg New York, pp 102–115
43. Baandrup U, Olsen EGJ (1981) Critical analysis of endomyocardial biopsies from patients suspected of having cardiomyopathy. I Morphological and morphometric aspects. Br Heart J 45: 475–486
44. Baandrup U, Florio RA, Rehahn M, Richardson PJ, Olsen EGJ (1981) Critical analysis of endomyocardial biopsies from patients suspected of having cardiomyopathy. II Comparison of histology and clinical/haemodynamic information. Br Heart J 45: 487–493
45. Symons C, Fortune F, Greenbaum RA, Dandona P (1985) Cardiac hypertrophy, hypertrophic cardiomyopathy and hyperparathyroidism: an association. Br Heart J 54: 539–542
46. Lewis JF, Maron BJ (1989) Elderly patients with hypertrophic cardiomyopathy: a subset with distinctive left ventricular morphology and progressive clinical course late in life. J Am Coll Cardiol 13: 36–45
47. Somerville J, Bonham-Carter RE (1972) The heart in lentigenosis. Br Heart J 34: 58–66
48. Smith ER, Sangalang VE, Hefferman LP, Welch JP, Flemington CS (1977) Hypertrophic cardiomyopathy: the heart disease of Friedreich's ataxia. Am Heart J 94: 428–434
49. Leading Article (1978) Cardiac involvement in Friedreich's ataxia. Br Med J 1: 261

50. Symons C, Richardson PJ, Feizi O (1974) Hypertrophic cardiomyopathy and hyperthyroidism: a report of 3 cases. Thorax 29: 713–719
51. Bell R, Barber PV, Bray C, Beton DC (1979) Incidence of thyroid disease in cases of hypertrophic cardiomyopathy, Br Heart J 40: 1306–1309
52. Olsen EGJ, Symons C, Hawkey CM (1977) The effect of TRIAC on the developing heart. Lancet 2: 221–223
53. Hawkey CM, Olsen EGJ, Symons C (1981) Production of cardiac muscle abnormalities in offspring of rats receiving triiodothyroacetic acid (Triac) and the effect of beta adrenergic blockade. Cardiovasc Res 15: 196–205
54. Maron BJ, Roberts WC, MacAllister HA, Rosing DR, Epstein SE (1980) Sudden death in young athletes. Circulation 62: 218–229
55. Maron BJ, Nichols PF III, Pickle LW et al. (1984) Patterns of inheritance in hypertrophic cardiomyopathy: assessment by M mode and two dimensional echocardiography. Am J Cardiol 53: 1087–1094
56. Olsen EGJ (1980) The pathology of the heart, 2nd edn. Macmillan, London, pp 324–325

CHAPTER 8

Clinical Investigation: Current Approaches

P. J. Richardson and H. J. F. Why

With Special Section on Echocardiography and Doppler by M. J. Monaghan

Definition

Hypertrophic cardiomyopathy is "ventricular hypertrophy in the absence of any obvious cause", but it is far more complex than this [1], with characteristic distribution of hypertrophy to the septum (asymmetric septal hypertrophy, ASH), abnormal systolic motion of the mitral valve apparatus (SAM) and particular myocardial features which include myofibrillar disarray [2]. It most frequently occurs in isolation, but it may also be associated with many other heart disorders, both congenital and acquired. The commonest of these are atherosclerotic coronary artery disease, systemic hypertension and aortic valve stenosis.

The clinical investigation of hypertrophic cardiomyopathy relates to the areas of abnormality already discussed (see Chap. 6). The features, which have been described in Chaps. 6 and 7 are:

1. Massive ventricular hypertrophy
2. Myofibrillar disarray and fibrosis
3. Occlusive changes in the intramural coronary arteries
4. Systolic pressure gradients in the outflow tract
5. Impaired relaxation of the left ventricle
6. Marked tendency for sudden death

A striking feature of systolic function is the rapid powerful ejection of the left ventricle, which expels 80% of the stroke volume in the first half of systole [3, 4]. The contraction is so powerful and the emptying so complete that the cavity of the left ventricle is virtually eliminated before the end of systole except for the immediate subvalvar portion. In addition to the powerful contraction of the ventricle, the extensive hypertrophy and reduced systolic volume of the ventricle produce apposition of the ventricular walls. The powerful contraction of the left ventricle slams the anterior papillary muscle apparatus against the hypertrophied septum and accounts for the impingement plaque, and for the systolic anterior motion of the valve shown on echocardiography. Mid-systolic closure of the aortic valve and systolic anterior motion of the mitral valve are features of hypertrophic cardiomyopathy, especially in patients with outflow tract gradients.

Systolic gradients are present in at least 50% of patients. They may vary from a few millimeters of mercury to well over 100 mmHg and tend to be variable, sometimes only occurring on provocation with exercise or positive inotropic agents. Gradients are produced or exaggerated by isoprenaline, by tachycardia, exercise and reduction in left ventricular volume, and they can be reduced or abolished by β-adrenergic blockade, bradycardia and increase in ventricular volume. The importance of gradients has been much debated. Those who believe that they represent true obstruction to outflow quote the abolition of gradients by the operation of septal resection [5, 6]. The variability of the gradients, overemptying of the left ventricle, the lack of correlation between level of gradient and prognosis, the ability to induce gradients in the normal heart by positive inotropic stimulation and the tendency for gradients to disappear as the left ventricle dilates with advance of the diesase, all suggest that gradients do not indicate true obstruction. Furthermore, flow velocity studies show that ejection is early and rapid and similar in patients with and without gradients. Recent work using Doppler with 2D echocardiography and radionuclide cineangiography with technetium-99m indicates that, in 75% of patients with gradients, ventricular cavity elimination is the explanation, but that in 25% there is true obstruction to outflow. Diastolic function is severely affected. The stiffness of the hypertrophied and fibrotic left ventricle is increased. Both left ventricular filling and time-to-peak filling times are prolonged. In many, though not all, cases the degree of diastolic abnormality depends upon the site and extent of the pathological lesions. In some patients ventricular filling may be rapid in early diastole [6]. Mitral valve opening is delayed and peak left ventricular filling rate correlates inversely with this delay [7, 8]. Thus, the normal sequence of events in diastole is completely disorganised. The isovolumic relaxation period of the left ventricle is usually, but not invariably, prolonged, as is the rapid relaxation period. Rapid deceleration of blood occurs and the fast flow is halted by the stiff, unyielding muscle. This may explain the third heart sound.

Abnormal Vasodilator Response

In some patients with hypertrophic cardiomyopathy hypotension occurs on effort due to inappropriate vasodilatation in non-exercising vascular beds. This response is associated with a family history of sudden death and may be implicated as prognostic feature. This aspect will be further discussed in Chap. 9.

Sudden Death

The mechanisms of sudden death are several and can be broadly divided into arrhythmic and haemodynamic. Arrhythmic causes are likely to be episodes of sustained ventricular tachycardia leading to ventricular fibrillation. Ventricular arrhythmias are set up in areas of myofibrillar disarray, ischaemia or fibrosis, probably by local re-entry mechanisms or by enhanced local automaticity. Atrial fibrillation with a very rapid ventricular rate which greatly reduces the time available for filling the ventricle may result in a catastrophic fall in stroke volume, minute volume and coronary perfusion and lead to ventricular fibrillation. Of the haemodynamic causes, shutdown of the outflow tract has been evoked, but a more likely mechanism is reduced diastolic filling resulting from decreased venous return due to peripheral vasodilatation, and reduced filling time resulting from tachycardia or catecholamine stimulation. A combination of increased resistance to ventricular filling with cavity elimination or resistance to outflow could halt the circulation completely. The presence of nerve endings in the ventricle that may be activated by cardiac distension or by vigorous rapid contraction has led to the suggestion that sudden cardiac death might be caused in this way [9, 10]. While ventricular arrhythmia is probably the commonest cause of sudden death and may occur without associated haemodynamic disorder, haemodynamic disturbance may cause arrest of effective circulation without any arrhythmia. McKenna et al. [11] reported a patient who was monitored during a syncopal attack; the left ventricular outflow tract murmur disappeared and the blood pressure became unrecordable, but there was no electrocardiographic evidence of significant arrhythmia. All these features suggested a primary haemodynamic mechanism as a cause of the circulatory arrest (see Chaps. 6, 7 and 9).

The possibility that myocardial ischaemia might be the cause of sudden death cannot be ignored. Transmural myocardial infarction without significant atherosclerosis of the large extramural coronary arteries has been reported [12]. In the majority of such patients, marked narrowing of the intramural coronary arteries and areas of subendocardial fibrosis have been found. Another possible mechanism for arrhythmias could be occlusive changes in the artery to the atrioventricular node that have been described in hypertrophic cardiomyopathy patients who died suddenly (see Chap. 6).

Investigations

The Role of Echocardiography and Doppler

No other non-invasive technique can provide such detailed anatomical, functional and haemodynamic information about the heart as echocardiography. This technique is the diagnostic tool of first choice. Since it is non-invasive it can also be used to screen the first degree relatives of patients who present with hypertrophic cardiomyopathy [13], and serial examination can be performed safely.

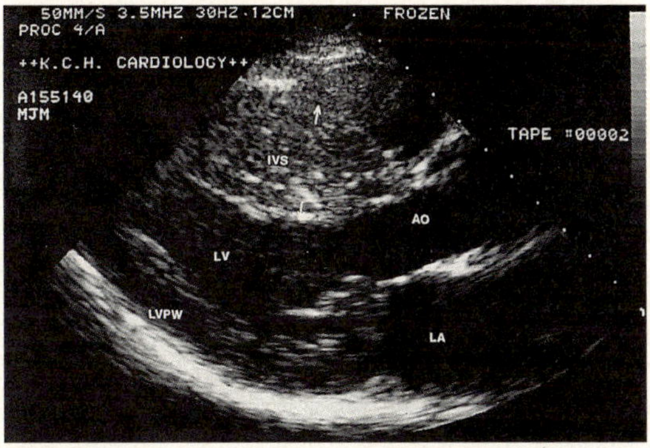

Fig. 8.1. Long axis view in a patient with a classical appearance of hypertrophic cardiomyopathy. There is extensive septal hypertrophy extending from the mitral valve towards the ventricular apex. The hypertrophy extends not only into the left ventricle, but also into the right ventricle. The left ventricular cavity is small. The *arrow* indicates the anterior side of the septum. *IVS*, interventricular septum; *AO*, aorta; *LA*, left atrium; *LV*, left ventricle; *LVPW*, left ventricular posterior wall

In the majority of patients myocardial wall thickness can be evaluated to a resolution of <1 mm. One of the hallmarks of hypertrophic cardiomyopathy is asymmetric septal hypertrophy [14]. An example of this is illustrated in Fig. 8.1. Here disproportionate hypertrophy of the interventricular septum is seen and there is the classical appearance of a small left ventricular cavity with septal hypertrophy. The protrusion of the septum into both left and right ventricles is visualised. In real time 2D images the septum is also usually relatively immobile. This is believed to be due to myocardial fibre disarray which results in no net uniform septal contraction [15]. The systolic cavity of the left ventricle is small and frequently elimination of part of the cavity may be seen [16].

The finding of asymmetric septal hypertrophy with a ratio of septal thickness to posterior wall thickness of greater than 1.5 has been considered to be diagnostic of this condition [17]. However, there are many other conditions, including aortic stenosis, hypertension, right ventricular hypertrophy and posterior wall infarction, which can all lead to a similar ratio. Therefore this diagnostic criterion cannot be taken in isolation and should be viewed in the context of the overall echocardiographic and Doppler appearances.

The M-mode echocardiogram as illustrated in Fig. 8.2 also shows the classical features of asymmetric hypertrophy in hypertrophic cardiomyopathy.

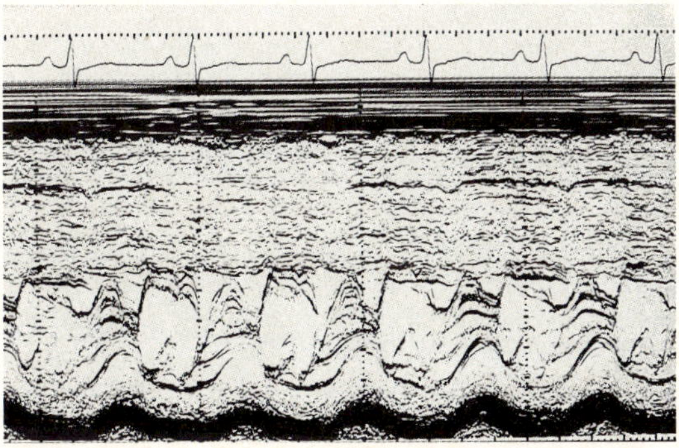

Fig. 8.2. M-mode recording at mitral valve level illustrating significant asymmetric septal hypertrophy. The septum is also akinetic and there is a small systolic cavity. Systolic anterior motion of the mitral valve leaflets is seen and the valve leaflets co-apt. with the ventricular septum during systole

However, it may be difficult to determine the true anteroseptal surface on an M-mode echo. The septum is also akinetic and there is exaggerated motion of the posterior left ventricular wall. The systolic cavity dimension is reduced.

Systolic anterior motion of the mitral valve as visualised on the M-mode recording is another classical feature of hypertrophic cardiomyopathy. This phenomenon is present particularly when there is a left ventricular intracavitary pressure gradient [18]. Figure 8.2 also illustrates this phenomenon and the mitral valve leaflets can be seen moving in an anterior direction towards the ventricular septum during systole. The exact mechanism for this phenomenon is unknown. However, it has been postulated that it occurs secondary to a Venturi effect when high-velocity blood in the left ventricular outflow tract creates a negative pressure which draws the mitral valve leaflets towards the septum [19]. It is also conceivable that the hypertrophied papillary muscles push the mitral valve apparatus and chordae out into the left ventricular outflow tract within the very small ventricular cavity. The exact relationship between this phenomenon and an intracavity gradient is, however, rather variable. If the mitral valve apparatus touches the interventricular septum for more than 30% of systole then this may indicate true "obstruction" [20].

Another indirect indicator of a pressure gradient is premature closure of the aortic valve leaflets [21]. Again this is a feature which may be appreciated relatively easily on the M-mode recording. As flow through the aortic valve leaflets is diminished by obstruction, the valve leaflets close partially and may exhibit coarse systolic fluttering. Doppler echocardiography provides a more precise and reliable method of determining the site of obstruction, and enables measurement of the gradient within the ventricular cavity in patients with hypertrophic cardiomyopathy [22]. In these patients the systolic flow velocity

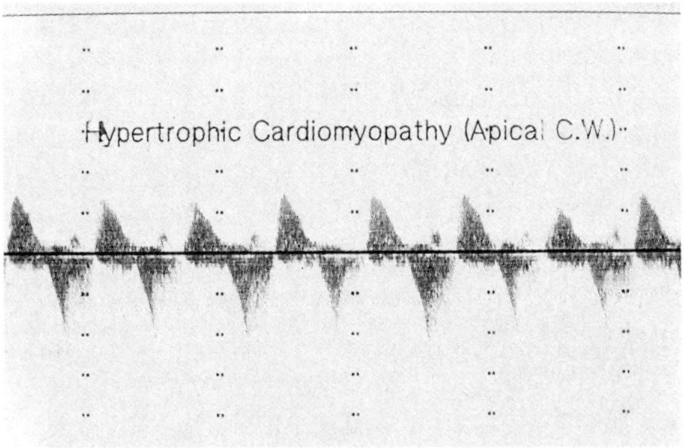

Fig. 8.3. Continuous wave Doppler recording from the cardiac apex in a patient with ventricular outflow tract obstruction. Diastolic flow into the left ventricle is seen moving towards the transducer and displayed above the zero line. In systole high flow velocity of approximately 3.5 m/s is detected. This has the classical concave appearance with delayed upstroke as seen in patients with dynamic obstruction. From the Bernoulli equation the intacavitary gradient of approximately 50 mmHg can be calculated

within the cavity or left ventricular outflow tract will be increased and the gradient may be calculated using the Bernoulli equation. An example of this is seen in Fig. 8.3. Here the flow velocity during systole is approximately 3.5 m/s, which suggests an intracavitary gradient of approximately 50 mmHg. In hypertrophic cardiomyopathy we are dealing with a dynamic obstruction which may vary during systole. This leads to a classical Doppler appearance with a delayed rise in peak systolic pressure so that the initial portion of the systolic flow profile has a concave appearance. In patients with true fixed obstruction, such as that found in aortic stenosis, the rise in systolic flow velocity is very rapid and abrupt. Continuous wave Doppler is necessary to record the highest velocities. However, it does not allow the identification of the exact site where obstruction is occuring. This can be evaluated by using pulsed wave Doppler and moving the pulsed Doppler sample volume throughout the left ventricular cavity, so that the point where a rapid increase in velocity occurs can be determined. Similar information can be obtained by colour flow mapping; aliasing of the colour flow signal occurs within the ventricular cavity at the point of obstruction and indicates a change from low-velocity laminar flow to high-velocity turbulent flow.

In Fig. 8.4 high-velocity turbulent flow is illustrated in the left ventricular outflow tract by the presence of aliasing and also green coloration within the colour flow signal. This image has utilised a variance colour map to highlight turbulent flow by the use of green colour marking. Within the left atrium a jet of mitral regurgitation can also be visualised. Mitral regurgitation is a common feature in patients with systolic anterior motion of the mitral valve. Its severity may be assessed by using Doppler techniques [23] and careful examination of the shape of the Doppler flow profile, as previously described, will allow separation of the mitral regurgitatant jet from the high-velocity systolic flow caused by "obstruction".

The left atrium is also frequently enlarged in hypertrophic cardiomyopathy and this may be due to mitral regurgitation, as previously described. Other contributing factors may be the impaired diastolic filling of the ventricle and the elevated left ventricular end-diastolic pressure, both of which can result in raised left atrial pressure. Limited information about diastolic filling abnormalities can be obtained from echo Doppler studies [24]. By positioning the pulsed Doppler sample volume within the mitral valve leaflets as illustrated in Fig. 8.5, the pattern and velocity of early and late diastolic filling can be studied. In normal patients the early diastolic filling velocity (E wave) is greater than the atrial component (A wave) which occurs in late diastole. In many patients with hypertrophic cardiomyopathy reversal of the E/A ratio may occur so that the E wave is lower in velocity than the A wave, as illustrated in Fig. 8.5. This finding, indicating abnormal diastolic filling, is not a diagnostic feature of hypertrophic cardiomyopathy since it frequently occurs in the hypertensive heart.

It is well known that in hypertrophic cardiomyopathy there is considerable variation in the distribution of hypertrophy within the ventricular walls. One of the major limitations of M-mode echocardiography in these patients is that it only evaluates the anterior septum and posterior left ventricular wall, therefore

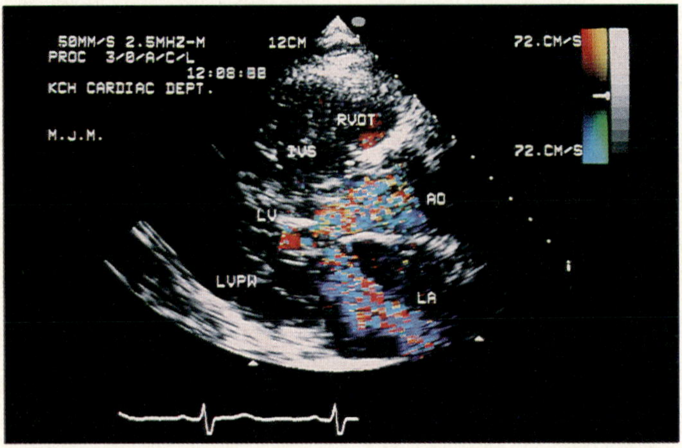

Fig. 8.4. Parasternal long axis colour flow image, illustrating high-velocity turbulent flow in the left ventricular outflow tract. Variance mapping is utilised in this example and therefore the turbulent flow can be detected not only by the presence of aliasing but also from the coloration within the left ventricular outflow tract. A jet of mitral regurgitation (predominantly blue) is seen within the left atrium. *AO*, aorta; *IVS*, interventricular septum; *LA*, left atrium; *LV*, left ventricle; *LVPW*, left ventricular posterior wall; *RVOT*, right ventricular outflow tract

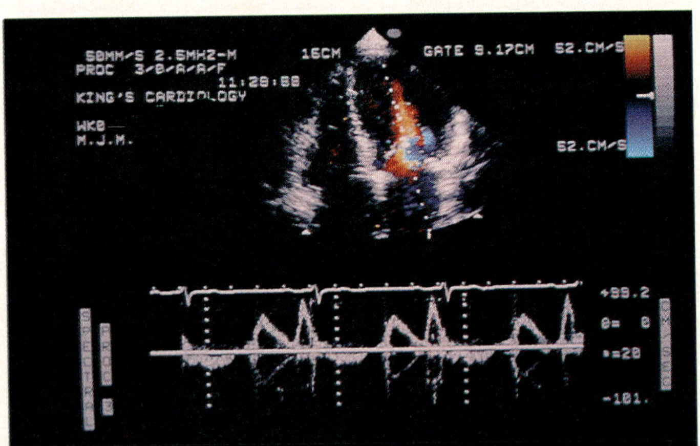

Fig. 8.5. Pulsed wave Doppler recording of left ventricular filling. Reversal of the normal filling pattern is illustrated. Early diastolic filling (E wave) is lower in velocity than the late diastolic atrial component (A wave). This reversal in the normal pattern may be seen in patients with impaired or abnormal diastolic filling and also in those with altered loading conditions

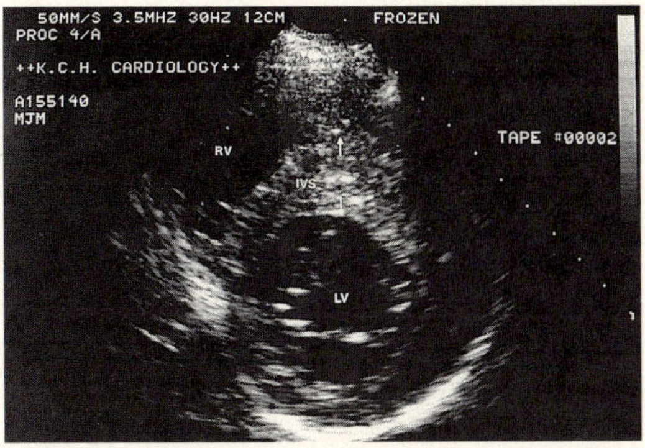

Fig. 8.6. Parasternal short axis view in a patient with hypertrophic cardiomyopathy. Extensive anteroseptal and posterior wall hypertrophy is visualised. However, the medial septal and posterior left ventricular wall are of normal thickness. The *arrows* indicate the width of the anterior intraventricular septum. *IVS*, interventricular septum; *LV*, left ventricle; *RV*, right ventricle

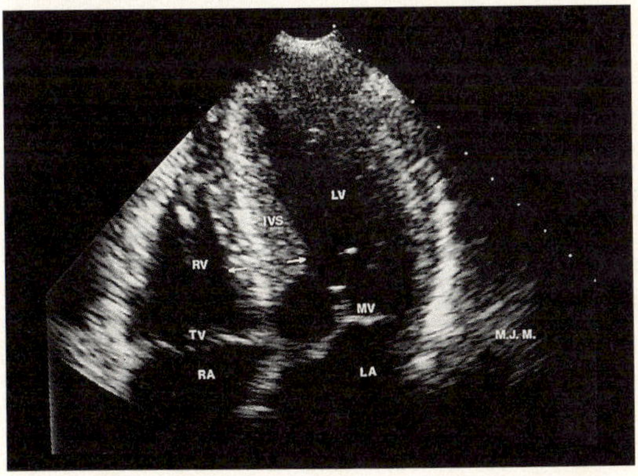

Fig. 8.7. An apical four-chamber view illustrating extensive hypertrophy of the interventricular septum at the base of the ventricle near the mitral valve leaflets and left ventricular outflow tract. Some hypertrophy extends down the septum towards the apex valve; *RA*, right atrium; *IVS*, interventricular septum, *LA*, left atrium; *LV*, left ventricle; *MV*, mitral valve; *RV*, right ventricle; *TV*, tricuspid valve

careful examination of the heart using multiple 2D imaging planes is essential when investigating these patients.

Examples of the varying distribution of hypertrophy are illustrated in Figs. 8.6–8.8. In Fig. 8.6 which is a parasternal short axis view, hypertrophy can be visualised within the anterior septum and lateral wall of the ventricle. The medial septum is relatively normal in thickness. In Fig. 8.7, an apical four-chamber view illustrates septal hypertrophy which is at its greatest near the left ventricular outflow tract, although clearly some hypertrophy extends down the septum towards the apex. Sometimes the standard M-mode echocardiogram may be entirely normal because septal and posterior wall thickness at the base of the left ventricle are within normal limits. This may particularly occur in patients with apical hypertrophic cardiomyopathy. Here again, careful 2D echo examination is vital. Figure 8.8 illustrates an example of a patient with apical hypertrophic cardiomyopathy. This is a subcostal four-chamber view showing gross hypertrophy of the interventricular septum and lateral wall at the cardiac apex. The left ventricular cavity is completely eliminated and has a slit-like appearance.

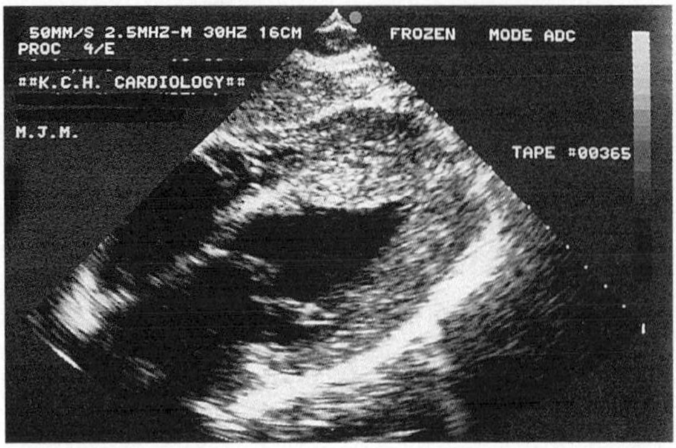

Fig. 8.8. A subcostal four-chamber view in a patient with apical hypertrophic cardiomyopathy. Gross hypertrophy of the interventricular septum and lateral wall is seen at the apex of the left ventricle. Some hypertrophy also extends into the right ventricular apex. The left ventricular cavity and right ventricular cavity are completely obliterated at the apex and have a slit-like appearance. Normal myocardial wall thickness is seen at the base of the heart

Some hypertrophy can also be seen in the right ventricular apex. However, the septal thickness at mitral valve level is entirely normal.

It is especially important to assess the exact distribution of hypertrophy if the patient is being considered for myectomy [25]. Where it is believed that extensive septal hypertrophy in the left ventricular outflow tract may be contributing to left ventricular outflow tract obstruction, resection of part of the septum may be useful. Obviously, if the hypertrophy is further down in the ventricle then surgical resection may not be so appropriate. Many surgeons now utilise intra-operative echocardiography from either the epicardial or transoesophageal approaches to study the heart during surgery [26]. It can provide precise evaluation of exactly where resection should be performed and how much myocardium should be removed.

An abnormal "granular" myocardial texture is also frequently present in hypertrophic cardiomyopathy [27]. Alternatively, the myocardium may simply appear as highly reflective. An example is illustrated in Fig. 8.9 and this appearance is probably due to increased fibrosis within the myocardium, and/or the myocardial fibre disarray which results in many acoustic interfaces and therefore increased ultrasound reflection from these tissues.

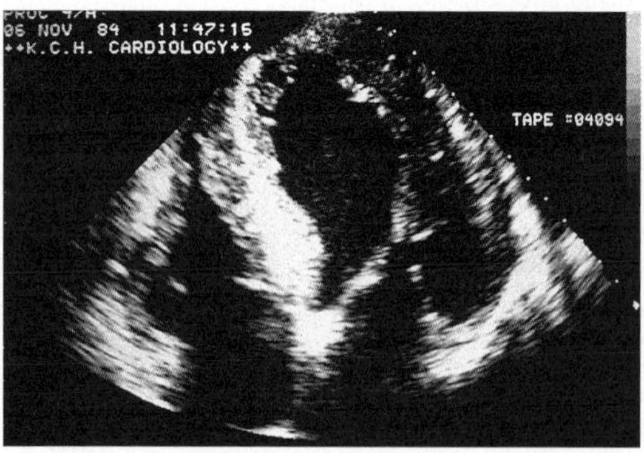

Fig. 8.9. In this apical four-chamber view very bright septal echoes are seen. These are probably the result of increasing fibrosis within the interventricular septum, and/or myocardial fibre disarray causing multiple acoustic interfaces. Such bright myocardial echoes, often with a granular appearance, are frequently seen in hypertrophic cardiomyopathy

None of the features described above should be taken in isolation as diagnostic of hypertrophic cardiomyopathy. For example, features suggestive of hypertrophic cardiomyopathy may be found in hypertensive heart disease, although demonstration of systolic anterior motion of the mitral valve and/or mid-systolic closure of the aortic valve by M-mode echocardiography strongly suggest a diagnosis of hypertrophic cardiomyopathy [28]. The latter features, coupled with information on extent and distribution of hypertrophy from 2D imaging, have contributed to the acceptance of echocardiography as the means of diagnosis in the majority of patients.

Ambulatory Electrocardiographic Monitoring

Electrocardiographic monitoring has little part to play in the diagnosis of hypertrophic cardiomyopathy. In patients with proven hypertrophic cardiomyopathy, however, 24-h or 48-h ambulatory electrocardiographic monitoring is frequently performed in order to detect either symptomatic or asymptomatic ventricular arrythmias. Studies have shown that the presence of non-sustained ventricular tachycardia on Holter monitoring is the strongest singler marker for identifying adult patients at risk of sudden death [29, 30]. Serial Holter monitoring has been employed to assess the effects of antiarrythmic therapy on the incidence of ventricular tachycardia in hypertrophic cardiomyopathy and to compare the efficacy of different agents. Currently, the agent of choice appears to be amiodarone, which leads to a reduction in asymptomatic ventricular arrythmias associated with an improvement in survival. Unfortunately these data seem to have little relevance to children, in whom the incidence of arrythmias is low.

Cardiac Catheterisation and Left Ventriculography

The indications for cardiac catheterisation and coronary angiography in echocardiographically proven hypertrophic cardiomyopathy are: (1) severe stable angina resistant to medical therapy, (2) unstable angina, and (3) following documented myocardial infarction. It is apparent, therefore, that the principal reason for angiographic investigation is to examine the major coronary arteries in patients with chest pain.

If hypertrophic cardiomyopathy is unsuspected, however, the left ventriculogram may suggest the diagnosis at routine cardiac catheterisation. The left ventriculogram reveals characteristic appearances: the ventricle in diastole is angulated in its mid-portion due to the hypertrophy of the papillary muscles and the end-diastolic volume is normal. In systole the contraction is rapid and well co-ordinated. The ventricle usually empties completely with virtual elimination of the cavity at the end of systole. The apex of the left ventricle may be isolated from the outflow portion by apposition of the lateral wall to the septum. The enlarged papillary muscles project into the cavity. Sometimes, contrast medium may be seen in the interstices of the columnae carneae in the shape of a star. In many patients, usually those with a gradient, there is slight mitral regurgitation. Occasionally appearances suggestive of a left ventricular aneurysm are seen.

In a study of 100 patients with hypertrophic cardiomyopathy, the left ventricular angiograms were grouped according to the end-systolic shape of the left ventricle. Elimination of the cavity occurred in 41 patients, marked narrowing of the mid-portion of the cavity in 45; the shape was normal in 10. Dilatation of the left ventricular cavity was observed in only 4 patients, 2 of whom had severe mitral regurgitation while 2 had shown a gradual disappearance of pressure gradients over a period of years and had died suddenly. Advanced heart failure, severe mitral regurgitation or transmural myocardial infarction are also causes of left ventricular dilatation.

Sophisticated echocardiographic techniques have made haemodynamic measurements largely obsolete and the administration of drugs is rarely required. However, in about 50% of patients at rest, and a further 15%–20% on provocation with amyl nitrate, the Valsalva manoeuvre, ectopic beats or isoprenaline, withdrawal traces from the apex of the left ventricle show gradients in the mid-section of the left ventricle; there is no overshoot as may be found with catheter entrapment. The gradients occur in association with forward movement of the mitral valve apparatus towards the septum, which can be seen both on Doppler echocardiography and angiocardiography.

The end-diastolic pressure in the left ventricle is usually elevated at rest, though may rise only on exercise. The aortic pressure pulse shows rapid collapse and often a tidal wave on the downstroke. The percussion wave causes the peak pressure.

Endomyocardial Biopsy

Endomyocardial biopsy is not advised for the routine clinical diagnosis of hypertrophic cardiomyopathy because in well-documented series the typical histological features fulfilling the histological hypertrophic cardiomyopathy index (HHI) [31] are found in only 50% of patients. This may in part relate to the patchy nature of the myocardial changes including the myofibrillar disarray. These latter changes are confined to the septum in some patients but in others may occur anywhere within the myocardium. In addition, because of the distorted shape of the ventricles and the small cavity size, biopsy may be dangerous.

Differential Diagnosis

The final diagnosis of hypertrophic cardiomyopathy is dependent on a combination of clinical features and the results of investigations performed. Therefore the section on differential diagnosis in Chap. 9 is expanded here.

In patients with a systolic murmur, the differential diagnosis includes aortic valvar stenosis, discrete subaortic stenosis, pulmonary stenosis, ventricular septal defect and mitral regurgitation from causes other than hypertrophic cardiomyopathy.

In patients with heart failure the clinical picture and haemodynamic abnormalities may resemble cardiac amyloidosis. Although bright echoes may be seen in the ventricular muscle, the massive hypertrophy seen in hypertrophic cardiomyopathy is usually absent in amyloid disease. Prolapse of the mitral valve may be simulated if there is any early or mid-systolic click followed by a systolic murmur at the apex, and may occur in association with hypertrophic cardiomyopathy. In patients with particularly high left ventricular end-diastolic pressure and no gradient, the physical signs may be essentially those of severe pulmonary hypertension and an incorrect diagnosis of primary pulmonary hypertension or Eisenmenger's syndrome may be made. Right-sided hypertrophic cardiomyopathy with outflow tract gradient may be difficult or impossible to differentiate at the bedside from infundibular pulmonary stenosis. But the electrocardiographic evidence of left ventricular involvement in hypertrophic cardiomyopathy is absent in lone infundibular pulmonary stenosis, with which there is usually an associated ventricular septal defect. It is apparent that hypertrophic cardiomyopathy may mimic a number of other cardiac diseases and if the signs and symptoms of the conditions do not harmonise, the possibility of hypertrophic cardiomyopathy should always be considered, particularly in young people.

New Approaches

Magnetic resonance imaging (MRI) is being used both in the scanning mode and for spectroscopic analysis of myocardial substrates. The extent of the involvement of the septum, the site of the major hypertrophy and the extent of the involvement of the ventricular walls is well shown by this technique, which may come to be regarded as a useful adjunct to echocardiography [32]. In the majority of patients with hypertrophic cardiomyopathy routine echocardiography will prove diagnostic. However, when technical factors preclude adequate echocardiographic visualisation, it has been found that MRI will provide diagnostic images. This was particularly found to be the case in the apical variant of hypertrophic cardiomyopathy [33].

Magnetic resonance spectroscopy provide a non-invasive means of studying intracellular biochemistry by measuring the relative proportions of high-energy phosphates. Whilst this technique has not yet been applied in hypertrophic cardiomyopathy it has been applied in the assessment of the hypertrophied myocardium in patients with aortic valve disease. In these patients it was found that when myocardial failure was present it was associated with a low phosphocreatine/ATP ratio [34]. This novel technique will allow assessment of metabolism, and detection of similar changes in patients with hypertrophic cardiomyopathy might identify a subset of patients with metabolic alterations of prognostic importance.

Radionuclide techniques with thallium-201 have been used to study the left ventricle [35], and uptake of rubidium-82 has been found to be reduced in the septum as compared with the free wall of the left ventricle [36]. Gated blood pool studies have revealed that stroke volume ejected by the left ventricle in the first third of systole was greater in hypertrophic cardiomyopathy than in normal patients and did not vary according to the presence or absence of gradients in the hypertrophic patients.

The development of molecular biological techniques should permit the use of genetic codes to assist diagnosis of the disease before birth (see Chap. 16) and perhaps detect and treat abnormal catecholamine receptors in the fetal myocardium.

References

1. Maron BJ, Epstein SE (1980) Hypertrophic cardiomyopathy. Recent observations regarding the specificity of three hallmarks of the disease: asymmetric septal hypertrophy, septal disorganisation and systolic anterior motion of the anterior mitral leaflet. Am J Cardiol 45: 141–154
2. St. John Sutton MG, Lie JT, Anderson KR, O'Brien PC, Frye RL (1980) Histopathological specificity of hypertrophic obstructive cardiomyopathy: myocardial fibre disarray and myocardial fibrosis. Br Heart J 44: 433–443
3. Murgo JP, Alter DJF, Altobelli SA, McGranahan GM (1980) Left ventricular ejection dynamics in hypertrophic cardiomyopathy. In: Sekiguchi M, Olsen EGJ (eds) Cardiomyopathy. University of Tokyo Press, Tokyo, pp 45–65
4. Sugrue DD, McKenna WJ, Dickie S et al. (1984) Relation between left ventricular gradient and relative stroke volume ejected in early and late systole in hypertrophic cardiomyopathy: assessment with radionuclide angiography. Br Heart J 52: 602
5. Maron BJ, Merrill WH, Freier PA, Kent KM, Epstein SE, Morrow AG (1978) Long term clinical course and symptomatic status of patients after operation for hypertrophic subaortic stenosis. Circulation 57: 1205
6. Wigle ED, Sasson Z, Henderson MA et al. (1985) Hypertrophic cardiomyopathy: the importance of the site and the extent of hypertrophy—a review. Prog Cardiovasc Dis 28: 1
7. Sanderson JE, Gibson DG, Brown DJ, Goodwin JF (1977) Left ventricular filling in hypertrophic cardiomyopathy: an angiographic study. Br Heart J 39: 661
8. Sanderson JE, Traill TA, St. John Sutton MG, Brown DJ, Gibson DG, Goodwin JF (1977) Left ventricular relaxation and filling in hypertrophic cardiomyopathy: an echocardiographic study. Br Heart J 40: 596
9. Almquist A, Goldenberg IF, Milstein S et al. (1989) Provocation of bradycardia and hypotension by isoproterenol and upright posture in patients with unexpected syncope. N Engl J Med 320: 346–351
10. Abboud FM(1989) Ventricular syncope: is the heart a sensory organ? N Engl J Med 320: 390–392
11. McKenna WJ, Harris L, Deanfield J (1982) Syncope in hypertrophic cardiomyopathy. Br Heart J 47: 177
12. Maron BJ, Epstein SE, Roberts WC (1979) Hypertrophic cardiomyopathy and transmural myocardial infarction without significant atherosclerosis of the extramural coronary artery. Am J Cardiol 43: 1036
13. Maron BJ, Nichols PS, Pickle LW, Wesley YE, Muldihill JJ (1984) Patterns of inheritance in hypertrophic cardiomyopathy: assessment by M-mode and 2-dimensional echocardiography. Am J Cardiol 53: 1087–1094
14. Henry WL, Clark CE, Roberts WC, Morrow AG, Epstein SE (1974) Difference in distribution of myocardial abnormalities in patients with obstructive and non-obstructive asymmetric septal hypertrophy (ASH): echocardiographic and gross anatomic findings. Circulation 50: 447
15. Kaul S, Kay TEIC, Shah PM (1983) Interventricular septal and free-wall dynamics in hypertrophic cardiomyopathy. J Am Coll Cardiol 4: 1024–1030

16. Murgo JP, Alter BR, Dorethy JF, Altobelli SA, McGranahan GM (1980) Dynamics of left ventricular ejection in obstructive and non-obstructive hypertrophic cardiomyopathy. J Clin Invest 66: 1369
17. Epstein SE, Henry WL, Clark CE (1974) Asymmetric septal hypertrophy. Ann Intern Med 81: 650–680
18. Shah PM, Gramiak R, Adelman AG, Wigle ED (1977) Role of echocardiograhpy in diagnostic and haemodynamic assessment of hypertrophic sub-aortic stenosis. Circulation 44: 891–898
19. Lin C-S, Chen K-S, Lin M-C, Fu M-C, Tang S-M (1991) The relationship between systolic anterior motion of the mitral valve and the left ventricular outflow tract Doppler in hypertrophic cardiomyopathy. Am Heart J 122: 1671–1682
20. Pollick C, Rakowski H, Wigle ED (1984) Muscular sub-aortic stenosis: the quantitative relationship between systolic anterior motion and the pressure gradient. Circulation 69: 43–49.
21. Krajcer Z, Orzan F, Pechacek LW, Garcia E, Leachman RD (1978) Early systolic closure of the aortic valve in patients wilth hypertrophic sub-aortic stenosis and discrete sub-aortic stenosis: correlation with pre-operative and post-operative haemodynamics. Am J Cardiol 421: 823–829
22. Maron DJ, Gottdiemer JS, Arce J, Rosing DR, Wesley YE, Epstein SE (1985) Dynamic sub-aortic obstruction in hypertrophic cardiomyopathy: analysis by pulsed wave Doppler echocardiography. J Am Coll Cardiol 6: 1–15
23. Blumlein S, Bouchard A, Schiller NB et al. (1986) Quantitation of mitral regurgitation flow by Doppler echocardiography. Circulation 74: 306–314
24. Maron DJ, Spirito P, Green KJ, Wesley YE, Bonow RO, Arce J (1987) Non-invasive assessment of left ventricular diastolic function by pulsed Doppler echocardiography in patients with hypertrophic cardiomyopathy. J Am Coll Cardiol 10: 733–742
25. Shapira JN, Stemple DR, Martin RP, Rakowski H, Stinson EB, Popp RL (1978) Single and 2-dimensional echocardiographic visualisation of the effects of septal myectomy in idiopathic hypertrophic sub-aortic stenosis. Circulation 58: 850–860
26. Stewart WJ, Schiavone WA, Salcedo EE, Lever HM, Cosgrove DN, Gill CC (1987) Intra-operative Doppler echocardiography in hypertrophic cardiomyopathy: correlations with obstructive gradient. J Am Coll Cardiol 10: 327–335
27. Martin RP, Rakowski H, French J, Popp RL (1979) Idiopathic hypertrophic sub-aortic stenosis viewed by wide angled, phased array echocardiography. Circulation 59: 1206–1217
28. Doi YL, Deanfield JE, McKenna WJ, Dargie HJ, Oakley CM, Goodwin JF (1980) Echocardiographic differentiation of hypertensive heart disease and hypertrophic cardiomyopathy. Br Heart J 44: 395–400
29. Maron BJ, Savage DD, Wolfson JK, Epstein SE (1981) Prognostic significance of 24-hour ambulatory electrocardiographic monitoring in patients with hypertrophic cardiomyopathy: a prospective study. Am J Cardiol 48: 252–257
30. McKenna WJ, England D, Doi YL, Deanfield JE, Oakley CM, Goodwin JF (1981) Arrythmia in hypertrophic cardiomyopathy. I. Influence on prognosis. Br Heart J 46: 168–172
31. Van Nordern S, Olsen EGJ, Pearse AGE (1971) Hypertrophic obstructive cardiomyopathy: a histological, histochemical and ultrastructural study of biopsy material. Cardiovasc Res 5: 118–131
32. Been M, Kean D, Smith MA, Douglas RHB, Best JJK, Muir AL (1985) Nuclear magnetic resonance in hypertrophic cardiomyopathy. Br Heart J 54: 48–52
33. Mattioli AV, Fantini G, Modena MG, Bertolani M, Tirelli G, Romagnoli R (1989) Magnetic resonance imaging versus ultrasound in the evaluation of hypertrophic cardiomyopathy. Cardiovasc Imag 1: 37–42
34. Conway MA, Allis J, Ouwerkerk R, Nhoka T, Rajagopalan B, Radda GK (1991) Detection of low phosphocreatine to ATP ratio in failing hypertrophied human myocardium by ^{31}P magnetic resonance spectroscopy. Lancet 338: 973–976
35. Hanrath P et al. (1981) Myocardial thallium imaging in hypertrophic obstructive cardiomyopathy. Eur Heart J 2: 177
36. Sugrue D, Dickie S, Oakley CM, Lavender JP (1984) Hemodynamic significance of left ventricular gradients in hypertrophic cardiomyopathy. Br Heart J 51: 113

CHAPTER 9

Haemodynamic Disorders: Management and Prognosis

J. T. Stewart and W. J. McKenna

Introduction

Hypertrophic cardiomyopathy is defined as a heart muscle disorder of unknown origin that is characterised by hypertrophy of a non-dilated left ventricle. The first systematic description of the condition was made by the pathologist Donald Teare in 1958 [1], from the post-mortem appearances of the hearts of 9 adolescents and young adults, 8 of whom had died suddenly. Teare drew attention to the disproportionate thickness of the interventricular septum compared with the left ventricular free wall in his autopsy specimens, and commented on focal myocardial fibre disarray in histological sections of the interventricular septum.

The characteristic morphological feature of hypertrophic cardiomyopathy is asymmetrical hypertrophy of the interventricular septum, but large autopsy series have shown that the left ventricular free wall is also thicker than normal in most patients and, in about 30% of cases, left ventricular hypertrophy is symmetrical [2]. The standard diagnostic technique, cross-sectional echocardiography, has further demonstrated that left ventricular hypertrophy may have almost any distribution—asymmetric septal, symmetrical, or predominantly involve the distal ventricle—and that, in addition, there is right ventricular hypertrophy in over one third of patients [3–5].

The characteristic histological feature of hypertrophic cardiomyopathy is myocyte disarray, which is quantitatively different in hypertrophic cardiomyopathy to the appearances seen in other forms of hypertrophy [6]. Maron and his colleagues [7–9] have demonstrated myocyte disarray in more than 5% of the area of the interventricular septum in 90% of patients with definite hypertrophic cardiomyopathy. In patients with normal hearts, or other cardiac pathologies, less than 5% (and usually less than 1%) of the area of the septum showed myofibre disorganisation [9]. Myocyte disarray is also seen in the left and right ventricular free walls, although usually to a lesser extent than is seen in the septum.

Under the light microscope the disorganised muscle bundles have a characteristic whorled pattern, and are associated with an excess of loose connective tissue. Ultrastructural examination by electron microscopy has demonstrated that there is also disorganisation of the myofibrils within individual cells, and that the cells frequently contain increased amounts of Z-band material [10] (see Chap. 7).

A high proportion of patients with hypertrophic cardiomyopathy (greater than 50%) also have abnormal intramural intracoronary arteries, particularly in the interventricular septum [11, 12]. These arteries are thick-walled with a narrowed lumen resulting from increased numbers of smooth muscle cells and increased amounts of fibrous tissue in the intima and media. There are also increased deposits of acid mucopolysaccharide material within the arterial walls. These abnormalities of the intramural coronary arteries are not specific for hypertrophic cardiomyopathy, but are more marked than in other conditions. The arterial abnormalities do not appear to correlate with any clinical parameters, and their cause and significance are uncertain (see Chap. 7).

About 50% of affected patients present with symptoms (dyspnoea or chest pain and, less commonly, syncope), while in the remaining 50% diagnosis is made as a result of family screening or following the detection of abnormality during investigation for some other reason [13, 14]. The natural history of hypertrophic cardiomyopathy in the majority of patients is of slow progression of symptoms with a high superimposed incidence of sudden death. The annual mortality from sudden cardiac death is 2.5% in adults, and as high as 4%–6% in children [13, 15–17]. The identification and treatment of patients who are at increased risk of sudden death remains a difficult but important task for those involved in the management of hypertrophic cardiomyopathy (see Chap. 6).

Pathophysiology: Systolic and Diastolic Dysfunction

Hypertrophic cardiomyopathy is diagnosed in many more patients now, using sensitive methods of screening (particularly cross-sectional echocardiography), than was the case when the condition was first described. At least 50% of affected individuals are asymptomatic, and the presence or absence of symptoms does not correlate with the degree or distribution of left ventricular hypertrophy [13, 14]. There is also disagreement over the relationship of disordered left ventricular function to symptom generation; in turn it has been claimed that both systolic and diastolic left ventricular dysfunction are responsible. Currently our understanding of the pathophysiology of this condition is in a state of evolution, and different factors may have more or less relevance in a particular individual.

In the 1960s clinical features of hyperdynamic systolic function and the presence of a dynamic left ventricular outflow tract gradient were emphasised. It has since become apparent that only about 35% of individuals with hypertrophic cardiomyopathy have a resting or provocable left ventricular outflow tract gradient of > 30 mmHg [12–14]. Where present, the subaortic pressure gradient is due to contact between the anterior mitral leaflet and the hypertrophied interventricular system. In this case the pressure in the distal outflow tract is low and equal to aortic systolic pressure, but all other intraventricular pressure, including that in the inflow tract, are elevated.

In subaortic obstruction the pressure gradient develops in mid to late systole. There is still debate over its exact cause; it has been ascribed to the effect of Venturi forces acting on the mitral leaflets [18]. According to this theory the narrowing of the outflow tract, produced by hyperdynamic contraction of the hypertrophied septum, causes the ejection jet in early systole to pass close to the mitral leaflets, producing systolic anterior motion of the mitral valve (SAM). Recent work using a flow model of the left ventricular outflow tract, however, has cast doubt on this theory [19]. As a result of this work a structural abnormality of the submitral apparatus has been proposed as the cause of SAM. However it is produced, early and prolonged mitral leaflet–septal contact is associated with a high pressure gradient, prolongation of the ejection time and significant mitral regurgitation; a large proportion of the left ventricular stroke volume is ejected against the obstruction [18, 20–22]. In the majority of patients with systolic anterior movement of the mitral valve, however, the volume of blood remaining in the left ventricle at the onset of mitral leaflet–septal contact is usually $<25\%$ of total stroke volume, and overall stroke volume is not reduced [23]. Though such patients may have clinical features of an outflow tract gradient they cannot be considered to have true obstruction of left ventricular ejection. Lesser degrees of mitral leaflet–septal contact, occurring later in systole and for a shorter time, produce smaller pressure gradients and less regurgitation.

Nevertheless, genuine obstruction to left ventricular ejection does seem to occur in a subset of patients [24], and intuitively the combination of increased resistance to antegrade left ventricular ejection and mitral regurgitation should have metabolic and clinical sequelae. There is, however, little published evidence to show that large outflow tract pressure gradients are particularly associated with increased myocardial oxygen demand, myocardial ischaemia, or a worse prognosis. Indeed many patients have disabling symptoms in the absence of a pressure gradient [14], but in the subset of pateints who do have a gradient, symptom severity seems to relate its magnitude [21]. The apparent conflict in this area may relate to centres with a greater proportion of patients who do not have a gradient but who are very symptomatic. Where severe symptoms and a significant pressure gradient coexist, experience suggests that reduction of the gradient is beneficial [21, 25]. It is likely that the majority of patients with hypertrophic cardiomyopathy do not have true obstruction to outflow but that a minority do, due to massive hypertrophy and greatly enlarged papillary muscles and very small ventricular cavity. Work by Criley and Siegel [26] and Murgo and Miller [27], employing indices of flow velocity, echocardiographic and angiographic ventricular emptying data and intraluminal gradient, has suggested that ejection from the left ventricle is very rapid and almost complete, whether or not there is a gradient. Their findings argue against true "obstruction" (see Chaps. 6 and 8).

In most patients with hypertrophic cardiomyopathy left ventricular diastolic function, manifest as the ability of the left ventricle to fill with blood without a compensatory increase in left atrial pressure, is compromised [28–30]. Thus, at low pressures, left ventricular filling is slow, and may be imcomplete unless left atrial pressure increases. (This is similar in some ways to the pathophysiology of pure mitral stenosis.) At its mildest, diastolic dysfunction may be manifest as slow or delayed left ventricular relaxation and filling, with little increase in left ventricular pressure, but in more severe forms it may result in pulmonary venous congestion or frank pulmonary oedema, even in the presence of near-normal left ventricular systolic function.

Diastole is a complex phenomenon which is poorly understood, even in the normal heart. Brutsaert et al. [31] describe three separate components: (1) energy-dependent active sequestration of calcium by the sarcoplasmic reticulum, which is influenced by metabolic rate, energy substrate levels, and circulating levels of catechols and other harmones; (2) ventricular loading, the rebound or recoil of passive compressive–elastic elements in the myocardium following compression during systolic contraction (greatly influenced by the shape and volume of the heart), and the effect of the rapid filling of the expanding coronary bed in early diastole as the heart relaxes; and (3) non-uniformity of loading and unloading in time and space. All three factors may be abnormal in hypertrophic cardiomyopathy.

There is reduced distensibility of the left ventricle (increased chamber stiffness) which is due to a number of factors: left ventricular mass is increased (and the volume to mass ratio is abnormally low), myocardial stiffness is increased, and active myocardial relaxation is impaired. Increased left ventricular mass can adversely affect chamber stiffness by simple geometric mechanisms [32, 33], and the hypertrophied septum, with its catenoid shape resulting in isometric contraction of the septal fibres, is thought to have a significant effect on passive recoil of the myocardium [34, 35]. In addition, the fibre disarray again gives rise to isometric contraction and abnormal recoil characteristics [36]. Myocardial stiffness, an intrinsic mechanical property of myocardium, is increased by the increased content of abnormal connective tissue and fibrosis, as well as by myocardial disarray [37, 38].

Myocardial relaxation, the active, energy-dependent process of deactivation, is intimately related to the loading conditions of the ventricle and these interrelated factors are, in turn, modulated by neurohumoral factors and metabolic influences, such as ischaemia [39]. There may be a primary defect of cellular calcium handling in hypertrophic cardiomyopathy (impaired uptake by the sarcoplasmic reticulum [40, 41]), with delayed "switchilng off" of contraction. Such calcium currents are also very sensitive to myocardial ischaemia.

In addition to the foregoing influences on diastolic function, asynchronous left ventricular activation and contraction can slow isovolumic relaxation and reduce early diastolic filling rates [42, 43]. Detailed digital analysis of left ventricular angiograms and echocardiograms has shown such incoordination of contraction, relaxation and filling which suggests segmental abnormalities of all aspects of left ventricular function [29, 30]. These abnormalities may result from areas of ischaemia or fibrosis within the left ventricular wall, or may reflect asymmetric distribution of hypertrophied myocardium, with conduction delays giving rise to non-uniformity of activation and deactivation in time and space.

It seems likely that abnormalities of both systolic and diastolic function are important in hypertrophic cardiomyopathy, but to varying degrees in any individual. This may be illustrated by the results of our recent investigation into the mechanism of symptom limitation in 81 patients with hypertrophic cardiomyopathy [44]. Although there was no relationship between maximal oxygen uptake (VO_2 max) and the incidence and magnitude of resting left ventricular outflow tract pressure gradients (>30 mmHg), there was evidence of different mechanisms of exercise limitation according to the presence or absence of such a gradient. In the 22 patients with a resting pressure gradient, multivariate analysis demonstrated that the most-important indicators of reduced exercise capacity were impaired left ventricular systolic performance and atrial systolic failure. In 59 patients without a resting outflow tract gradient, similar analysis showed that diastolic dysfunction was a more important factor in the limitation of exercise.

Further difficulty in the understanding of the pathophysiology of the condition arises if too much emphasis is placed upon increased cardiac mass, even though the standard diagnostic criteria depend upon unexplained left ventricular hypertrophy. The *sine qua non* of hypertrophic cardiomyopathy is probably myocardial disarray, rather than increased cardiac mass, and it seems likely that the cellular disorganisation gives rise to electrical instability of the myocardium, and that it may contribute to the abnormalities of left ventricular function. We have seen patients in whom restrictive cardiac physiology led to transplantation, and in whom examination of the explanted heart showed myocyte disarray in the absence of hypertrophy. In addition we have recently described two families with the characteristic histological abnormalities, and many of the clinical features, of hypertrophic cardiomyopathy in the absence of left ventricular hypertrophy. In one family the clinical presentation was with sudden unexpected cardiac death in four family members; in the other presentation was with electrocardiographic repolarisation changes and abnormalities of left ventricular diastolic function [45].

Symptoms

The commonest symptoms in hypertrophic cardiomyopathy are dyspnoea, chest pain and syncope (see Chap. 6).

Dyspnoea

It is seldom possible to identify a single cause of dyspnoea in an individual patient. As discussed above, most patients have some degree of diastolic dysfunction, and probably raised left atrial and pulmonary venous pressure, to which left ventricular hypertrophy, ischaemia, mitral regurgitation and myocyte disarray may all contribute. The physical attributes of the abnormal left ventricle do not explain dyspnoea in all cases, however. In the study referred to above, there was no relationship between exercise capacity and left ventricular filling pressures, suggesting that there may be determinants of breathlessness other than cardiac factors alone [44]. The central perception of dyspnoea and the control of skeletal muscle blood flow may be as relevant to symptoms in hypertrophic cardiomyopathy as in cardiac failure [46].

Although dyspnoea has often been attributed to the presence of a left ventricular outflow tract gradient, Braunwald et al.'s [14] early clinical study showed no relationship between the presence or severity of a gradient and the patient's symptoms. Wigle et al. [24], however, has presented data showing that in those patients with genuine obstruction to left ventricular ejection ($< 50\%$ of the stroke volume ejected before the development of the outflow tract gradient) symptoms are related to the severity of the gradient and results from several centres make it clear that reduction of the gradient by either surgical or pharmacological means improves symptom status and may improve exercise tolerance [21, 25].

Chest Pain

Chest pain is also common, and is frequently difficult to treat satisfactorily. It is often related to exertion or emotion, and usually has the character of angina pectoris, with a sensation of retrosternal pressure or tightness which may radiate to the neck, jaw and arms. Unlike typical angina it may persist for hours without enzymatic evidence of myocardial necrosis, and it may occur at rest [47]. Nevertheless the nature and distribution of the chest pain suggests that myocardial ischaemia is probably responsible, but in most patients, certainly in those aged less than 40 years, the epicardial coronary arteries are normal (although non-atherosclerotic narrowing of the intramural arteries has been described [48]. Myocardial ischaemia is most likely to result from a mismatch between the increased oxygen demand of the hypertrophied myocardium and the supply of oxygen by the coronary circulation, although a primary abnormality of energy substrate use, or oxidative metabolism, at the cellular level, is possible.

The results of exercise stress testing in hypertrophic cardiomyopathy are often difficult to interpret because of resting electromyocardiographic abnormalities, and several groups have used thallum-201 scintigraphy to assess regional perfusion in patients with normal coronary arteries [49–54]. The results have been varied, but overall thallium perfusion defects are common, both in patients with and without chest pain. The exact significance of reversible thallium perfusion defects in hypertrophic cardiomyopathy is not yet known, but fixed thallium defects probably represent areas of myocardial scarring, and seem to be more common in patients with impaired left ventricular systolic function [52] and adverse prognostic features [53].

Evidence of myocardial ischaemia has also been sought in experiments using metabolic markers of anaerobic myocardial metabolism, such as lactate production. Although a relatively specific indicator of myocardial ischaemia, the demonstration of lactate production is quite insensitive, because of the mixture of venous effluent from different areas of myocardium, not all of which may be ischaemic [54]. Despite its shortcomings, studies of coronary sinus lactate concentration during incremental pacing or isoprenaline infusion have been performed to investigate the mechanisms or chest pain in patients with hypertrophic cardiomyopathy and normal epicardial coronary arteries. Incremental pacing or isoprenaline infusion has usually reproduced the symptoms in a majority of patients, and such studies have provided evidence of anaerobic myocardial metabolism during stress [55–60]. These studies indicate that in the majority of patients with hypertrophic cardiomyopathy who complain of anginal-type pain, the cause is myocardial ischaemia. Those in whom chest pain is not a prominent symptom do not seem to have an ischaemic metabolic response to pacing or isoprenaline stresses.

A number of the features of hypertrophic cardiomyopathy could contribute to an abnormal myocardial oxygen supply-and-demand relationship. Hypertrophied myocardium has a greater absolute oxygen requirement than normal myocardium. Although the hypertrophied muscle in hypertrophic cardiomyopathy is abnormal, and contains large amounts of connective tissue in which metabolic activity is low, the content of contractile proteins, which require oxidative metabolism to provide high-energy phosphate substrates for mechanical activity, is also increased. Coronary flow per unit mass has been normal in most studies [61–63], but the requirement for higher absolute flow rates at rest and during stress requires greater than normal vasodilatation of the intramyocardial autoregulatory arterioles. This reduces the capacity of the coronary bed to dilate further, such that hypertrophic cardiomyopathy is characterised by reduced coronary flow reserve [55–57, 64, 65]. The reduction in coronary flow reserve may be offset to some extent by the reduction in wall stress which results from increased wall thickness (Laplace's Law), but wall stress is probably still higher than normal in the subendocardial layers of the left ventricular wall in hypertrophic cardiomyopathy because ventricular pressures are increased.

There are also haemodynamic changes in hypertrophic cardiomyopathy which may adversely affect coronary blood flow. Under normal conditions most coronary flow occurs during diastole but some flow does occur during systole. Compression of the epicardial and septal perforating coronary arteries during systole is common in this group of patients [48, 66], and although it is not specific for hypertrophic cardiomyopathy, it may be partly responsible for reduced myocardial perfusion, particularly if vessel compression lasts into early diastole when intramyocardial blood flow is ususlly high. Even in the absence of systolic compression of the large coronary arteries, early diastolic flow is almost certainly abnormal in a majority of patients because of the abnormal diastolic function of the left ventricle itself. The raised intracavitary pressure, at the onset of and during diastole, must reduce the driving pressure for coronary perfusion, and the impaired relaxation of the ventricular myocardium will reduce the early diastolic filling of the myocardial microcirculation.

At a tissue level, it is probable that the distance over which oxygen must diffuse from the capillaries to the hypertrophied myocytes is increased in hypertrophic cardiomyopathy. The abnormal myocardial architecture (excess amounts of loose connective tissue and bizarrely shaped, abnormal aligned myocytes) is likely to have an adverse effect on the numbers of small vessels, the dilatory capacity of the vascular bed, and the distance over which diffusion must occur.

Finally, of course, atherosclerotic coronary artery disease may coexist with hypertrophic cardiomyopathy, particularly in the older age group. Since it is not possible from the history or from noninvasive investigations to exclude obstructive coronary disease, coronary arteriography is the only means of detecting coexisting coronary disease in symptomatic patients.

Syncope

Syncope occurs in 15%–25% of patients [13, 14] and is considered an ominous prognostic sign, particularly in the young. An individual with syncope is at increased risk of sudden death, although the absence of a history of syncope does not confer a low risk. Its mechanism must be individually explored because the origins of syncope are diverse, and many possible mechanisms of circulatory collapse exist in these patients.

Studies of Holter monitoring in hypertrophic cardiomyopathy do not suggest an increased incidence of sinoatrial disease or of atrioventricular nodal disease in patients with the condition [67–69]. Data from electrophysiological studies may be skewed by the fact that patients undergoing such studies tend to be those who are most symptomatic, or are considered for some reason to be at high risk of complications of the disease. In our own study of 17 patients with recurrent syncope or cardiac arrest and 17 controls with severe symptoms but no history of cardiac arrest or syncope, no patient had abnormalities of sinus node function. There were no cases of prolongation of the AH interval > 120 ms, but prolongation of the HV interval > 55 ms was shown in 4 (23.5%). In 3 of those 4, however, the mechanism of syncope was not impaired function of the His–Purkinje system; in 1 case syncope was associated with sustained monomorphic tachycardia, and in 2 cases with paroxysmal atrial fibrillation. The mechanism in the fourth patient was not difinitely established.

Fananapazir et al. [70] reported abnormalities of sinus node function in a majority of patients undergoing electrophysiological study; a prolonged sinoatrial conduction time (> 120 ms) was seen in 61 of 93 (66%), but only 6 of 82 (7%) patients had prolonged sinus node recovery time (> 1500 ms). They also discovered abnormalities of atrioventricular node function in a small number. The AH interval was delayed (> 120 ms) in 9 of 146 patients (6%), and His–Purkinje conduction was abnormal (HV interval > 55 ms) in 44 of 148 patients (30%). The significance of these findings is uncertain; the prevalence of conduction tissue abnormalities was similar in asymptomatic patients and in those with cardiac arrest, syncope or pre-syncope.

Individual case reports, however, have documented complete heart block, asystole, myocardial infarction and rapid conduction of a supraventricular tachycardia over an accessory pathway as causes of syncope [12, 15, 16]. A physiological tachycardia or a tachyarrhythmia may result in ischaemia, diastolic dysfunction, hypotension and ultimately ventricular fibrillation. This sequence of events was well illustrated by a young patient who underwent electrophysiological study following resuscitation from out-of-hospital cardiac arrest. Sustained atrial fibrillation was induced, with a ventricular rate of 170–190 beats/min in the absence of an accessory pathway. This rhythm was not associated with palpitations, but hypotension and myocardial ischaemia developed leading to the onset of ventricular fibrillation. Ventricular tachycardia could not be induced [71].

In our electrophysiological study of 17 patients with syncope and 17 matched controls with severe symptoms but no syncope, there were no patients with accessory atrioventricular connections but there was accelerated atrioventricular conduction (atrioventricular Wenckebach cycle length <300 m) in 2 of the syncopal patients. In one of these patients, however, syncope was due to primary ventricular fibrillation, and in the other to exertional hypotension without rhythm disturbance. Two patients from the syncopal group had dual atrioventricular nodal pathways, and in both cases syncope was associated with paroxysmal atrial fibrillation. In those without syncope, however, there were 4 with enhanced atrioventricular nodal conduction and 2 with dual atrioventricular nodal pathways.

In Fananapazir et al.'s [70] study there was evidence of accessory pathways in 7 (5%) of 155 patients undergoing electrophysiological study, 3 of whom presented with palpitations—1 with syncope, 1 with presyncope, and another had a strong family history of sudden cardiac death. The invesigators found dual atrioventricular nodal pathways in only 3 patients (1.9%), but did not comment on the presence of accelerated atrioventricular nodal conduction.

Hypotension may also develop during exercise without very rapid heart rates or evidence of myocardia ischaemia. We observed this mechanism of collapse in a patient who was wearing an ambulatory electrocardiographic recorder during an episode of exercise-induced syncope [72]. After the patient complained of palpitations and breathlessness, her pulse gradually became impalpable, her outflow tract murmur disappeared, and she lost consciousness. Spontaneous recovery of consciousness occurred after 90s, and was accompanied by the gradual restoration of peripheral pulses and the systolic murmur. The cardiac rhythm during this episode was sinus, with a gradually increasing rate from 70 beats virgule/min at baseline ot a maximum of 130 beats/min at the time she lost consciousness. There was no ST segment change to suggest myocardial ischaemia before syncope occurred.

As a result of this observation we have prospectively assessed this effect of exercise on cardiac output and systemic blood pressure, and have seen exercise-induced hypotension in 43 out of 129 patients (33%) studied during treadmill exercise [73]. Hypotension was not due to a reduction in cardiac output on exertion, because cardiac output rose normally in all individuals with increasing levels of exercise. Associated with hypotension, however, was an abnormal fall in systemic vascular resistance, suggesting inappropriate vasodilatation in non-exercising vascular beds. In a subsequent study of forearm blood flow during supine bicycle exercise, abnormal vascular responses implying vasodilatation of the forearm (either no change in blood flow with exercise, or increased blood flow) were seen in 39 of 103 consecutive patients (38%) with hypertrophic cardiomyopathy [74]. The significance of these findings is uncertain, particularly as most of the patients who were hypotensive during exercise had no symptoms of impaired consciousness at that time.

The relationship between syncope and sudden death will be further explored in "Mechanism of Sudden Death" below.

Natural History

The natural history of hypertrophic cardiomyopathy in adults is of a slow progression of symptoms, but with an annual mortality from sudden cardiac death of 2%–3% [13, 15]. Treatment of the condition may require drugs or surgery (myotomy/myectomy or mitral valve replacement) for the control of symptoms, although neither has been shown to improve prognosis); cardiac transplantation for uncontrollable symptoms (which may improve prognosis); low-dose amiodarone, regardless of symptom status, in those shown to be at high risk of sudden death; or the use of the implantable cardioverter–defibrillator. Of these, only low-dose amiodarone has been shown to improve prognosis [75].

Treatment of the condition in childhood poses particular problems, and the natural history may be more aggressive when hypertrophic cardiomyopathy presents in the very young. In particular, when it appears for the first time in infancy hypertrophic cardiomyopathy seems to behave differently form the disease in other age groups. The diagnosis is frequently missed at presentation, which may be with stillbirth, sudden infant death ("cot death") or a systolic murmur. Heart failure is the usual presentation in infancy. The correct diagnosis is more likely to be made when the presenting features are heart failure and cyanosis.

Few centres have much experience of treating very young children with the disease. Maron et al. [76] have reviewed the multicentre experience in 20 infants under the age of 1 year. The 5-year mortality was 50%, with cardiac failure the commonest mode of death; 9 of the 11 infants (82%) who presented in heart failure died [76]. These data suggest that when hypertrophic cardiomyopathy is diagnosed in the first year of life the prognosis is very poor and outcome is probably determined by left ventricular function.

In older children the presentation is more likely to be with chest pain and exertional dyspnoea, as is the case with adults. The clinical hallmark of the disorder, unexplained left ventricular hypertrophy, may develop during a growth spurt in childhood or adolescence; if already established, it may progress during a growth spurt [77]. Progression of hypertrophy has been well documented in young persons also and may be rapid within a few years, or even months [78].

Unfortunately, the prognosis in children, while not as bad as in infants, is worse than in adults, and the annual mortality from sudden cardiac death is 4%–6% [17]. Sudden death, in both children and adults, frequently occurs in patients whose symptoms are mild or who are asymptomatic. The detection of those at highest risk of sudden death, and their treatment, will be addressed in "Mechanism of Sudden Death" and "Treatment of Sudden Death" below (see also Chap. 6).

Management

Where possible therapy should be chosen to treat specific symptoms. In attempting to identify the best therapy for any particular individual it is desirable to know how important different aspects of impaired left ventricular function are to that individual, and the impact of any treatmemt strategy on the disordered physiology. For example, is there an important abnormality of ventricular emptying (outflow tract obstruction), and if so which drug would be most effective at reducing the gradient? Are ventricular relaxation (fall in pressure during isovolumic relaxation) or ventricular filling (diastolic compliance) the dominant abnormalities? Is there evidence of myocardia ischaemia? Are there important rhythm disturbances? There is no evidence that any of the currently available treatment regimens may cause regression of hypertrophy or alteration of the myocyte disarray, therefore all symptomatic treatments are palliative rather than curative.

Beta-Blocking Drugs

The greatest experience in the pharmacological treatment of hypertrophic cardiomyopathy has been with beta-adrenergic blockers, particularly with propranolol. In support of the use of beta-blocking drugs, an increased functional response of the left ventricle in hypertrophic cardiomyopathy to low-dose infusion of adrenaline has been observed [79]. The reason for the heightened sensitivity to adrenaline is not obvious; blood levels of noradrenaline are higher in hypertrophic cardiomyopathy than in controls but examination of tissue obtained at biopsy from hearts with and without hypertrophic cardiomyopathy has shown no difference in terms of beta receptor numbers, the proportion of $beta_1$ and $beta_2$ receptors, or in adenylate cyclase activity in response to stimulation [79, 80]. But calcium receptors have been claimed to be increased [81].

Soon after the first clinical description of hypertrophic cardiomyopathy, at the time when attention was focused on the hyperdynamic systolic function and the left ventricular outflow tract gradient, it was realised that the outflow tract gradient was a labile phenomenon which could be manipulated by physical and pharmacological intervention [82, 83]. Obstruction to left ventricular emptying is increased by manoeuvres which increase myocardial contractility, by a reduction in impedance to left ventricular ejection (aferload reduction), or by a reduction in left ventricular size at the onset of systole (decreased left ventricular filling). Beta-blockade has the potential to reduce the resistance or obstruction to left ventricular emptying on all these mechanisms. The negative inotropism of beta-adrenoceptor antagonists reduces the force and velocity of myocardial contraction, thereby reducing hyperdynamic systolic function. Blockade of the dilator $beta_2$-adrenoceptors in the peripheral vasculature reduces the control over the vasoconstrictor influence of the alpha-adrenoceptors, tipping the balance of sympathomimetic activity towards peripheral arteriolar constriction and increased left ventricular afterload. There is also a small venoconstricting effect of beta-blockers which increases left ventricular filling.

Thus, beta-adrenoceptor blockers have, at least on theoretical grounds, a beneficial effect on left ventricular emptying by a tripartite mechanism. Given the importance of the effects of such drugs on the peripheral vasculature as well as direct cardiac effects, it is probably better to use drugs which are not cardioselective. Indeed, for historical reasons, the greatest amount of experience has been gained with the earliest available beta-blocker, propranolol, which is non-selective. There is, in addition, some evidence gained in short-term experiments in the cardiac catheter laboratory that propranolol is more effective at reducing the outflow tract gradient than newer, cardioselective agents [83–85]. Propranolol also shows the heart rate at rest and blunts the rate response to exercise, thereby reducing myocardial oxygen demand (lower rate/pressure product for a given level of exercise), and can attenuate the rise in outflow tract obstruction which may accompany exercise [86].

Diastolic left ventricular function in patients with hypertrophic cardiomyopathy has been compared with that in controls (individuals with chest pain and normal coronary and left ventricular arteriography) using high fidelity catheter-tip micromanometer pressure studies [87]. The time constant of $\mathrm{d}P/\mathrm{d}T$ during the isovolumic relaxation phase of diastole was longer implying slower relaxation, and minimum $\mathrm{d}P/\mathrm{d}T$ was lower in the patients with hypertrophic cardiomyopathy. During pacing studies there were no differences in indices of relaxation between those patients with hypertrophic cardiomyopathy who became ischaemic (coronary sinus lactate production) and those who did not. In patients studied after propranolol administration there was a reduction in left ventricular end-diastolic pressure and in indices of contractility, but not in the time constant of relaxation. There was less evidence of ischaemia during pacing to the same heart after propranolol administration, but no improvement in ventricular relaxation.

If beta-blockade does not affect active myocardial relaxation, it may still improve diastolic function in other ways, particularly by its effect on passive left ventricular filling. By slowing the heart rate propranolol prolongs diastole, increasing the time available for ventricular filling. Ventricular filling, however, is a complex phenomenon, and the effect of beta-blockade seems to be due to more than just its effects on heart rate and venoconstriction. Early catheter studies of ventricular filling in hypertrophic cardiomyopathy showed that in the majority of symptomatic patients the left ventricular end-diastolic pressure was elevated at rest, and that it rose further with exercise and isoprenaline infusion. Pacing to the same heart rate, however, showed little increase in end-diastolic pressure, and sometimes a reduction [88–90]. Acute administration of a beta-blocker showed a fall in end-diastolic pressure and an increase in end-diastolic volume which was not related to change in heart rate alone but suggested a beneficial direct effect on left ventricular compliance [89, 90]. More detailed follow-up studies looking at pressure–volume relationships throughout diastole have produced conflicting data. In one study the pressure–volume loop was consistently shifted down and to the right, suggesting an increase in distensibility or compliance of the left ventricle [85]. In another, however, a minority of the patients studied showed this pattern but in majority beta-blockade had no effect on compliance [91]. A more recent study [92] has shown improvement in diastolic function with beta-adrenergic blockade. Left ventricular filling has also been assessed non-invasively by echocardiography and Doppler echocardiography. A number of indices derived from the echocardiogram have been assessed in hypertrophic cardiomyopathy with and without beta-blockade; peak rate of change of left ventricular dimension during early rapid filling, peak early and late diastolic transmitral flow velocity, the ratio of late to early peak velocity, and the deceleration of early diastolic flow. In patients with hypertrophic cardiomyopathy and no mitral regurgitation these indices are usually abnormal, but they tend to normalise in the presence of mitral regurgitation [93–95]. Since the presence and degree of mitral regurgitation may vary from day to day, and is influenced by drug therapy, sequential studies of diastolic function which rely on these indices must be viewed cautiously.

The effect of beta-blockade on left ventricular filling in hypertrophic cardiomyopathy may be summarised by saying that there appears to be improved left ventricular compliance in some individuals. How the effect in those individuals is mediated is not known, since an acute change in the viscoelastic properties of abnormal myocardium seems unlikely; nor is it known why beta- blockers do not have the same effect in all patients.

The previously discussed effects of beta-blockers on left ventricular emptying, on the heart rate at rest and in response to exercise or emotional stress, and on diastolic function are all likely to reduce the myocardial oxygen demand. Furthermore, the prolongation of diastole and the lowering of the left ventricular end-diastolic pressure should improve myocardial perfusion, and hence act beneficially on the supply side of the myocardial oxygen supply-and-demand relationship. Thus, the use of beta-blocking agents should be beneficial in the treatment of ischaemic cardiac pain in hypertrophic cardiomyopathy. Propranolol has been shown, in short-term haemodynamic and metabolic studies, to reverse the abnormalities induced by isoprenaline infusion and to increase coronary sinus flow [60]. In clinical practice, beta-blockers are effective in controlling chest pain in hypertrophic cardiomyopathy in the majority of patients. It is unlikely that beta-blocking drugs can reduce myocardial hypertrophy in hypertrophic cardiomyopathy, but a recent study suggests that regression of hypertrophy may occur with high doses of propranolol (7–18 mg/kg) [96]. Regression of hypertrophy with fibrous replacement of myocardium, which is probably spontaneous, may occur. This gives a reduction in electrocardiographic measurement of wall thicknesss. Fibrous replacement of the myocardium is associated with a deterioration in left ventricular performance and mild increase in cavity dimensions.

There are no good controlled data on the effect of propranolol on mortality, although one non-randomised trial using very high doses of the drug showed good symptomatic control and no mortality over a 5-year period [97]. Our own experience suggests that while propranolol is a useful drug for the control of symptoms, it does not prevent sudden death. During a mean follow-up of 6 years, 18 out of 164 patients (11%) taking a mean dose of 280 mg propranolol daily died suddenly [13]. Nevertheless propranolol is usually well tolerated, its safety record is good, and in Britain and the United States it is the first-line drug for the treatment of symptoms.

Calcium Channel Blockers

The other main class of drugs used to treat the symptoms of hypertrophic cardiomyopathy is the calcium channel blockers, particulary verapamil [99]. Recent work has shown an increase in calcium antagonist receptors in the ventricular and atrial myocardium of 33% of patients with hypertrophic cardiomyopathy [81]. Animal work has shown that when pregnant rats were subjected to increased calcium their offspring developed myofibrillar disarray which could be prevented by verapamil [98]. Overall the experience of these drugs is less than with propranolol, but in many European centres, particularly in Germany, verapamil is used as the drug of first choice in symptomatic patients. The effects of verapamil on left ventricular systolic function are similar to those of propranolol, although the mode of action is different. In addition, however, there is some evidence that it can exert a beneficial effect on disordered ventricular relaxation (which is dependent upon calcium uptake into the sarcoplasmic reticulum). When given acutely by intravenous bolus, verapamil slows conduction through the atrioventricular node (which is calcium dependent), and slows impulse formation in the sinus node, thus tending to slow heart rate. Its effect on the peripheral vasculature may override this effect; by its vasodilator action in the peripheral circulation verapamil causes a fall in systolic blood pressure which, through baroreceptor reflexes, may cause an increased heart rate [100, 101]: Like propranolol, verapamil is negatively inotropic causing a reduction in the force and velocity of myocardial contraction, the effect of which is to reduce any pressure gradient in the left ventricular outflow tract [100, 101]. There is also evidence of a direct effect on delayed and incoordinate left ventricular relaxation and early diastolic filling [102–105].

The exact mechanism by which verapamil improves ventricular relaxation is not clear, but it is thought to be related to a reduction in myocyte cytosolic calcium concentration, which serves to increase the speed of relaxation. Some evidence has been presented, however, from experiments assessing left ventricular cycle efficiency (a measure of synchronicity of contraction and relaxation) which suggests that the speed of relaxation is increased by an improvement in regional asynchrony, rather than by changes in cytosolic calcium concentration [105]. Other workers have shown improvement in asynchronous left ventricular wall motion, assessed by radionuclide ventriculography, following the intravenous administration of verapamil [106].

What do not appear to change with verapamil administration are the passive elastic properties of the left ventricular myocardium [107]. These, of course, are a function of the cellular architecture of the myocardium, and will be influenced both by myocyte disarray and by the excessive amounts of connective tissue present; it is unlikely that the abnormal myocardium could suddenly change its viscoelastic properties.

In long-term use, verapamil is associated with an improvement in functional class in most patients with symptomatic hypertrophic cardiomyopathy [108]. This is associated with a reduction in the magnitude of the left ventricular outflow tract gradient, where one is present, and improved left ventricular emptying. Indeed verapami in high doses has been shown to produce a significantly greater reduction in the outflow tract gradient than does propranolol [12, 100, 101, 103].

There is also a profound effect on diastolic left venticular function, and the filling characteristics of the left ventricle. During chronic verapamil usage the left ventricular end-diastolic volume, measured angiographically, has been shown to increase, with little or no change in the left ventricular end-diastolic pressure—an observation which suggests improved distensibility [109]. The exact mechanism of this action is uncertain; it probably cannot be explained solely on the basis of altered loading, although in the case of verapamil the issue of altered ventricular loading versus improved myocardial inactivation has not been addressed directly. The negative inotropism of verapamil may also play a role, and it has been suggested that an improvement in the oxygen supply-and-demand relationship of the hypertrophied myocardium may reduce the stunning effect of recurrent subendocardial ischaemia [99, 110]. Correction of abnormal myocardial cytosolic calcium transients, with a beneficial effect on diastolic relaxation and filling, is another attractive hypothesis. All of these hypotheses remain unproven, but there is a correlation between ventricular asynchrony, filling rate, functional class and symptom status [111], and verapamil can improve asynchrony, increase the early diastolic filling rate and compliance, and improve symptoms.

There is debate about whether or not long-term verapamil therapy can induce regression of hypertrophy in hypertrophic cardiomyopathy. Some workers have claimed a reduction in angiographic left ventricular mass [109], but this has not been confirmed using other techniques, particularly echocardiography [108]. The influence of verapamil on prognosis is also debatable. Those studies which claim to have shown improved survival in patients treated with verapamil compared with those who received either no treatment or treatment with beta-blockade (propranolol) have, on the whole, included very small numbers of patients [101, 105]. It is probably safer to conclude that verapamil is an effective drug for the relief of symptoms in hypertrophic cardiomyopathy but that it does not have a significant effect on survival. Indeed, its use can be associated with serious complications [112]. It can suppress impulse formation in the sinus node and adversely affect conduction through the atrioventricular node, as noted above. It has been associated with the development of complete heart block in patients with pre-existing, but unsuspected, conduction disease. The combination of conduction disturbance, negative inotropism and vasodilator properties has caused pulmonary oedema and death in some patients [112]. Verapamil must not be given with a beta-blocking agent.

Other newer calcium channel blockers which have slightly different spectra of activity to verapamil (more intense vasodilatation, less effect upon conducting tissue) have been used less often. In particular, the use of nifedipine has been disappointing. The results of initial experiments with the acute administration of sublingual nifedipine suggested that the drug had haemodynamic effects which were likely to be beneficial in hypertrophic cardiomyopathy. Delayed left ventricular relaxation is improved and early diastolic filling enhanced with, in addition, downward displacement of the pressure–volume loop suggesting improved left ventricular compliance [113–115]. However nifedipine also causes intense peripheral vasodilatation, with a decrease in systolic blood pressure, a reflex increase in heart rate and a decreased cavity size—effects which may be deleterious [113–115]. Indeed in some patients there has been a substantial increase in the magnitude of the outflow tract gradient, particularly if the initial resting gradient was high [116]. Acute nifedipine administration may cause a reduction in the outflow tract gradient, but the potential of this drug to adversely affect hyperdynamic systolic function and left ventricular emptying must be recognised. On the other hand, its effect on diastole, the mechanism of which remains uncertain, should improve left ventricular function. It may be due solely to the intense vasodilatation observed (and thereby a reduction in left ventricular afterload), particularly in those in whom baseline blood pressure and systemic vascular resistance are high, or to a direct effect on myocyte inactivation. Paulus et al. [114] studied the effect of acute administration of nifedipine and sodium nitroprusside (a powerful arterial vasodilator with no direct cardiac action) on haemodynamic indices and diastolic function in 10 patients with hypertrophic cardiomyopathy. There was much greater improvement in left ventricular relaxation and filling indices with nifedipine than with nitroprusside, and the pressure–volume loop was moved down and to the right by nifedipine but not nitroprusside. These findings suggest that only the calcium blocker had a beneficial effect on left ventricular distensibility, and that the overall effect on diastolic function cannot be due solely to changes in ventricular loading.

In this study, and in one other, the time constant of ventricular relaxation appeared to decrease, and the rate of early diastolic lengthening appeared to increase after sublingual nifedipine administration [113, 114]. It was suggested that the beneficial effect of nifedipine on relaxation and diastolic filling, like that of verapamil, was due either to a direct myocardial effect, by altering calcium content or transport in the hypertrophied myocardium, or to a reduction in the level of subendocardial ischaemia. Unlike similar experiments with verapamil, however, regional left ventricular wall motion was not assessed, so it is not clear whether an improvement in regional asynchrony after nifedipine administration may have been responsible for the improved diastolic function.

Initial enthusiasm for the use of nifedipine, based on these results, has not been borne out by clinical practice. In a direct double-blind, placebo-controlled comparision with verapamil, nifedipine was effective in controlling symptoms in only 22% of patients,whereas verapamil improved symptoms in 48%. Exercise tolerance improved in 36% of patients treated with verapamil, and only 18% of those treated with nifedipine [116]. Overall, any increase in left ventricular compliance and improvement in diastolic function have been overshadowed by the complications of the intense peripheral vasodilatation. After an early report of the possible benificial effect obtained by using a combination of nifedipine and propranolol, this regimen was evaluated in 15 patients whose response to verapamil had been suboptimal. Over a mean follow-up period of 18 months, symptomatic improvement was seen in only 2 patients. In 5 others there was no change in symptomps, and in 8 patients there was a frank deterioration in symptom status [117]. This combination cannot be recommended.

Less is known about diltiazem. Acute intravenous or oral administration is associated with haemodynamic changes similar to those seen with verapamil and nifedipine: peripheral vasodilatation with a fall in systolic blood pressure and a reflex increase in heart rate, and an improvement in delayed relaxation and early diastolic filling [115, 118, 119]. The effect on heart rate is offset to some extent by the direct inhibitory effect of diltiazem on the sinus node, although this is less powerful than that seen with verapamil.

In the short term, the effect of diltiazem on symptom status and haemodynamic variables in hypertrophic cardiomyopathy appears to be comparable to that of verapamil. In a double-blind cross-over comparison between the two, performed in Japan, there was symptomatic improvement in 83% of patients receiving diltiazem and 71% of patients treated with verapamil [118]. In the one study of long-term usage of diltiazem for which results are known, initial improvement in symptom status was seen in 8 out of 10 patients and was maintained in 7, during mean follow-up of 3.2 years [120]. Exercise duration improved by 32% during short-term use of diltiazem, and by 16% when treatment was maintained in the long term. No change has been reported in left ventricular wall thickness during long-term diltiazem administration.

Adverse effects are seen more commonly with calcium channel blockers than with propranolol, although discontinuation of the drug has been required infrequently. As alluded to in the discussion of nifedipine, the vasodilatory action of the calcium channel blockers, particularly nifedipine and diltiazem, has the potential to increase considerably any outflow tract gradient, and increase obstruction to left ventricular ejection. A 7% incidence of pulmonary oedema, and some deaths, with verapamil use have been reported by one group [112].

The exact cause is not clear, but is probably a combination of the effect of reduced afterload with increased outflow tract obstruction, and negative inotropism.

The potential of verapamil, in particular, to cause conduction disturbances has been alluded to, and it may unmask pre-existing, but unsuspected conduction tissue disease. The combination of a beta-blocker and verapamil is particularly dangerous, with a high risk of producing complete atrioventricular block. In 120 patients treated with oral verapamil, profound sinus bradycardia with junctional escape rhythm was seen in 11%, second-degree atrioventricular block occurred in 4%, and there was sinus arrest in 2% [112]. The risk of acute symptomatic deterioration in patients who have a profound bradycardia,increased obstruction to left ventricular ejection and depressed myocardial contractility is obviously high.

Other Drugs

Sototol, which has action similar to amiodarone and beta-blockade, has been used as a substitute for amiodarone.

Cardiac Pacing

A report from Dublin [121] suggested that dual chamber pacing could increase effort tolerance and decrease symptoms in severe hypertrophic cardiomyopathy. The reason for improvement is not fully explained. In some patients outflow tract gradients diminished while another study from the same group [122] showed a shorter time to peak ventricular filling rate during dual chamber pacing, suggesting an improvement in diastolic ventricular function. Further work is clearly necessary before dual chamber pacing can be unreservedly recommended.

Cardiac Surgery

The use of cardiac surgery for the relief of symptoms and improvement of prognosis in hypertrophic cardiomyopathy is contentious. Cardiac surgery for this condition developed in the era when it was believed that the primary abnormality in hypertrophic cardiomyopathy was hyperdynamic systolic function, and that intraventricular pressure gradients, particularly of the outflow tract, were responsible for symptoms. Experience of surgical treatment is limited in most centres, although over 1000 cases have been reported world-wide. The first operations were designed to "relieve" hypertrophy of the subaortic portion of the muscular septum. Beginning with the simple transaortic approach of Cleland and Morrow [123–125], the technique employed has become more complex and extensive, and usually consists of myotomy/myectomy of the interventricular septum (removal of a segment of the upper anterior septum), with or without replacement of the mitral valve via a transaortic, transventricular or left transatrial approach. Early surgical results suggested that myotomy/myectomy alone could improve the degree of mitral regurgitation [126], but later surgeons have advocated mitral valve replacement as well, and in some cases mitral valve replacement without myectomy [127]. Good results for mitral valve replacement have been obtained in the relatively small number of patients whose condition is complicated by severe mitral regurgitation. A low-profile valve is required.

The majority of patients submitted to surgery have not responded to medical therapy, or have had deteriorating symptoms and impaired exercise tolerance after showing a good initial response to either beta-blockade or to calcium channel blockers. Because of the significant morbidity and mortality of surgery, most centres require that patients are at least in New York Heart Association (NYHA) functional class III, despite medical therapy, before surgery will be considered. Usually the patients will have a significant resting or provokable left ventricular outflow tract pressure gradient as well.

The stated aims of one centre with considerable experience of surgical treatment of hypertrophic cardiomyopathy, in Dusseldorf, Germany are: geometric correction of left ventricular cavity angulation by subvalvar septal myectomy (performed by the transaortic approach), leading to enlargement of the outflow tract, and abolition or significant reduction of the resting or provokable outflow tract gradient [128]. This is claimed to improve diastolic function also, and to reduce the degree of mitral regurgitation.

To ensure optimal results, these workers perform a detailed haemodynamic assessment when the patient is on the operating table with the chest open, but before cardiopulmonary bypass has been instituted. Right atrial and right ventricular pressures are measured simultaneously to exclude tricuspid regurgitation and any degree of right ventricular outflow tract stenosis. Simultaneous left atrial and left ventricular pressures are recorded at rest and after volume loading and pacing (or inotropic) stress to assess the severity of mitral regurgitation, and the left ventricular to aortic pressure gradient is measured at rest and after provocation to determine the severity of the left ventricular outflow tract gradient. A deep intraventricular myectomy is then performed, any fibrous connections of the papillary muscle apparatus to the ventricular wall are excised, the aortic root and left ventricle are vented to remove any air bubbles, and the aortotomy is closed. The meticulous haemodynamic assessment is repeated before the chest is closed after discontinuation of bypass.

Between 1963 and 1988, 248 patients with hypertrophic cardiomyopathy complicated by refractory symptoms and outflow tract "obstruction", and 6 patients with relatively little functional impairment but a malignant family history of sudden death and/or recurrent syncope and cardiac arrest, underwent such surgery. In the 1960s, early postoperative mortality was 25%; this had fallen to 2.7% by the 1980s. The improved mortality rates are related to better patient selection (no patients in NYHA functional class IV in the 1980s) and improved surgical technique. The commonest mode of death in the early postoperative period was intractable cardiac failure; surgical mortality was increased by additional procedures, particularly mitral valve replacement (27.8% early mortality).

The reduction in left ventricular outflow tract gradient and pulmonary artery pressure was impressive, and most of those who survived the operation had an improvement in symptom status of at least one functional class, which seemed to be maintained during follow-up for a mean of 4.5 years. Their uncontrolled results also seem to demonstrate an improvement in survival over patients treated medically, with a disease-related mortality of 1.1% per annum, although patients dying from myocardial infarction were excluded from analysis.

These results, and others like them, show that there is no doubt that myotomy/myectomy can significantly improve symptoms in some patients who are difficult to manage medically, but that abolition of the outflow tract gradient is not necesarily the explanation of its success. An influence on myocardial innervation, vascular reflexes, the effect of pericardiotomy and the negatively inotropic effect of cardiopulmonary bypass may all profoundly influence symptoms. These results also demonstrate that the early surgical mortality is still higher than for other types of cardiac surgery. Notwithstanding the most recent results of the Dusseldorf group, the overall perioperative mortality of myotomy/myectomy is 5%–10% [129]. A recent report of the use of intraoperative echocardiography to direct surgery suggests that the perioperative mortality can be reduced by this technique [130]. The transventricular approach carries a particularly high risk of late death due to cardiac failure.

Cardiac transplantation has been advocated in hypertrophic cardiomyopathy both for the treatment of intractable symptoms and in situations where the risk to the individual of sudden cardiac death is very high. Provided that severe and irreversible changes in the pulmonary vascular bed secondary to left ventricular dysfunction have not occurred, transplantation may be a very useful treatment option.

Arrhythmias and Antiarrhythmic Drug Therapy

Supraventricular Arrhythmias

Approximately 5% of patients have established atrial fibrillation at the time of diagnosis, and an additional 10% will develop this arrhythmia during the subsequent 5 years [67, 68, 131]. A poor prognosis after the development of atrial fibrillation has often been assumed, supported by invasive haemodynamic studies during atrial fibrillation and after the restoration of sinus rhythm, and by isolated case reports indicating that its acute onset was poorly tolerated and potentially fatal [71, 132]. Existing natural history studies, however, have provided little support for this pessimistic view, and we have recently published a retrospective review of outcome in patients with hypertrophic cardiomyopathy and atrial fibrillation [133] in which the outcome in 52 patients with atrial fibrillation was compared with that in a matched group of patients who remained in sinus rhythm.

Symptomatic deterioration (usually new or worse chest pain and dyspnoea, associated with the acute onset of atrial fibrillation) was seen in patients with impaired left ventricular function, but the majority of such patients were restored to their previous functional class by treatment, even if they remained in atrial fibrillation. Thus, after the development of acute atrial fibrillation, symptoms are common and are related not only to the ventricular response but also to impairment of left ventricular systolic and diastolic function. Furthermore, the development of atrial fibrillation did not adversely affect prognosis in this study [133].

Short episodes of paroxysmal atrial fibrillation, or other supraventricular tachycardia, do not warrant treatment, as the patients are usually unaware of them and their prognostic significance is uncertain. Sustained paroxysms (30 or longer) of atrial fibrillation may cause a rapid ventricular response and are associated with an important risk of embolisation as well as haemodynamic collapse [71, 132, 133]. Such patients should be fully anticoagulated.

In the majority atrial fibrillation has little effect on functional status provided that the ventricular rate is controlled, as discussed above. This is probably because in most patients who develop chronic atrial fibrillation there has been a gradual reduction in the contribution made by atrial systole to stroke volume, as ventricular compliance has diminished and atrial distension has increased with time. In such patients atrial systole results in a pressure wave without much forward flow, producing a palpable atrial impulse in the absence of a fourth heart sound. Thus, by the time atrial fibrillation develops, atrial transport has ceased to be of much haemodynamic importance.

Class I agents, in particular disopyramide and propafenone, have been used with success to control the heart rate in atrial fibrillation, and to produce "chemical cardioversion" back to sinus rhythm. Their role in maintaining sinus rhythm has not been systematically assessed. Amiodarone has proved itself a useful drug in the context of sustained paroxysms of atrial fibrilation. It is effective in preventing the episodes and, if breakthrough does occur, it will attenuate the ventricular rate response. It has now been shown that the use of amiodarone to treat paroxysmal atrial fibrillation can retard the development of sustained atrial fibrillation [133].

Amiodarone was introduced into clinical cardiology as an anti-anginal agent, but it has a wide spectrum of antiarrhythmic effects and is a non-competitive sympathetic antagonist [134]. Its use in high doses is associated with a significant incidence of side effects ranging from the relatively trivial (corneal deposits) through the troublesome (sleep disturbance and photosensitisation) to the life threatening (pulmonary fibrosis). These adverse effects are generally seen with plasma amiodarone concentrations in excess of 2 mg/l [135]. Fortunately there is now evidence that the suppression of supraventricular arrhythmias in hypertrophic cardiomyopathy can be obtained with plasma concentrations of 0.5–1.5 mg/l [136]. Significant adverse effects are seldom seen at these levels. Impairment of thyroid function (hyper and hypo), abnormality of liver function tests and peripheral neuropathy also occur. Thyroid and liver disturbance is usually only biochemical with low-dose treatment. Photosensitisation leads to flushing and, if protection is inadequate, irreversible pigmentation can occur. The role of this drug in the prevention of sudden cardiac death in hypertophic cardiomyopathy, and the potential mechanisms of its action, will be discussed later.

Usually atrial fibrillation develops because of atrial distension, a consequence of raised filling pressure in a stiff, hypertrophied left ventricle. In a minority, atrial fibrillation may develop in the absence of atrial distension and with normal filling pressures, because of involvement of atrial tissue in the disease process. Such patients may depend on atrial transport for a considerable fraction of their stroke volume, and the restoration and maintenance of sinus rhythm in such individuals is very important. In them every effort should be made to restore sinus rhythm by cardioversion, under anticoagulant cover, supported by treatment with amiodarone.

If sinus rhythm cannot be restored, either chemically or by DC conversion, or if it cannot be maintained, digoxin is an appropriate agent for the control of the ventricular rate, as it is in atrial fibrillation of other causes. One should perhaps be cautious in its use in patients with hyperdynamic systolic left ventricular function and a significant outflow tract gradient, because it may possibly worsen obstruction to left ventricular emptying. Most patients in atrial fibrillation, however, have impaired systolic function and do not suffer any deleterious haemodynamic consequences as a result of digoxin use. Digoxin should not be given to patients with pre-excitation because if atrial fibrillation occurs impulses may be shunted down the accessory pathway and cause ventricular fibrillation. The effect of digoxin is potentiated by amiodarone.

Ventricular Arrhythmias

Clinical sustained monomorphic ventricular tachycardia is rare in hypertrophic cardiomyopathy, with only a handful of cases reported in the literature [137, 138]. In a study published recently, 51 patients out of more than 200 had ventricular tachycardia detected by ambulatory monitoring, but sustained ventricular tachycardia (>30 beats at ≥ 120 beats/min) associated with symptomatic deterioration was seen in only 2 [138]. In both patients the relatively rare finding of a left ventricular aneurysm in the presence of normal epicardial coronary arteries was demonstrated by angiography. Electrophysiological testing was undertaken in both: in 1 the tachycardia was non-inducible; in the other it could be induced and was mapped to the edge of the aneurysm. Treatment with class I agents and verapamil was unsuccessful in both patients, but the tachycardias were suppressed by amiodarone and both patients remain well after more than 5 years of follow-up.

Inducible monomorphic ventricular tachycardia is also uncommon. In a series of 7 consecutive patients investigated because of syncope, sustained monomorphic ventricular tachycardia was induced at the electrophysiological study in 3, but spontaneous ventricular tachycardia was not documented. Two patients were treated with class I agents and the third received amiodarone, with apparent relief of symptoms in all 3, but the follow-up period was short (median 7 months) [139]. In our own experience, 2 of 17 patients (12%) investigated because of syncope had sustained monomorphic ventricular tachycardia on electrophysiological testing minomorphic venricular tachycardia had previously been documented as the cause of syncope in one. In 17 controls without syncope there were no cases of spontaneous sustained monomorphic ventricular tachycardia, and none could be induced on electrophysiological testing, although non-sustained polymorphic ventricular tachycardia was induced in 4 patients and ventricular fibrillation was induced in 1.

Non-sustained ventricular tachycardia, on the other hand, is common in hypertrophic cardiomyopathy, and can be detected in about 25% of adult patients [67, 68]. This arrhythmia may appear benign; it is invariably asymptomatic, and the rate is usually slow (the mean heart rate in more than 400 episodes in 52 patients was 142 beats/min). Non-sustained ventricular tachycardia frequently follows a period of relative bradycardia, and is not associated with ST segment changes or alteration in the QT interval. Analysis of different episodes in the same patients has shown considerable variation in the QRS morphology, suggesting multiple sites of origin [69], which is in keeping with a disease process which is diffuse and generalised.

The importance of non-sustained ventricular tachycardia is that it has been clearly demonstrated, in work from two independent centres, to be the single best predictor of risk of sudden death in adult patients [67, 140]. Treatment of these patients with low-dose amiodarone significantly improves survival in the short term [75], and the indications are that this benefit is sustained during long-term therapy. This will be amplified in "Prevention of Sudden Death" below.

The Role of Electrophysiological Studies

The role of electrophysiological studies in the assessment of symptoms and the evaluation of prognosis in hypertrophic cardiomyopathy has not yet been established. Electrophysiological studies have been undertaken in an attempt to understand the mechanisms of syncope in an individual, and to try to detect those at high risk of sudden death.

Fananapazir's group [70] included programmed ventricular stimulation (PVS) in their electrophysiological evaluation of 155 patients, referred to earlier. PVS produced non-sustained ventricular tachycardia (3–30 beats at a rate of ≥120 beats/min) in 14% and sustained ventricular tachycardia (defined as a tachycardia >30 beats, or a tachycardia that required termination because of haemodynamic instability) in 43%. The significance of these findings is uncertain because the stimulation protocol was very aggressive (up to three premature stimuli in two right ventricular sites and one left ventricular site, with three different paced ventricular drive-cycle lengths of 600, 500 and 400 ms), and sustained monomorphic ventricular tachycardia was seen in only 16 of the 155 patients (10%). In the other 50 patients (32% of the total or 76% of those inducible) the response (polymorphic ventricular tachycardia in 48 and ventricular fibrillation in 2) would be considered non-specific and uninterpretable in patients with other cardiac dieseases such as coronary artery disease. In the group studied there was an association between inducibility of sustained ventricular arrhythmia and clinical presentation; it was more common in those with cardiac arrest, syncope or pre-syncope than in those who were asymptomatic. Fractionated pacing of the right ventricle using two sequences and a high-pass filtered electrogram has suggested that electrophysiological quantification of myofibrillar disarray may help to predict the risk of ventricular arrhythmia [141].

The combined European experience is in general agreement with the incidence of induced ventricular arrhythmias in relation to the aggressiveness of the stimulation protocol. What is different is that the patients with inducible polymorphic ventricular tachycardia have not experienced the adverse outcome which the National Institutes of Health study would have predicted for them [142, 143]. In those rare cases with clinical sustained ventricular tachycardia, the approach to therapy should be the same as the approach to the treatment of ventricular tachycardia in other conditions. Although such patients may be difficult to resuscitate from arrhythmias which cause haemodynamic embarrassment, treatment should be guided by electrophysiological study, with a "stepped" approach to therapy. If drug therapy fails, electro-physiologically-guided surgical resection of the focus or aneurysm would be appropriate. In the event of failure of surgery, the patient could be fitted with an automatic implantable cardioverter–defibrillator.

Treatment Options

In the treatment of congestive symptoms due to a stiff, non-compliant ventricle, the aim of treatment is to reduce pulmonary and systemic venous pressure, but the left ventricular diastolic pressure–volume curve in hypertrophic cardiomyopathy is steep, and a small change in volume can produce a large change in pressure. It is important, therefore, to avoid excesive preload reduction as this may lead to systemic hypotension; special care is needed if there is an important left ventricular outflow tract gradient with obstruction to ventricular emptying. On the whole, diuretics are best avoided in hypertrophic cardiomyopathy unless there is frank pulmonary oedema or congestive heart failure. If preload reduction is deemed necessary, then nitrates are probably the best agents and have the added advantage of their anti-ischaemic effect.

When dyspnoea is the dominant symptom in patients who show slow filling throughout diastole, prolongation of the filling time by slowing the heart rate, with either propranolol or verapamil, is appropriate. Conversely those who show a "restrictive" pattern of diastolic dysfunction, with rapid early filling, probably benefit from a relative tachycardia. In such patients negatively chronotropic agents should be avoided, and a beta-blocker with intrinsic sympathomimetic activity (ISA) should be considered. Where there is dyspnoea in association with definite outflow tract obstruction (50% or more of the left ventricular stroke volume within the ventricular cavity at the onset of the gradient), very high dose verapamil may be effective in reducing both the degree of obstruction and the symptoms. If this fails, myotomy/myectomy may produce an improvement in haemodynamic indices and improvement in symptom status and functional class.

Although systolic anterior movement of the mitral valve and the resulting outflow tract gradient are usually associated with some degree of mitral regurgitation, this is rarely severe in volume terms. Rarely, the degree of mitral regurgitation may be sufficiently severe to cause dyspnoea in its own right. Mitral valve replacement is obviously appropriate in such patients, but meticulous angiographic and Doppler echocardiographic assessment of mitral regurgitation are necessary before proceeding to surgery. An elevated pulmonary capillary wedge pressure with a prominent "v" wave may be seen in the absence of severe regurgitation if the atria are themselves diseased and non-compliant. Mitral valve replacement is frequently difficult, however, because of the small left ventricular cavity.

Chest pain in the presence of normal epicardial coronary arteries probably still represents ischaemia in the majority of patients, and usually responds to treatment with verapamil or propranolol. When choosing between them, propranolol is the safer drug, but patients with severe or refractory symptoms may not respond to propranolol. Though verapamil may be effective in this group, it is precisely these patients who are most at risk from its adverse effects (inhibition of impulse formation in the sinus node, delayed atrioventricular nodal conduction, reduction of the force and velocity of myocardial contraction, and peripheral vasodilatation). In such cases therapy with verapamil should be initiated slowly, and in hospital. The same comments probably apply to diltiazem.

If chest pain is related to definite outflow tract gradient, and is refractory to medical therapy, myectomy may be useful. Coronary arteriography should be performed in patients over the age of 40 who complain of chest pain. Atherosclerotic coronary artery disease can coexist with hypertrophic cardiomyopathy, and the results of coronary artery bypass surgery combined with myectomy are good [144]. In the last resort, cardiac transplantation should be considered for intractable symptoms (see Chaps. 6 and 8).

Symptomatic tachycardias should be treated in the same way as in other forms of cardiac disease. Troublesome ventricular or supraventricular ectopic activity may respond to simple therapy, such as low-dose propranolol. Paroxysmal or sustained atrial fibrillation carries a substantial risk of systemic thromboembolism, and patients with such rhythm disturbances should be anticoagulated. Probably the best drug for converting atrial fibrillation to sinus rhythm, and maintaining sinus rhythm, is amiodarone. Symptomatic ventricular tachycardia is very rare; when present it should be treated conventionally in a "stepped care" fashion, ideally with therapy guided by electrophysiological investigation.

Although not strictly symptomatic treatment, patients with hypertrophic cardiomyopathy are at high risk of infective endocarditis, particularly if there is systolic anterior movement of the mitral valve and mitral regurgitation. Vegetations usually form on the anterior mitral leaflet, which is frequently thickened and abnormal, at the point where it strikes the interventricular septum, or on the septum itself. There is usually a fibrotic plaque on the septum at the point of mitral leaflet–septal contact, which can be involved in the development of vegetations. All patients with miral regurgitation or turbulent blood flow in the left ventricular outflow tract should receive antibiotic prophylaxis for dental work and other procedures likely to cause bacteraemia.

Prognosis

Although the natural history of hypertrophic cardiomyopathy in adults is of a slow progression of symptoms over many years, survival data from referral centres indicate that there is an annual disease-related mortality of 2%–3% from sudden unexpected cardiac death which is not reduced by symptomatic treatment [15.145, 146]. Indeed sudden death is often the initial presentation of hypertrophic cardiomyopathy, and the risk of sudden death is not related to the severity of symptoms, or to functional class. In children and adolescents the natural history appears to be more aggressive, and the annual disease-related mortality from sudden death is 4%–6% in this age group [131].

Identification of the Patient at Risk of Sudden Death

The identification of patients at highest risk of sudden death, and the modification of that risk, is one of the most demanding problems in the management of patients with hypertrophic cardiomyopathy. Analysis of outcome in large series of patients indicates that those features which best predict the risk of sudden death are: diagnosis in childhood or adolescence, a family history of hypertrophic cardiomyopathy and sudden death, and syncopal episodes [69]. The predictive accuracy of the risk of sudden death of clinical, haemodynamic and angiographic characterisation, including the assessment of left ventricular outflow tract gradients, is low (sensitivity 70%, specificity 68%, positive predictive accuracy 24%).

The single best marker of the high-risk adult is still the identification of non-sustained ventricular tachycardia on ambulatory electrocardiographic monitoring, which is probably a marker of cellular disarray and electrical instability, and is associated with a seven-fold increase in the incidence of sudden death [67, 140]. In adults, the finding of non-sustained ventricular tachycardia represents a sensitive (> 70%) and specific (> 80%) marker of increased risk of sudden death. The negative predictive accuracy is high (97%), but the positive predictive accuracy is relatively low (23%), reflecting the fact that the majority of patients with non-sustained ventricular tachycardia do not die during short-term (3-year) follow up.

Since the negative predictive accuracy of non-sustained ventricular tachycardia is high, asymptomatic adults who do not have this marker probably do not require further investigation in terms of risk assessment. The low positive predictive accuracy of this finding, however, means that some patients with non-sustained ventricular tachycardia are at higher risk of sudden death than others. Further work is required to improve risk stratification in this group. In particular, the role of electrophysiological investigation in refining the risk assessment of those patients who do have features of increased risk (syncope, "malignant family history", exertional hypotension and non-sustained ventricular tachycardia) requires definition. Such patients should undergo assessment at referral centres with a particular interest in the condition. Electrophysiological testing should be undertaken with a view to detecting conduction tissue disease, accelerated atrioventricular conduction (either intranodal or via an accessory pathyway) and inducible monomorphic ventricular depolarisation and repolarisation, may aid in further risk factor stratification. Although for the moment this is speculative, such information could be particularly valuable in young patients, for whom the mortality is highest and the ability to predict an adverse outcome is worst.

Mechanism of Sudden Death

The mechanisms of sudden death in most patients are not known and the association with non-sustained ventricular tachycardia does not mean that this arrhythmia is the initiating mechanism. Several potential initiating mechanisms, which may be interrelated, exist (including haemodynamic collapse and rhythm disturbances) and may lead to the terminal event, which is ventricular fibrillation in most patients. For example, a supraventricular tachycardia, usually atrial fibrillation, whether or not associated with a very rapid ventricular response, may lead to haemodynamic colapse and ventricular fibrillation [71]. Primary haemodynamic collapse, for which many potential mechanisms exist [12, 15, 16, 72–74], may produce myocardial ischaemia, arrhythmias and ventricular fibrillation. If either primary haemodynamic collapse or a supraventricular tachycardia were the initiating event, then the outcome (survival versus sudden death) might be determined by the electrical stability of the myocardium, which itself is probably a function of myocardia disarray. Support for this hypothesis comes from the observation that there is greater cellular disarray in the hearts of adolescents who die suddenly than in adults who die suddenly. Adult patients who die of other causes have the least disarray [15, 69] (see Chap. 6).

A history of recurrent syncope and a bad family history are ominous features in the young patient with hypertrophic cardiomyopathy, but the majority of those who die suddenly do not have these markers. The incidence of sudden death in children and adolescents is 4%–6%, but the occurrence of non-sustained ventricular tachycardia on ambulatory monitoring is rare, and it is not a useful prognostic indicator [17]. It is of interest, however, that symptoms of impaired consciousness were generally absent in the younger patients with exertional hypotension during treadmill exercise. The absence of warning about exertional hypotension may allow the development of regional myocardial ischaemia in such cases. It is possible that exercise hypotension may prove to be a useful marker of risk in this group, but longer follow-up studies are required to establish whether or not this is so.

Prevention of Sudden Death

There is no good evidence that symptomatic therapy with propranolol or verapamil can influence the prognosis in hypertrophic cardiomyopathy. The enthusiasm of the proponents of a surgical approach to therapy, and the possibility that survival in patients with significant left ventricular outflow tract obstruction who survive the operation of myotomy/myectomy may be greater than in patients with obstruction who do not undergo surgery, must be tempered by the perioperative mortality, and the knowledge that patients with significant obstruction are a minority. Most of those who die suddenly do not have left ventricular outflow tract obstruction. Many of those who die suddenly, particularly among children and adolescents, have no symptoms beforehand. Surgical treatment, with the exception of mitral valve replacement for severe mitral regurgitation, and cardiac transplantation do not appear to improve survival.

As discussed earlier, patients with sustained spontaneous ventricular tachycardia should be treated in the same way as patients with ventricular tachycardia associated with other cardiac conditions. Management should be guided by electrophysiological study, using conventional therapeutic options. The automatic implantable cardioverter–defibrillator may find a place in the treatment of patients with documented sustained tachyarrhythmias who fail on medical therapy—those who have recurrent episodes of ventricular tachycardia/ ventricular fibrillation, or episodes of collapse due to sustained tachycardia, despite medical therapy. Its use in other high-risk patients, even those with recurrent syncope, has not been justified. In most cases the initiating mechanism of syncope is not clear (supraventricular arrhythmia, myocardial ischaemia, peripheral vasodilatation or acute obstruction of the left ventricular outflow tract are all potential mechanisms in an individual) and the rationale for defibrillation is uncertain. The device might restore sinus rhythm (if this were not the rhythm anyway), without restoring cardiac output.

Even in patients with one episode of out-of-hospital ventricular fibrillation, the use of the automatic implantable cardioverter–defibrillator may be controversial. A series of 33 survivors of cardiac arrest was reported recently [147]. The 18 patients with a resting or provocable left ventricualr outflow tract gradient underwent surgery (septal myotomy/myectomy in 17, and mitral valve replacement in 1), and all but 2 received anti-arrhythmic therapy with a class I agent postoperatively; the remaining 17 received medical therapy alone (a class I agent in II, and amiodarone in 4). Five patients survived more than one cardiac arrest, 4 of whom were in the medical group, and there were 11 deaths (8 disease-related) during follow-up for a mean of 7 years. Four patients, 2 in each group, died suddenly and 4, all in the surgical group, died of progressive heart failure. Actuarial survival for the whole group was 97% at 1 year, 74% at 5 years and 61% at 10 years, which is not significantly different from survival for a group of patients with hypertrophic cardiomyopathy who have not experienced cardiac arrest.

Thus, in hypertrophic cardiomyopathy aborted episodes of sudden death may not carry the same ominous prognosis with which they are associated in coronary artery disease, but such patients represent a difficult management problem and more information about them is needed. The projected availability of the automatic implantable cardioverter–defibrillator with electrocardiographic monitoring capability may provide the data to assess the initiating mechanism, which would help to determine appropriate therapy.

Non-sustained ventricular tachycardia is still the best marker of the adult patient at increased risk of sudden death, but since it is not usually associated wiht symptoms treatment is not required on symptomatic grounds. Treatment of these patients with low-dose amiodarone does, however, significantly improve survival in the short and medium term [75]. No such marker has been identified in children, and there is a natural reluctance to commit children to an indefinite period of treatment with amiodarone because of the potential side effects. Nevertheless, encouraging results have been seen in an uncontrolled study with very low doses of amiodarone (plasma concentration 0.5 mg/l) in a group of high-risk children with an expected annual mortality of at least 8%. Although confirmation of benefit is required, no deaths occurred over a 3-year period in a cohort of 15 patients [131].

A clinical study of the use of high-dose amiodarone in patients with refractory symptoms and arrhythmias reported several sudden deaths, particularly during a prolonged high-dose loading period [148]. The mode of action of amiodarone in preventing sudden death at low dose, particularly in the absence of sustained spontaneous arrhythmias, is speculative. Prevention of primary arrhythmias, supraventricular tachycardias in particular, raising the threshold for ventricular fibrillation, or an effect on the control of peripheral blood flow may all be relevant.

References

1. Teare RD (1958) Asymmetrical hypertrophy of the heart in young adults. Br Heart J 20: 1–8
2. Roberts CS, Roberts WC (1989) Hypertrophic cardiomyopathy: morphologic features. In: Zipes DP, Rowlands DJ (eds) Progress in cardiology, vol 2/2. Lea and Febiger, Philadelphia, pp 2–32
3. McKenna WJ, Kleinebenne A, Nihoyannopoulos P, Foale RA (1988) Echocardiographic measurement of right ventricular wall thickness in hypertrophic cardiomyopathy: relation to clinical and prognostic features. J Am Coll Cardiol 11: 351–358

4. Maron BJ, Gottdiener JS, Epstein SE (1981) Patterns and significance of distribution of left ventricular hypertrophy in hypertrophic cardiomyopathy: a wide angle, two dimensional echocardiographic study of 125 patients. Am J Cardiol 48: 418–428
5. Shapiro LM, Kleinebenne A, McKenna WJ (1985) The distribution of left ventricular hypertrophy in hypertrophic cardiomyopathy: comparison to athletes and hypertensives. Eur Heart J 6: 967–674
6. Davies MJ (1984) The current status of myocardial disarray in hypertrophic cardiomyopathy. Br Heart J 51: 361–363
7. Maron BJ, Clark CE, Henry WL, Fukuda T, Edwards JE, Mathews EC, Redwood DR, Epstein SE (1977) Prevalence and characteristics of disproportionate ventricular septal thickening in patients with acquired or congenital heart diseases: echocardiographic and morphologic findings. Circulation 55: 489–496
8. Maron BJ, Roberts WC (1979) Quantitative analysis of cardiac muscle cell disorganization in ventricular septum of patients with hypertrophic cardiomyopathy. Circulation 59: 689–706
9. Maron BJ, Anan TK, Roberts WC (1981) Quantitative analysis of the distribution of cardiac muscle cell disorganisation in the left ventricular wall of patients with hypertrophic cardiomyopathy. Circulation 63: 882–894
10. Ferrans VJ, Morrow AG, Roberts WC (1972) Myocardial ultrastructure in idiopathic hypertrophic subaortic stenosis: a study of operatively excised left ventricular outflow tract muscle in 14 patients. Circulation 45: 769–792
11. Maron BJ, Wolfson JK, Epstein SE, Roberts WC (1986) Intramural "small vessel" coronary artery disease in hypertrophic cardiomyopathy. J Am Coll Cardiol 8: 545–557
12. Maron BJ, Bonow RO, Cannon RO III, Leon MB, Epstein SE (1987) Hypertrophic cardiomyopathy: interrelations of clinical manifestations, pathophysiology and therapy (parts 1 and 2). N Engl J Med 316: 780–789, 844–852
13. McKenna WJ, Deanfield J, Faruqui A, England D, Oakley CM, Goodwin JF (1981) Prognosis in hypertrophic cardiography: role of age, and clinical, electrocardiographic and hemodynamic features. Am J Cardiol 47: 532–538
14. Braunwald E, Lambrew C, Rockoff S, Ross J, Morrow AG (1964) Idiopathic hypertrophic subaortic stenosis. I. Description of the disease based upon an analysis of 64 patients. Circulation 29 Suppl IV. 3–119
15. Loogen F, Kuhn H, Krelhaus W (1978) The natural history of hypertrophic cardiomyopathy and the effect of therapy. In: Kaltenbach M, Loogen F, Olsen EGJ (eds) Cardiomyopathy and myocardial biopsy. Springer, Berlin Heidelberg New York, pp 268–299
16. McKenna WJ (1988) The natural history of hypertrophic cardiomyopathy. In: Brest AN, Shaver JA (eds) Cardiovascular clinics. Davis, Philadelphia, pp 135–148
17. McKenna WJ, Deanfield JE (1984) Hypertrophic cardiomyopathy:an important cause of sudden death. Arch Dis Child 59: 971–975
18. Wigle ED, Adelman AG, Silver MD (1971) Pathophysiological considerations in muscular subaortic stenosis. Ciba Found Study Group 47: 63
19. Cape EG, Simons D, Jimoh A, Weyman AE, Yoganathan AP, Levine RA (1989) Chordal geometry determines the shape and extent of systolic anterior mitral motion: in vitro studies. J Am Coll Cardiol 13: 1438–1448
20. Pollick C, Rakowski H, Wigle ED (1984) Muscular subaortic stenosis: the quantitative relationship between systolic anterior motion and the pressure gradient. Circulation 69 Suppl 1: 43–49
21. Wigle ED, Sasson Z, Henderson MA, Ruddy TD, Fulop J, Rakowski H, Williams WG (1985) Hypertrophic cardiomyopathy: the importance of the site and extent of hypertrophy. A review. Prog Cardiovasc Dis 28: 1–83
22. Gilbert BW, Pollick C, Adelman AG, Wigle ED (1980) Hypertrophic cardiomyopathy: subclassification by M-mode echocardiography. Am J Cardiol 45: 861–872
23. Yonezawa Y, Dickie S, Nihoyannopoulos P, McKenna WJ (1987) The significance of left ventricular gradients in hypertrophic cardiomyopathy (Abstr). Br Heart J 57: 581

24. Wigle ED, Rakowski H (1987) Evidence for true obstruction to left ventricular outflow in obstructive hypertrophic cardiomyopathy (muscular or hypertrophic subaortic stenosis). Z Kardiol 76 Suppl 3: 61–68
25. Wigle ED, Auger P, Marquis Y (1967) Muscular subaortic stenosis: the direct relation between the intraventricular pressure gradient and left ventricular ejection time. Circulation 36: 36–44
26. Criley JM, Siegel RJ (1985) A non-obstructive view of hypertrophic cardiomyopathy: In Goodwin JF (ed) Heart muscle disease. MTP Press, Lancaster, p 157
27. Murgo JP, Miller JW (1985) Haemodynamic, angiographic and echocardiographic evidence against impeded ejection in hypertrophic cardiomyopathy. In: Goodwin JF (ed) Heart muscle disease. MTP Press, Lancaster, p 187
28. Stewart S, Mason DT, Braunwald E (1968) Impaired rate of left ventricular filling in idiopathic hypertrophic subaortic stenosis and valvular aortic stenosis. Circulation 37: 8–14
29. Sanderson JE, Gibson DG, Brown DJ, Goodwin JF (1977) Left ventricular filling in hypertrophic cardiomyopathy: an angiographic study. Br Heart J 39: 661–670
30. Sanderson JE et al. (1978) Left ventricular relaxation and filling in hypertrophic cardiomyopathy: an echocardiographic study. Br Heart J 40: 596–601
31. Brutsaert DL, Rademakers FE, Sys SU, Gillebert TC, Housmans PR (1985) Analysis of relaxation in the evaluation of ventricular function of the heart. Prog Cardiovasc Dis 28: 143–163
32. Gaasch WH, Levine HJ, Quinones MA, Alexander JK (1976) Left ventricular compliance: mechanisms and clinical implications. Am J Cardiol 38: 645–653
33. Glantz SA, Parmley WW (1978) Factors which affect the diastolic pressure–volume curve. Circ Res 42: 171–180
34. Hutchins GM, Bulkley BH (1978) Catenoid shape of interventricular septum: possible cause of idiopathic hypertrophic subaortic stenosis. Circulation 58: 392–397
35. Silverman KL, Hutchins GM, Weiss JL, Moore GW (1982) Catenoidal shape of the interventricular septum in idiopathic subaortic stenosis: two dimensional echocardiographic confirmation. Am J Cardiol 49: 27–32
36. Perloff JK (1981) Pathogenesis of hypertrophic cardiomyopathy: hypothesis and speculation. Am Heart J 101: 219–226
37. Tanaka M, Fujiwara H, Onodera T, Wu DJ, Hamashima Y, Kawai L (1986) Quantitative analysis of myocardial fibrosis in normals, hypertensive hearts, and hypertrophic cardiomyopathy. Br Heart J 55: 575–581
38. Unverferth DV, Baker PB, Pearce LI, Lautman J, Roberts WC (1987) Regional myocyte hypertrophy and increased interstitial myocardial fibrosis in hypertrophic cardiomyopathy. Am J Cardiol 59: 932–936
39. Gaasch WH, Stauffer J-C (1989) Hypertrophic cardiomyopathy: diastolic dysfunction. In: Zipes DP, Rowlands DJ (eds) Progress in cardiology Vol 2/2. Lea and Febiger, Philadelphia, pp 87–96
40. Pearce PC, Hawkey C, Symons C, Olsen EG (1985) Role of calcium in the induction of cardiac hypertrophy and myofibrillar disarray: experimental studies of a possible cause of hypertrophic cardiomyopathy. Br Heart J 54: 420–427
41. Gwathmey JK, Warren S, Briggs GM, Copelas L, Feldman MD, Callahan M, Schoen F, Grossman W, Morgan JF (1988) Direct evidence for intracellular Ca^{++} overload in working myocardium from patients with hypertrophic cardiomyopathy. Quoted in: Braunwald E (Ed.) Heart disease: a textbook of cardiovascular medicine, 3rd edn. Saunders, Philadelphia, p 1421
42. Zile MR, Blaustein AS, Shimizu G, Gaasch WH (1987) Right ventricular pacing reduces the rate of left ventricular relaxation and filling. J Am Coll Cardiol 10: 702–709
43. Brutsaert DL (1987) Nonuniformity: a physiologic modulator of contraction and relaxation of the normal heart. J Am Coll Cardiol 9: 341–348
44. Chikamori T, Counihan PJ, Dickie S, Stewart JT, Frenneaux MP, McKenna WJ (1992) Mechanisms of exercise limitation in hypertrophic cardiomyopathy. J Am Coll Cardiol 19: 507–512
45. McKenna WJ, Stewart JT, Nihoyannopoulos P, McGinty F, Davies MJ (1990) Hypertrophic cardiomyopathy without hypertrophy: two families with myocardial disarray in the absence of increased myocardial mass. Br Heart J 62: 287–290

46. Woodcock AA, Gross ER, Gellert A, Shah S, Johnson M, Geddes DM (1981) Effects of dihydrocodeine, alcohol and caffeine on breathlessness and exercise tolerance in patients with chronic obstructive lung disease and normal blood gases. N Engl J Med 305: 1611–1616
47. Frank S, Braunwald E (1968) Idiopathic hypertrophic subaortic stenosis: clinical analysis of 126 patients with emphasis on the natural history. Circulation 37: 759–788
48. Brugada P, Bar FWHM, de Zwaan C, Roy D, Green M, Wellens HJJ (1983) "Sawfish" systolic narrowing of the left anterior descending coronary artery: an angiographic sign of hypertrophic cardiomyopathy. Circulation 67: 191–197
49. Pitcher D, Wainwright R, Maisey M Curry P, Sowton E (1980) Assessment of chest pain in hypertrophic cardiomyopathy using exercise thallium -201 myocardial imaging. Br Heart J 44: 650–656
50. Rubin KA, Morrison J, Padnick MB, Binder AJ, Chiaramida S, Margouleff D, Padnanabhan VT, Gulotta SJ (1979) Idiopathic hypertrophic subaortic stenosis: evaluation of anginal symptoms with thallium-201 imaging. Am J Cardiol 44: 1040–1045
51. Hanrath P, Mathey D, Montz R, Thiel U, Vorbinger H, Kupper W, Schneider C, Bleifeld W (1981) Myocardial thallium-201 imaging in hypertrophic obstructive cardiomyopathy. Eur Heart J 2: 177–185
52. O'Gara PT, Bonow RO, Damske BA, van Lingen A, Bacharach SL, Larsen SM, Epstein SE (1987) Myocardial perfusion abnormalities in patients with hypertrophic cardiomyopathy: assessment with thallium-201 emission computed tomography. Circulation 76: 1214–1223
53. Takata J, Chikamori T, Counihan PJ, Gane JN, Hunter GJ, McKenna WJ (1991) Thallium-201 perfusion defects in hypertrophic cardiomyopathy. Br Heart J 66: 59
54. Gorlin R (1969) Evaluation of myocardial metabolism in ischemic heart disease. Circulation 40 Suppl 4: 155–167
55. Thompson DS, Naqvi N, Juul SM, Swanton RH, Coltart DJ, Jenkins BS, Webb-Peploe MM (1980) Effects of propranolol on myocardial oxygen consumption, substrate extraction, and haemodynamics in hypertrophic cardiomyopathy. Br Heart J 44: 488– 498
56. Pasternac A, Noble J, Streulens Y, Elie R, Henschke C, Bourassa MG (1982) Pathophysiology of chest pain in patients with cardiomyopathies and normal coronary arteries. Circulation 65: 778–789
57. Cannon RO, Schenke WH Maron BJ, Tracey CM, Leon MB, Brush JE, Rosing DR, Epstein SE (1987) Differences in coronary flow and myocardial metabolism at rest and during pacing between patients with obstructive and patients with nonobstructive hypertrophic cardiomyopathy. J Am Coll Cardiol 10: 53–62
58. Cannon RO, Brush J, Tracey CM (1987) Contribution of left ventricular contractility and outflow gradient to ischemia in hypertrophic cardiomyopathy (Abstr). J Am Coll Cardiol 9: 230A
59. Ogata Y, Hiyamuta K, Terasawa M, Ohkita Y, Bekki H, Koga Y, Toshima H (1986) Relationship of exercise or pacing induced ST segment depression and myocardial lactate metabolism in patients with hypertrophic cardiomyopathy. Jpn Heart J 27: 145–148
60. Cuccurullo F, Mezzetti A, Lapenna D, Tomassetti V, Porreca E, Poggiopollini G, Guglielmi MD, Mancini M, Merzio L, Lenzi S (1987) Mechanism of isoproterenol-induced angina pectoris in patients with obstructive hypertrophic cardiomyopathy and normal coronary arteries. Am J Cardiol 60: 667–673
61. Brink AJ, Lewis CM, can Heerden PDR (1967) Coronary blood flow and myocardial metabolism in obstructive cardiomyopathy: observations before and after treatment with a beta adrenergic blocking agent. Am J Cardiol 19: 548–555
62. Rudolph W, Schinz A (1973) Studies on myocardial blood flow, oxygen consumption and myocardial metabolism in patients with cardiomyopathy. In: Bajusz E, Rona G (eds) Recent advances on cardiac structure and metabolism: Cardiomyopathies. Vol. 2. Baltimore University Park Press, pp 739
63. Weiss MB, Ellis K, Sciacca RR, Johnson LL, Schmidt DH, Cannon PJ (1976) Myocardial blood flow in congestive and hypertrophic cardiomyopathy: relationship to peak wall stress and mean velocity of circumferential fibre shortening. Circulation 54: 484–494
64. Shimamatsu M, Toshima H (1987) Impaired coronary vasodilatory capacity after dipyridamole administration in hypertrophic cardiomyopathy. Jpn Heart J 28: 387–401

65. Cannon RO, Rosing DR, Maron BJ et al. (1985) Myocardial ischemia in hypertrophic cardiomyopathy: contribution of inadequate vasodilator reserve and elevated left ventricular filling pressures. Circulation 71: 234–243
66. Pichard AD, Meller J Teichholz LE, Lipnick S, Gorlin, R Herman MV (1977) Septal perforator compression (narrowing) in idiopathic hypertrophic subarotic stenosis. Am J Cardiol 40: 310–314
67. McKenna WJ, England D, Doi YL, Deanfield JE, Oakley CM, Goodwin JF (1981) Arrhythmia in hypertrophic cardiomyopathy. I. Influence on prognosis. Br Heart J 46: 168–172
68. Savage DD, Seides SF, Maron BJ, Myers DM, Epstein SE (1979) Prevalence of arrhythmia during 24 hour electrocardiographic monitoring and exercise testing in patients with obstructive and onobstructive cardiomyopathy. Circulation 59: 866–875
69. McKenna WJ, Alfonso F (1988) Arrhythmias in the cardiomyopathies and mitral valve prolapse. In: Zipes D, Rowlands D (eds) Progress in cardiology. Lea and Febiger, Philadelphia pp 59– 75
70. Fananapazir L, Tracy C, Leon MB, Winkler JB, Cannon RO, Bonow RO, Maron BJ, Epstein SE (1989) Electrophysiologic abnormalities in patients with hypertrophic cardiomyopathy: a consecutive analysis of 155 patients. Circualtion 80: 1259–1268
71. Stafford WJ, Trohman RG, Bilsker M, Zaman L, Castellanos A, Myerburg RJ (1986) Cardiac arrest in an adolescent with atrial fibrillation and hypertrophic cardiomyopathy. J Am Coll Cardiol 7: 701–704
72. McKenna WJ, Harris L, Deanfield J (1982) Syncope in hypertrophic cardiomyopathy. Br Heart J 47: 177–179
73. Frenneaux MP, Counihan PJ, Caforio ALP, Chikamori T, McKenna WJ (1990) Abnormal blood pressure response during exercise in hypertrophic cardiomyopathy. Circulation 82: 1995–2002
74. Counihan PJ, Frenneaux MP, Webb DJ, McKenna WJ (1992) Abnormal vascular responses to supine exercise in hypertrophic cardiomyopathy. Circulation 84: 686–696
75. McKenna WJ, Oakley CM, Krikler DM, Goodwin JF (1985) Improved survival with amiodarone in patients with hypertrophic cardiomyopathy and ventricular tachycardia. Br Heart J 53: 412–416
76. Maron BJ, Tajik AJ, Ruttenberg HD et al. (1982) Hypertrophic cardiomyopathy in infants: clinical features and natural history. Circulation 65: 7–17
77. Maron BJ, Spirito P, Wesley Y, Arce J (1986) Development and progression of left ventricular hypertrophy in children with hypertrophic cardiomyopathy. N Engl J Med 315: 610–614
78. Shem-Tov AA, Harpaz D, Cooley DA (1991) Hypertrophic cardiomyopathy: a report of a case with rapidly progressive hypertrophy and surgical intervention. Cardiology 78: 64–67
79. Koga Y, Itaya M, Toshiya H (1985) Increased cardiovascular response to epinephrine in hypertrophic cardiomyopathy. Jpn Heart J 26: 727–740
80. Golf S, Myhre E, Abdelnoor M, Anderson D, Hansson V (1985) Hypertrophic cardiomyopathy characterized by beta-adrenoreceptor density, relative amount of beta-adrenoreceptor subtypes, and adenylate cyclase activity. Cardiovasc Res 19: 693– 699
81. Wagner JA, Sax SG, Weisman HE, Porterfield J, Mclntosh C, Weisdfeldt MD, Snyder FH, Epstein SE (1989) Calcium antagonist receptors in the atrial tissue of patients with hypertrophic cardiomyopathy. N Engl J Med 320: 755
82. Braunwald E, Morrow AG, Cornell WP, Augen MM, Hilbish TF (1960) Idiopathic hypertrophic subaortic stenosis: clinical, hemodynamic and angiographic manifestations. Am J Med 29: 924–945
83. Goodwin JF et al. (1964) The clinical pharmacology of hypertrophic obstructive cardiomyopathy. Ciba Found Symp 81: 189– 213
84. Braunwald E, Lambrew CT, Harrison DC, Morrow AG (1964) The hemodynamic effects of circulatory drugs in patients with idiopathic subaortic stenosis. Ciba Found Symp 81: 172–188
85. Swanton RH, Brooksby IAB, Jenkins BS, Webb–Peploe MM (1977) Hemodynamic studies of beta-blockade in hypertrophic obstructive cardiomyopathy. Eur J Cardiol 5/4: 327–334

86. Cohen LS, Braunwald E (1967) Amelioration of angina pectoris in idiopathic hypertrophic subaortic stenosis with beta-adrenergic blockade. Circulation 35: 847–851
87. Thompson DS, Wilmshurst P, Juul SM, Waldron CB, Jenkins BS, Coltart DJ, Webb-Peploe MM (1983) Pressure-derived indices of left ventricular relaxation in patients with hypertrophic cardiomyopathy. Br Heart J 49: 259–267
88. Swan DA, Bell B, Oakley CM, Goodwin JF (1971) Analysis of the symptomatic course and prognosis and treatment of hypertrophic cardiomyopathy. Br Heart J 33: 671–685
89. Webb-Peploe MM, Oakley CM, Croxson RS, Goodwin JF (1971) Cardioselective beta-adrenergic blockade in hypertrophic obstructive cardiomyopathy. Postgrad Med J 47 Suppl: 93–97
90. Webb-Peploe MM (1974) Management of hypertrophic obstructive cardiomyopathy by beta-blockade. Ciba Found Symp 37: 103
91. Speiser KW, Krayenbühl HP (1981) Reappraisal of the effect of acute beta-blockade on left ventricular filling dynamics in hypertrophic obstructive cardiomyopathy. Eur Heart J 2: 21–29
92. Alvares RF, Shaver JA, Gamble WH, Goodwin JF (1984) Isovolumic relaxation period in hypertrophic cardiomyopathy. J Am Coll Cardiol 3: 71
93. Takenaka K, Dobestani A, Gardin JM, Russell D, Clark S, Allfie A, Henry WL (1986) Left ventricular filling in hypertrophic cardiomyopathy: a pulsed Doppler echocardiographic study. J Am Coll Cardiol 7: 1263–1271
94. Maron BJ, Spirito P, Green KJ, Wesley YE, Bonow RO, Arce J (1987) Non-invasive assessment of left ventricular diastolic function by pulsed Doppler echocardiography in patients with hypertrophic cardiomyopathy. J Am Coll Cardiol 10: 733–742
95. Bryg RJ, Pearson AC, Williams AG, Labovitz AJ (1987) Left ventricular systolic and diastolic flow abnormalities determined by Doppler echocardiography in obstructive hypertrophic cardiomyopathy. Am J Cardiol 58: 925–931
96. Ostman-Smith I (1991) Regression of cardiac hypertrophy achieved by high dose propranolol treatment in children and adults with hypertrophic cardiomyopathy. Br Heart J 66: 76
97. Frank MJ, Abdulla AM, Canedo MI, Saylors RE (1978) Long-term medical management of hypertrophic obstructive cardiomyopathy. Am J Cardiol 42: 993–1001
98. Pearce PC, Hawkey C, Symons C, Olsen EGJ (1985) Role of calcium in the induction of cardiac hypertrophy and myofibrillar disarray: experimental studies of a possible cause of hypertrophic cardiomyopathy. Br Heart J 54: 420
99. Lorell BH (1985) Use of calcium channel blockers in hypertrophic cardiomyopathy. Am J Med 78 Suppl 2B: 43–54
100. Rosing DR, Kent KM, Borer JS, Seides SF, Maron BJ, Epstein SE (1979) Verapamil therapy: a new approach to the pharmacologic treatment of hypertrophic cardiomyopathy. I. Hemodynamic effects. Circulation 60: 1201–1207
101. Rosing DR, Kent KM, Maron BJ, Epstein SE (1979) Verapamil therapy: a new approach to the pharmacologic treatment of hypertrophic cardiomyopathy. II. Effects on exercise capacity and symptomatic status. Circulation 60: 1208–1213
102. Hanrath P, Mathey DG, Siegert R, Bleifeld W (1980) Left ventricular relaxation and filling patterns in different forms of left ventricular hypertrophy: an echocardiographic study. Am J Cardiol 45: 15–23
103. Bonow RO, Rosing DR, Bacharach SL, Green MV, Kent KM, Lipson LC, Maron BJ, Leon MB, Epstein SE (1981) Effects of verapamil on left ventricular systolic function and diastolic filling in patients with hypertrophic cardiomyopathy. Circulation 64: 787–796
104. Hasin Y, Lewis BS, Lewis N, Weiss AT, Gotsman MS (1982) Long-term effect of verapamil in hypertrophic cardiomyopathy. Int J Cardiol 1: 243–251
105. Hess OM, Murakami T, Krayenbühl HP (1986) Does verapamil improve left ventricular relaxation in patients with myocardial hypertrophy? Circulation 74: 530–543
106. Bonow RO, Vitale DF, Maron BJ, Bacharach SL, Frederick TM, Green MV (1987) Regional left ventricular asynchrony and impaired global left ventricular filling in hypertrophic cardiomyopathy: effect of verapamil. J Am Coll Cardiol 9: 1108–1116

107. Hess OM, Grimm J, Krayenbuhl HP (1983) Diastolic function in hypertrophic cardiomyopathy: effects of propranolol and verapamil on diastolic stiffness. Eur Heart J 4 Suppl F: 47–56
108. Rosing DR, Condit JR, Maron BJ, Kent KM, Leon MB, Bonow RO, Lipson LC, Epstein SE (1981) Verapamil therapy: a new approach to the pharmacologic treatment of hypertrophic cardiomyopathy. Effects of long-term administration. Am J Cardiol 43: 545–553
109. Kaltenbach M, Hopf R, Kober G, Bussmann WD, Keller M, Petersen Y (1979) Treatment of hypertrophic obstructive cardiomyopathy with verapamil. Br Heart J 42: 35–42
110. Bonow RO, Ostrow HG, Rosing DR, Cannon RO, Lipson LC, Maron BJ, Kent KM, Bacharach SL, Green MV (1983) Effects of verapamil on left ventricular systolic and diastolic function in patients with hypertrophic cardiomyopathy: pressure–volume analysis with a nonimaging scintillation probe. Circulation 68: 1062–1073
111. Bonow RO, Dilsizian V, Rosing DR, Maron BJ, Bacharach SL, Green MV (1985) Verapamil-induced improvement in left ventricular diastolic filling and increased exercise tolerance in patients with hypertrophic cardiomyopathy: short- and long-term effects. Circulation 72: 853–864
112. Epstein SE, Rosing DR (1981) Verapamil: its potential for causing serious complications in patients with hypertrophic cardiomyopathy. Circulation 64: 437–441
113. Lorell BH, Paulus WJ, Grossman W, Wynne J, Cohn PF (1982) Modification of abnormal left ventricular diastolic properties by nifedipine in patients with hypertrophic cardiomyopathy. Circulation 65: 499–507
114. Paulus WJ, Lorell BH, Craig WE, Wynne J, Murgo JP, Grossman W (1983) Comparison of the effects of nitroprusside and nifedipine on diastolic properties in patients with hypertrophic cardiomyopathy: altered left ventricular loading or improved muscle inactivation? J Am Coll Cardiol 2: 879–886
115. Suwa M, Hirota Y, Kawamura K (1984) Improvement in left ventricular diastolic function during intravenous and oral diltiazem therapy in patients with hypertrophic cardiomyopathy: an echocardiographic study. Am J Cardiol 54: 1047–1053
116. Rosing DR, Cannon RO, Watson RM, Kent KM, Lakatos E, Epstein SE (1982) Comparison of verapamil and nifedipine effects on symptoms and exercise capacity in patients with hypertrophic cardiomyopathy (Abstr). Circulation 66 Suppl 2: 24
117. Hopf R, Thomas J, Klepzig H, Kaltenbach M (1987) Behandlung der hypertropischen Kardiomyopathie mit Nifedipin und Propranolol in Kombination. Z Kardiol 76: 469–478
118. Toshima H, Koga Y, Nagata H, Toyomasu K, Itaya K, Matoba T (1986) Comparable effects of oral diltiazem and verapamil in the treatment of hypertrophic cardiomyopathy. Jpn Heart J 27: 701–715
119. Iwase M, Sotobata I, Takagi S, Miyaguchi K, Jing HX, Yokotu M (1987) Effects of diltiazem on left ventricular diastolic behaviour in patients with hypertrophic cardiomyopathy: evaluation with exercise pulsed Doppler echocardiography. J Am Coll Cardiol 9: 1099–1105
120. Nagata H, Koga M, Toyomasu K, Ikeda H, Haya K, Koga Y, Ikeda H, Utsu F, Toshima H (1985) The effects of long-term diltiazem administration on hypertrophic cardiomyopathy (Abstr). Jpn Circ J 49: 803
121. McDonald K, McWilliams E, O'Keefe B, Maurer B (1988) Functional assessment of patients treated with permanent dual chamber pacing as primary treatment for hypertrophic cardiomyopathy. Eur Heart J 9: 893–898
122. Erwin J, McWilliams E, Gearty G, Maurer B (1986) Haemodynamic assessment of dual chamber pacing in hypertrophic cardiomyopathy using a radionuclide ventriculography (Abstr). Br Heart J 55: 507
123. Goodwin JF, Hollman A, Cleland WP, Teare D (1960) Obstructive cardiomyopathy simulating aortic stenosis. Br Heart J 22: 403–414
124. Morrow AG, Brockenbrough EC (1961) Surgical treatment of idiopathic subaortic stenosis: technique and hemodynamic results of subaortic ventriculotomy. Ann Surg 154: 181–189
125. Cleland WP (1963) The surgical management of obstructive cardiomyopathy. J Cardiovasc Surg 4: 489–491
126. Brauwald E, Lambrew CT, Rockoff DS, Ross J, Morrow AG (1964) Idiopathic hypertrophic subaortic stenosis. Circulation 30 Suppl 4: 1–119

127. Cooley DA, Wukasch DC, Leachman RD (1976) Mitral valve replacement for idiopathic subaortic stenosis: results in 27 patients. J Cardiovasc Surg 17: 380–387
128. Schulte HD, Bircks W, Losse B (1989) Surgical treatment of hypertrophic obstructive cardiomyopathy (HOCM): early and late results. In: Zipes DP, Rowlands DJ (eds) Progress in cardiology vol 2/2. Lea and Febiger, Philadelphia, pp 195–215
129. Maron BJ, Merrill WH, Freier PA et al. (1978) Long–term clinical course and symptomatic status of patients after operation for hypertrophic subaortic stenosis. Circulation 57: 1205–1213
130. McIntosh C, Maron BJ (1988) Current operative treatment of obstructive hypertrophic cardiomyopathy. Circulation 78: 487–495
131. McKenna WJ, Franklin RCG, Nihoyannopoulos P, Robinson KR, Deanfield JE (1988) Arrhythmia and prognosis in infants, children and adolescents with hypertrophic cardiomyopathy. J Am Coll Cardiol 11: 147–153
132. Glancy Dl, O'Brien KP, Gold HK, Epstein SE (1970) Atrial fibrillation in patients with Idiopathic Hypertrophic Subaortic Stenosis. Br Heart J 32: 652–659
133. Robinson K, Frenneaux MP, Stockins B, Karatasakis G, Poloniecki JD, McKenna WJ (1990) Atrial fibrillation in hypertrophic cardiomyopathy: a longitudinal study. J Am Coll Cardiol 15: 1279–1285
134. Marcus F, Fontaine GH, Frank R, Grosgogeat Y (1981) Clinical pharmacology and therapeutic applications of the antiarrhythmic agent, amiodarone. Am Heart J 101: 480–493
135. Harris L, McKenna WJ, Rowland E, Krikler DM (1983) Side effects of long-term amiodarone therapy. Circulation 67: 45–51
136. McKenna WJ, Harris L, Rowland E, Kleinebenne A, Krikler DM, Oakley CM, Goodwin JF (1984) Amiodarone for long-term management of patients with hypertrophic cardiomyopathy. Am J Cardiol 54: 802–810
137. Geibel A, Brugada P, Zehender M, Stevenson W, Waldecker B, Wellens HJJ (1987) Value of programmed electrical stimulation using a standardized ventricular stimulation protocol in hypertrophic cardiomyopathy. Am J Cardiol 60: 738–739
138. Alfonso F, Frenneaux M, McKenna WJ (1989) Clinical sustained monomorphic ventricular tachycardia in hypertrophic cardiomyopathy: association with left ventricular apical aneurysm. Br Heart J 61: 178–181
139. Kowey PR, Eisenberg R, Engel TR (1984) Sustained arrhythmias in hypertrophic obstructive cardiomyopathy. N Engl J Med 310: 1566–1569
140. Maron BJ, Savage DD, Wolfson JK, Epstein SE (1981) Prognostic significance of 24 hour ambulatory electrocardiographic monitoring in patients with hypertrophic cardiomyopathy: a prospective study. Am J Cardiol 48: 252–257
141. Saumarez RC, Camm AJ, Panagos A, Stewart JT, Simpson IA, McKenna W, de Belder M (1990) Ventricular fibrillation in hypertrophic cardiomyopathies is associated with increased fractionation of paced right ventricular electrocardiogram. Circulation 86: 464–474
142. Kuck K-H, Kunze K-P, Schluter M, Nienaber CA, Costard A (1988) Programmed electrical stimulation in hypertrophic cardiomyopathy: results in patients with and without cardiac arrest or syncope. Eur Heart J 9: 177–185
143. Borgreffe M, Podczeck A, Breithardt G (1986) Electrophysiologic studies in hypertrophic cardiomyopathy (Abstr). Circulation 74 Suppl 2: II–1922
144. Cokkinos DV, Krajcer Z, Leachman RD (1985) Coronary artery disease in hypertrophic cardiomyopathy. Am J Cardiol 55: 1437–1438
145. Maron BJ, Lipson LC, Roberts WC, Savage DD, Epstein SE (1978) "Malignant" hypertrophic cardiomyopathy: Identification of a subgroup of families with unusually frequent premature death. Am J Cardiol 41: 1133–1140
146. Maron BJ, Roberts WC, Epstein SE (1982) Sudden death in hypertrophic cardiomyopathy: a profile of 78 patients. Circulation 65: 1388–1394
147. Cecchi F, Maron BJ, Epstein SE (1989) Long-term outcome of patients with hypertrophic cardiomyopathy successfully resuscitated after cardiac arrest. J Am Coll Cardiol 13: 1283–1288
148. Fananapazir L, Leon MB, Bonow RO, Tracy CM, Cannon RO, Epstein SE (1991) Sudden death during empiric amiodarone therapy in symptomatic hypertrophic cardiomyopathy. Am J Cardiol 67: 169–174

Part IV
Restrictive Cardiomyopathy

CHAPTER 10

Clinical Aspects

J. F. Goodwin

[See also Chapter 13]

Restrictive cardiomyopathy is a form of diastolic heart disease, which may be defined as "cardiac disease initially and predominantly of diastolic rather than systolic function". It does not include the commonest cause of impairment of diastolic function; that is, preceding impairment of systolic function.

Normal diastolic function has been defined as sufficient filling of the left ventricle to produce a cardiac output sufficient for the normal bodily function at a mean pulmonary capillary venous pressure of less than 12 mmHg [1]. Diastolic function involves both active and passive phases in the ventricle. Isovolumic relaxation occurs after closure of the aortic valve and involves both active relaxation and change in shape of the left ventricle. When the mitral valve opens, rapid ventricular filling commences. The late stages fo the rapid filling phase are passive events, but active relaxation consumes energy [2].

Restriction has been defined as "organic interference with filling of the ventricles from endomyocardial disease with rapid early filling and slow late filling (see Chap. 1).

Diastolic heart disease refers to all conditions that primarily effect diastolic function. Important members of this group are constrictive pericarditis, restrictive cardiomyopathy, hypertrophic cardiomyopathy and amyloid disease. The mechanisms by which various members of the group of diastolic heart disease impair diastolic function differ; for example, external compression is the cause in constrictive pericarditis while resistance to filling by stiff, poorly compliant, irregularly relaxing ventricular myocardium is the cause in hypertrophic cardiomyopathy [3]. Involvement of the endocardium tends to reduce ventricular volume and is an important aspect of diastolic heart disease. In diastolic heart disease or diastolic heart failure, the ventricle is incompletely filled so that stroke volume is reduced despite compensatory tachycardia; cardiac output is correspondingly reduced (Fig. 10.1, Table 10.1).

Causation

Causes of Restrictive Cardiomyopathy

The commonest cause of restrictive cardiomyopathy is eosinophilic endomyocardial disease consisting of tropical endomyocardial fibrosis and Löffler's endo-

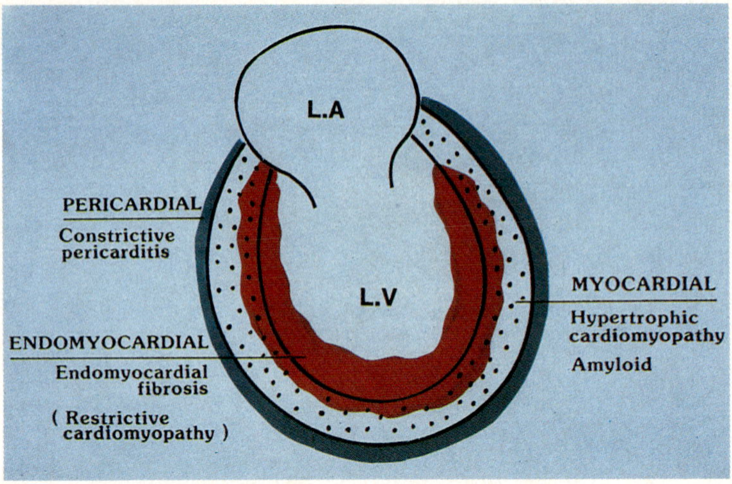

Fig. 10.1. Diagram to show the distribution of conditions causing diastolic heart disease. *LA*, left atrium; *LV*, left ventricle

Table 10.1. Clinical clues to diastolic heart disease

	Jugular verous pressure	Paradoxical pulse	Heart size	Third heart sound	Murmurs
Constrictive pericarditis	↑	+	Small	+	0
Endomyocardial fibrosis	↑	+	Small unless mitral regurgitation	+	Mitral regurgitation
Amyloid disease	↑	±	Small or large	0	±
Hypertrophic cardiomyopathy	'a'	Jerky arterial	Atrial Beat, left ventricular hypertrophy	±	Late systolic murmur, mid-diastolic murmur or none

carditis parietalis fibroplastica [4]. Other groups are: cryptogenic endomyocardial fibrosis without eosinophilia, haemochromatosis and Fabry's disease [5]. Amyloid disease, while an example of diastolic heart disease, is not a typical restrictive cardiomyopathy because filling is slow throughout diastole and the typical restrictive features of early rapid filling followed by slower late filling do not occur. Because of this, and because it is poised provocatively between the "cardiomyopathy" and "specific heart muscle disease" groups, amyloid disease deserves a class of its own (see Chap. 13).

Table 10.2. Causes of eosinophilia in patients with Löfflers endomyocardial disease

1. Myeloproliferative disorders with eosinophilia
   a) Chronic myeloid leukaemia
   b) Myelofibrosis
   c) Acute transformation of chronic myeloid leukaemia
2. Acute eosinophilic leukaemia
3. Vasculitic diseases with eosinophilia
   a) Polyarteritis nodosa
   b) Hypersensitivity vasculitis
   c) Granulomatous angitis
4. Parasitic and infectious diseases with eosinophilia
   a) Filariasis
   b) Trichinosis
   c) Syphilis
   d) Tuberculosis
   e) Amoebiasis
   f) Malaria
5. Malignant disease with eosinophilia
   a) Acute (T) lymphatic leukaemia
   b) Hodgkin's disease and lymphomas
   c) Carcinomas of the lung
   d) Melanoma

Causes of Eosinophila in Endomyocardial Disease

The causes of eosinophilia in endomyocardial disease are set out in Table 10.2. It should be noted that in most cases of eosinophilic endomyocardial disease the cause of the eosinophilia is unknown. Conversely, eosinophilic heart disease does not always produce endomyocardial fibrosis. For example, in the Churg-Strauss syndrome the heart is dilated and systolic ventricular function is impaired without endocardial disease. Pericardial effusion may be present, often in association with asthma. Hypersensitivity as a basis for the eosinophilia seems possible. Eosinophilic endomyocardial disease is part of the spectrum of the hypereosinophilic syndrome [6] in which hypereosinophilia of unknown cause is associated with cardiac and other complications.

Hypereosinophilia, the Hypereosinophilic Syndrome and Their Relation to Endomyocardial Fibrosis

In the majority of patients with endomyocardial fibrosis there is good reason to suppose that the eosinophils actively damage the endomyocardium. Persisting eosinophil counts are usually over 1.5×10/litre. Many eosinophils are qualitatively abnormal showing vacuolation and degranulation. If more than 20%

of eosinophils contain vacuoles and more than 15% are degranulated, biopsy will show endomyocardial disease even if cardiac disease is not in evidence clinically. [7, 8]. Degranulation is an important and constant feature. Increase in Fc receptors causes more effective binding to IgG and C3B coated particles, which could produce a cytotoxic response [7, 8]. Exocytosis of cationic proteins (which are thrombogenic) from the cell may damage the endocardium. In addition, the eosinophils may infiltrate the heart muscle and degranulate there, causing localised lesions., But studies have shown that neutrophils as well as eosinophils can damage myocytes [9]. However, eosinophilic granular protein has been deposited on acute necrotic and thrombotic myocardial lesions in acute necrotising eosinophilic myocarditis, emphasising the relation between eosinophilic granular protein and myocardial injury. Of course it is possible that viral or other stimuli might cause both the myocardial damage and the eosinophilia [8] (see Chaps. 11 and 12).

What Ails the Rogue Eosinophil?

Evidence suggesting that eosinophilic endomyocardial disease is really a blood disorder begs the question as to the cause of the abnormality. It seems that an infection by a virus could be responsible, but studies in Nigeria did not reveal any significant antibodies to Coxsackie B6 or other virus, and there was no difference between endomyocardial fibrosis patients and controls. However, all of 8 patients with endomyocardial fibrosis had high antibody titres to *Toxoplasma gondii* [10]. The probability of a virus infection damaging the eosinophils is enhanced by the appearance of the endomyocardium in the acute stage, in which masses of abnormal eosinophils pack the lesions; evidence of active myocarditis is present [11], which, since it is a non-specific inflammatory reaction, could be due to causes other than infection. Many patients with hypereosinophilia do not develop myocardial disease, but 95% of those with sufficient abnormal eosinophils do [6].

The Presumed Identity of Löffler's Eosinophilic Endomyocardial Disease and Tropical Endomyocardial Fibrosis

Tropical endomyocardial fibrosis (EMF) was first described in East Africa [12, 13]. Since then a wealth of literature has appeared documenting the epidemiological, clinical, pathological and haemodynamic features. The most notable epidemiological data have been the concentration of cases in humid, tropical zones in East, West and Central Africa, South America and South India, corresponding to a belt extending 5% north and south of the equator. In West Africa the onset of the disease seems to be related to climate, the majority of cases appearing in the wet season [14].

The natural history of both EMF in the tropics and Löffler's disease is similar but with certain differences that could be accounted for by local environmental and genetic factors, especially perhaps differences in immunological reactions betweeen black and white peoples. Most striking of all is the close identity of the pathological changes in both conditions. It is thus understandable that they should be regarded as the same disease [7, 15]. An apparent striking difference has been the absence of abnormal eosinophils in tropical EMF, although many Africans have eosinophilia that is due to parasites and other causes. However, recent studies in India and Africa, with appropriate techniques of examining the eosinophils, have revealed characteristic changes in a few patients; but in one study in India, evidence of eosinophilic toxic damage to the endocardium was not significant, though a high incidence of filariasis and infection was found in 16% of patients. Tropical EMF and Löffler's disease together are now termed eosinophilic endomyocardial disease [16].

It is natural to assume, in the light of recent knowledge, that the endomyocardial disease is due to the effects of disordered eosinophils. The causes of eosinophil disease being unknown, causes may differ according to geographical, climatic, genetic and environmental factors. The well-documented reports of EMF in Europeans living in the tropics harmonises with an infective cause, but Africans may have an increased susceptibility since the disease is rare even in white persons living for many years in the tropics. It seems likely, therefore, that some toxic or infective agent damages the eosinophil which in turn affects the heart and, in temperate climates, other organs as well. There is a suggestion that cardiotrophic viral infection may initiate the disease.

Since the causes of eosinophilia are not known, it is inappropriate to categorise Löffler's endomyocardial disease as a specific heart muscle disease [11]; it should remain within the definition of cardiomyopathy as "Heart muscle disease of unknown aetiology".

Clinical Features of Tropical Endomyocardial Fibrosis

Symptoms

These symptoms are usually those of developing heart failure: lassitude, cough, dyspnoea. Atrial fibrillation is common, and together with thrombosis constitutes an important cause for embolism. Non-specific symptoms may occur—further evidence that the disorder may be more widespread in the body than the heart, and that the rogue eosinophil may damage other organs.

Signs

In EMF recurrent fever, heart failure and atrial fibrillation are common features. In patients in Africa (who are often seen late) raised jugular venous pressure,

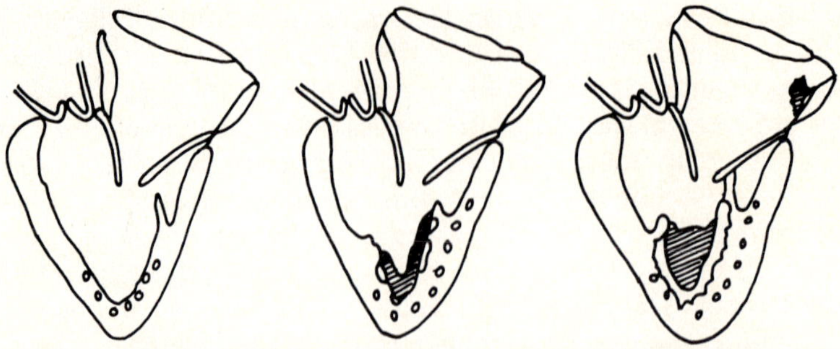

The acute necrotic stage	The later thrombotic stage	The late fibrotic stage
• Grossly normal • Rare areas of myocardial pitting • Intense myocarditis full of eosinophils • Occasional vessel lesions	• Cavity thrombus and myocardial pitting • Thrombi superimposed and in small vessels • Less myocarditis	• Endocardial fibrosis some thrombus, and valve involvement • Hypertrophy • Layers of fibrosis • Less myocarditis • Mild vessel changes

Fig. 10.2. Endomyocardial fibrosis. The acute necrotic stage produces the clinical syndrome of malaise, fever, transient atrial fibrillation and heart failure. The later thrombotic stage produces embolism and heart failure. The late fibrotic stage is associated with obliteration of the ventricular cavity producing severe diastolic impairment due to reduced ventricular volume. Heart failure and embolism are common.

ascites and hepatomegaly are usual [14]. In the early stages, however, fever, tachycardia and a rash support the concept of an "active" phase of the disease that would harmonise with the early inflammatory endomyocardial lesion [17] (Fig. 10.2). A prominent 'a' wave in the jugular venous pulse with steep 'x' and 'y' descents is usual. A puffy face, accentuation of pulmonary valve closure and an enlarged liver are seen. The chronic fibrothrombotic phase (Fig. 10.3, Table 10.3) without evidence of active inflammation in the endomyocardium would correspond to the later "chronic" clinical phase. In this stage, studies in Africa [17] have documented clinical features very similar to constrictive pericarditis: a very high jugular venous pressure, marked 'a' and 'v' waves with sharp 'x' and 'y' descents, grossly distended ascites, hepatomegaly with presystolic pulsation, proptosis (Fig. 10.4) and oedema of the eyelids. In the late stages in right-sided EMF, pericardial effusion is often present also.

The jugular venous pressure may be too high and the external jugular veins too distended for analysis of the characteristic wave form, particularly as there may be a prominent systolic wave due to tricuspid regurgitation, especially when atrial fibrillation is present. The heart may be massively enlarged due partly to an enormous right atrium and partly to a large pericardial effusion.

The clinical signs are influenced by the extent of the disease and the involvement of the atrioventricular valves. In purely right-sided EMF the dominant features are those of severe right ventricular failure and tricuspid regurgitation.

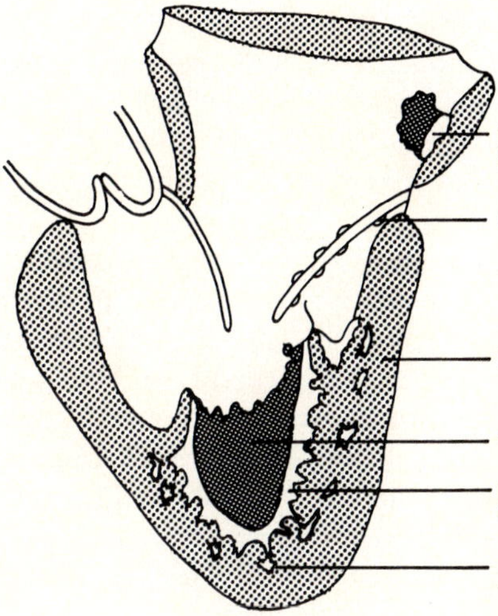

Fig. 10.3. The severe endomyocardial fibrosis damages diastolic function which is further affected by fibrothrombotic obliteration of the cavity. The fibrin deposits on the mitral valve cusps contribute to mitral regurgitation caused by the involvement of the chordae and papillary muscles in the endomyocardial fibrosis. The plaque on the left atrial wall adds to the risk of embolism. From [7] with permission of the authors and publishers

Table 10.3. Causes of congestive heart failure in EMF

Myocardial fibrosis
Restriction of ventricular filling by endocardial disease
Mitral and/or tricuspid regurgitation
Atrial fibrillation

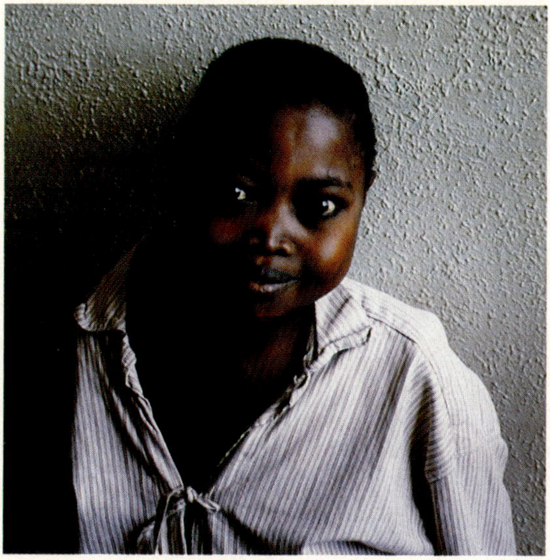

Fig. 10.4. Ugandan boy with severe right-sided EMF. The face is puffy and there is proptosis due to the very high central venous pressure. Despite the extensive involvement of the right heart, he was ambulant and reasonably happy

The fibrotic stage in the right ventricle may reduce the volume of the cavity to a mere vestige, the right atrium becoming huge. Tricuspid regurgitation is manifest by a pansystolic murmur heard in the tricuspid area, which increases on ispiration. Despite these formidable disorders, patients are often able to continue on their feet although effort tolerance is restricted and fatigue easily induced.

When the left ventricle is involved, dyspnoea is present and pulmonary oedema may occur as a result of increased left ventricular diastolic pressure consequent upon reduced volume and compliance of the left ventricle and the development of mitral regurgitation when the mitral valve is involved. The signs of left ventricular EMF include left ventricular enlargement, but the cardiac impulse, while left ventricular in character, is not strikingly abnormal. There is usually a third heart sound and pulmonary valve closure is accentuated because of the high pulmonary artery pressure. A fourth heart sound is commonly heard, while summation gallop tends to occur because of the tachycardia. Mitral regurgitaion is revelaed by a pansystolic murmur at the apex which, because the anterior mitral valve chordae and cusp are usually spared by the disease, diminishes in late systole as the competent components of the mitral valve control and limit the mitral regurgitation. Frank right heart failure may develop as a result of the severe pulmonary hypertension caused by left-sided disease, and there may be coexistent involvement of both ventricles with EMF. Biventricular EMF is common in tropical areas. The extreme degrees of right ventricular fibrosis seen in the tropics appear not to be so common in temperate zones. Signs of systemic and pulmonary embolism are frequent as a result of large and multiple intraventricular thrombi.

In Löffler's disease the signs and symptoms are very similar to trophical EMF though the early active inflammatory stage is more clear-cut in Löffler's disease large pericardial effusions are unusual and embolism more common. Evidence of enlargement of organs other than the heart is usually lacking in tropical EMF.

In a personal series of 15 patients with the hypereosinophilic syndrome, 11 had endomyocardial disease, 2 with pericarditis. Skin lesions, lymph node and splenic enlargement, arthralgia, psychiatric disturbances and focal cerebral lesions were common. The commonest presenting symptoms were nocturnal sweating, coughing, anorexia and loss of weight in addition to cardiovascular symptoms. The mean age of onset was 36 years and only 2 patients were female. Serum immunoglobulin levels were raised in 50% [8].

Chest Radiography

The heart is usually enlarged and in the tropics right-sided EMF can produce an enormous heart shadow on the chest radiograph due to pericardial effusion and the large right atrium. When right-sided disease is dominant the lung fields may be clear, but pleural effusion is common and signs of pulmonary infarction can be present. In left-sided disease there are signs of increased left atrial pressure with horizonal costophrenic lines and diversion of blood flow from the bases to the apices of the lungs. An important finding in the tropics is linear calcification in a thrombus, seen as a thin curving shadow within the silhouette of the left ventricle. This appearance is highly suggestive of EMF, but is apparently less common in cases in temperate climates.

Electrocardiography

The electrocardiogram is not specific. Atrial fibrillation is often present. In right-sided EMF in sinus rhythm there is evidence of right atrial enlargement with high-voltage peaked P waves; the PR interval may be increased, and atrioventricular block, right bundle branch block and fascicular blocks may be seen. Pericardial effusion will reduce QRS and T wave voltage. In left-sided disease there is usually evidence of left ventricular hypertrophy and in sinus rhythm the P wave is often notched and widened due to left atrial hypertension. Ventricular arrhythmias may occur in the late stage and may be related more to heart failure than to electrical disorder of the fibrotic process [18–20].

Cardiac Catheterisation and Angiocardiography

The characteristic, haemodynamics and angiographic features are described under "Differential Diagnosis" below (Figs. 10.5, 10.7 and 10.9).

Echocardiography

Echocardiography is described in Chap. 12.

Differential Diagnosis of Restrictive Cardiomyopathy/Diastolic Heart Disease

Constrictive Pericarditis

The clinical features may be quite similar with regard to the characteristic elevation of jugular venous pressure with its appropriate "square wave" form, third heart sound and systemic congestive features. The heart is usually smaller in constrictive pericarditis; signs of a raised atrial pressure are absent and murmurs are uncommon, though mitral regurgitation occasionally occurs. Chest radiography may show pericardial calcification in constrictive pericarditis and endomyocardial calcification in EMF. The atria are usually small in constrictive

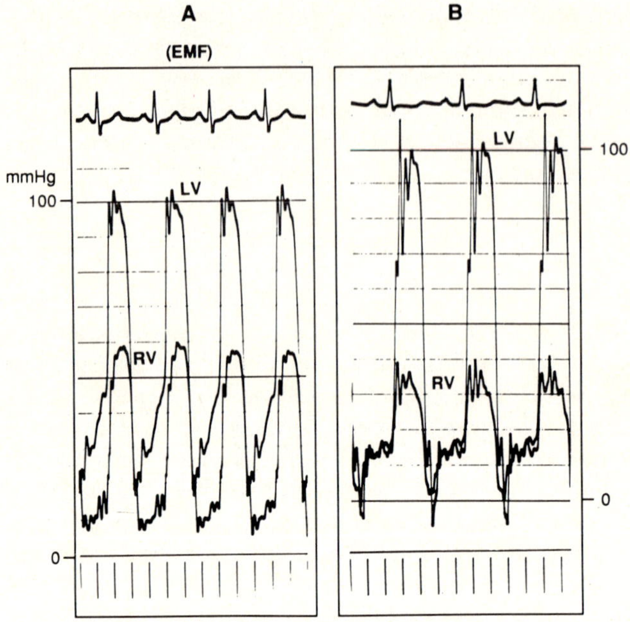

Fig. 10.5. **A** Right (*RV*) and left (*LV*) ventricular pressure pulses in EMF. The diastolic pressures are different and the early diastolic pressures in both ventricles are above zero. The right ventricular systolic pressure is above normal. **B** Constrictive pericarditis. The right and left ventricular diastolic pressures are identical, the early diastolic pressures fall below zero and the late diastolic plateau is clearly seen. The right ventricular systolic pressure is normal

pericarditis, but may be greatly enlarged in EMF. The main differences between the two conditions are the result of the different distribution of the restrictive forces. Constrictive pericarditis is a generalised disease involving the whole heart, thus left and right ventricular diastolic pressures are usually equal (Fig. 10.5). This prevents development of pulmonary congestion and hypertension. By contrast, EMF is patchy process and does not involve both sides of the heart equally. Therefore, pressures in diastole in the two ventricles differ and in EMF the end-diastolic pressure is elevated above zero and pulmonary hypertension is common (Fig. 10.5). The general symptom involvement of other organs in EMF in a temperate climate is absent in constrictive pericarditis in which there is no eosinophilia. Differentiation in difficult cases may depend upon echocardiography, computed tomography or magnetic resonance imaging (MRI), which demonstrate the thickened pericardium in constrictive pericarditis (see Chap. 12).

Other Forms of Heart Muscle Disease Producing Restrictive Features

Haemochromatosis, beta thalassaemia major and daunorubicin toxicity can usually be differentiated by the characteristics of the disorder in other organs, such as raised serum iron, iron binding and serum transfers in haemochromatosis, and evidence of anaemia and iron overload in thalassaemia major. In all such cases, as in EMF, endomyocardial biopsy can usually confirm the diagnosis.

EMF without eosinophilia or evidence of disease in other organs is seen from time to time. The cardiac features are those of Löffler's disease and the cause is unknown; perhaps a viral infection is the most likely explanation.

Amyloid Disease of the Heart

Amyloid disease of the heart may occur with amyloid disease elsewhere, involving the tongue (Fig. 10.6), mucous membranes, palmar fascia and rectus sheath, or be confined to the heart. Amyloid heart disease is not usually seen in association with involvement of lever and kidneys. The jugular venous pulse tends to show the characteristic wave form of restriction. The heart is not usually grossly enlarged, murmurs are absent and there is no gallop rhythm [21] because ventricular fillng is slow throughout diastole so there is no early rapid filling phase, the termination of which causes sudden tension of the papillary muscles that produces the 3rd sound, as in constrictive pericarditis and true restrictive cardiomyopathy (Fig. 10.7). In the late stages of amyloid disease the heart enlarges and congestive heart failure develops. Bilateral orbital haemorrhages (Fig. 10.8) can be a striking feature. The electrocardiogram is usually non-

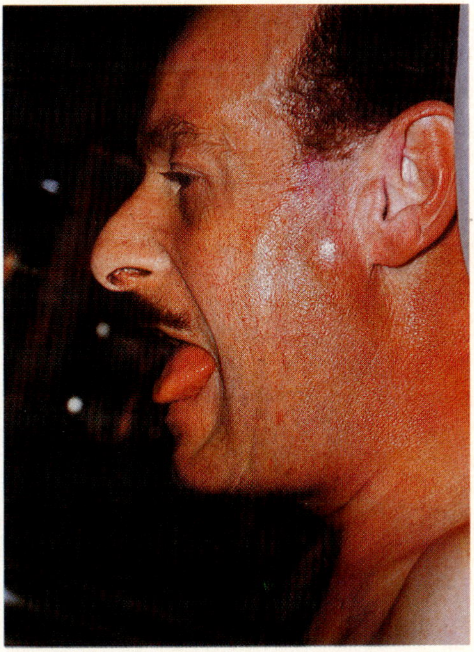

Fig. 10.6. Man with amyloid disease involving heart, rectus sheath, palmar fascia, and mucous membranes and tongue, which is enlarged stiff and restricted in movement (See Chap. 13)

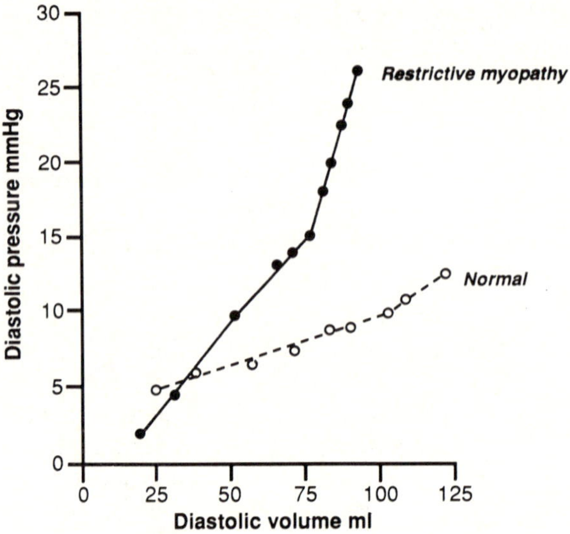

Fig. 10.7. Pressure–volume curves in restrictive cardiomyopathy and normal left ventricle. In the restrictive curve here is a rapid increase in diastolic pressure and volume in the first half of diastole, indicating the early rapid filling period. Subsequently there is little increase in volume with marked increase in pressure consistent with minimal ventricular filling in late systole. The normal curve shows a steady increase in volume throughout diastole with a minimal increase in pressure due to normal compliance and relaxation.
(Courtesy of Dr. C. Oakley)

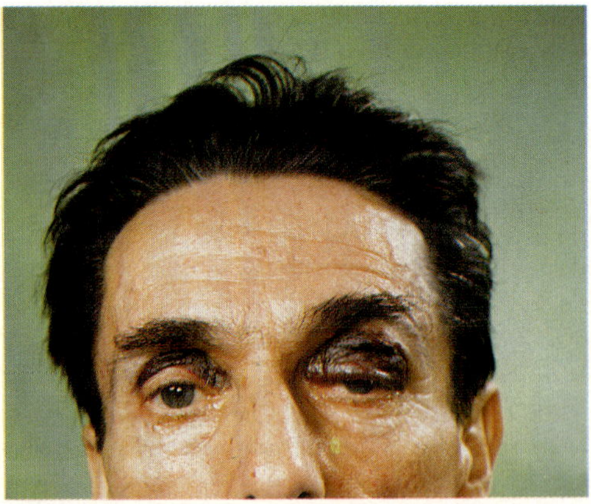

Fig. 10.8. Bilateral orbital haematomata in a man with amyoid heart disease (see Chap. 13)

specific, but may show Q waves suggesting myocardial infarction. Low voltage is common. The chest radiograph is not diagnostic. Diagnosis often depends largely upon echocardiography confirmed by endomyocardial biopsy (see Chaps. 12 and 13).

Hypertrophic Cardiomyopathy

Hypertrophic cardiomyopathy may cause difficulty in differential diagnosis because of the pronounced diastolic abnormalities of impaired relaxation, increased stiffness and poor compliance of the left ventricle. The characteristic jugular venous pulse of restriction is not usually seen, and clinical signs of hypertrophic cardiomyopathy are often present (see Chap. 6). However, in the late stages of hypertrophic cardiomyopathy with heart failure, amyloid disease may be suggested because of the very high jugular venous pressure and evidence of diastolic failure. In sinus rhythm the left atrial beat is an important sign of hypertrophic cardiomyopathy not seen in amyloid disease. Occasionally, amyloid disease and hypertrophic cardiomyopathy may coexist (see Chaps. 11 and 13).

Treatment of Restrictive Cardiomyopathy and Diastolic Heart Disease

In haemochromatosis repeated venesection can be of value, while iron chelation therapy is appropriate for some patients and for those with thalassaemia major. There is no consistently effective treatment for cardiac amyloidosis except cardiac transplantation (see Chap. 13). The treatment of hypertrophic cardiomyopathy is dealt with in Chap. 9. Pericardial resection is the only effective treatment for constrictive pericarditis.

Table 10.4. Medical and surgical treatment of congestive heart failure in EMF

Acute inflammatory stage
Anti-inflammatory agents
Digitalis if atrial fibrillation (anticoagulants)
Diuretics
? Pericardial tap
Chronic fibrotic stage
Digitalis if atrial fibrillation
Diuretics
Anticoagulants
Endocardectomy
Atrioventricular valve replacement
Transplantation

Treatment of Löffler's Endomyocardial Disease (Table 10.4)

In the initial necrotic stage the aim of treatment is to reduce the acute inflammatory reaction, prevent the progression of the disease and discourage embolism. In the chronic fibrotic stage control of congestive heart failure and prevention of embolism are the main aims. Surgical methods consist of endocardectomy, valve replacement or transplantation.

Medical Methods

No treatment has yet been entirely successful in arresting the progress of the disease, though steroids may slow its progression. Prednisolone, 60 mg daily initially follwed by tapering doses, has been used [19, 20]. It has been suggested that prednisolone should regularly be used in the acute necrotic phase to attempt to prevent the development of the late fibrotic stage and atrioventricular valve involvement. Hydroxyurea and prednisolone have been tried with variable success [22]. Vincristine has been successful to some extent when there is thrombocytopenia and anaemia [7]. Attempts to produce haematological remission are not likely to succeed. A recent report suggests that interferon may be effective [23].

Probably the most important aspect of treatment (with the possible exception of steroids) is discouragement of thrombosis and prevention of embolism. Anticoagulants (wafarin) and antiplatelet agents (dipyridamole) may be combined with steroids. Warfarin is especially important when atrial fibrillation is present. Since eosinophilia and cationic protein activate the coagulation system and heparin can neutralise this effect, its use has been suggested [19]. Thus the mainstay of treatment is steroids, warfarin and dipyridamole in the acute stage, but there is no evidence that steroids benefit the chronic stage. The progress of treatment may have to be guided by serial biopsy or echocardiography.

Bone marrow transplantation is considered if there is evidence of disease of eopsinophil precursors in the marrow suggesting a leukaemic process [8]. Leucophoresis and plasma exchange to remove large numbers of eosinophils when the count is high and blood viscosity increase have been effective for a short period [8].

In the chronic fibrotic–thrombotic stage anticoagulants must be continued and diuretics will often be required when congestive heart failure sets in, but over-diuresis must be avoided since depletion of circulating blood volume may lead to hypotension and circulatory collapse. Atrial fibrillation will require digitalis for control of ventricular rate and amiodarone may be considered. The use of digitalis or any angent that produces bradycardia needs to be monitored with great care in sinus rhythm since tachycardia is necessary to maintain adequate preload and stroke volume. Tachycardia is also helpful when severe mitral regurgitation is present as it limits the time available for reflux to occur.

The wisdom of giving vasodilator agents such as nitrates, hydralazine and angiotensin converting enzyme inhibitors is uncertain. When ventricular volume is restricted and a high filling pressure preload is essential, reduction of afterload may impair cardiac output by reducing preload, but if ventricular dilatation has occurred then vasodilator agents may be appropriate.

Surgical Treatment (Figs. 10.9, 10.10)

Surgical treatment has been carried out since 1971 [24–26]. In the chronic stage endocardectomy is of definite, though not usually sustained, value. It should be combined with tricuspid valve and/or mitral valve replacement when indicated

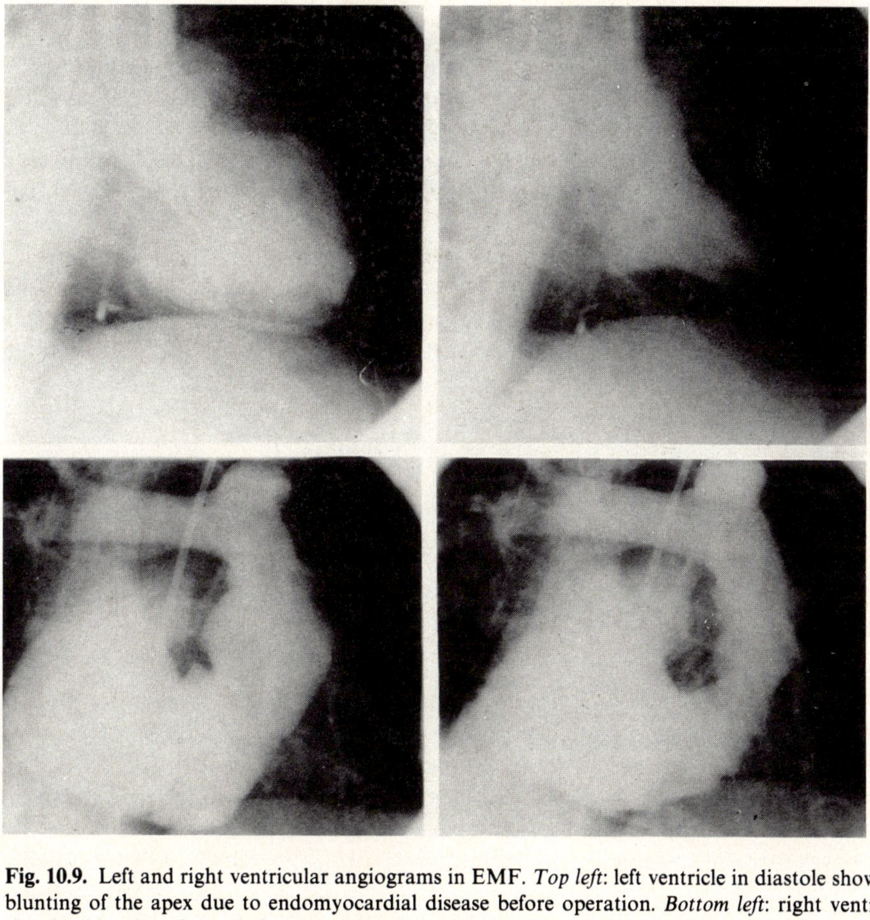

Fig. 10.9. Left and right ventricular angiograms in EMF. *Top left*: left ventricle in diastole showing blunting of the apex due to endomyocardial disease before operation. *Bottom left*: right ventricle showing blunting of apex before operation. *Top right*: left ventricle in systole after operation. *Bottom right*: right ventricle after operation showing improvement

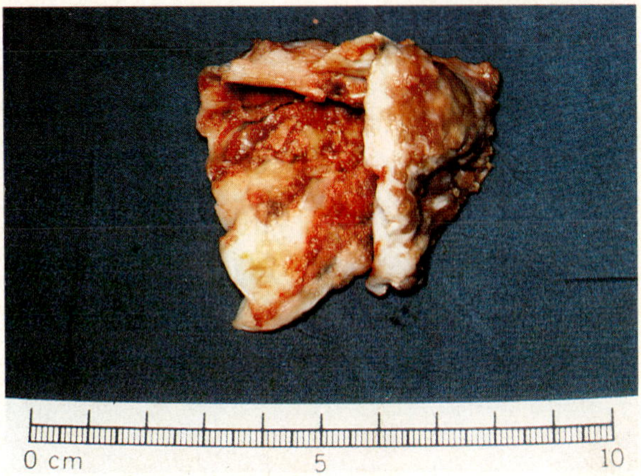

Fig. 10.10. Cast of right ventricular fibrosis with overlying thrombus removed at operation. (Courtesy of Mr. R Sapsford)

by appreciable atrioventricular valvar regurgitation. In 1980, 2 patients with severe EMF underwent surgery at Hammersmith Hospital, London, with initial improvement, though 1 relapsed with chronic heart failure due to impaired diastolic function [27]. A review of 22 other patients showed encouraging results overall without recurrence of endocardial lesions or progression of the disease for up to 7 years [19].

A new technique from Brazil for complete removal of fibrous tissue and preservation of mitral and tricuspid valves has been described in 9 patients with encouraging results [28].

It seems likely that where appropriate, valve replacement is the most effective surgical approach other than transplantation. This should be considered, but despite encouraging results caution should be shown in assuming that lasting benefit will occur, since the underlying disease is that of the eosinophil, and other organs may be involved. Cardiac surgical procedures will not affect these basic problems.

Prognosis

EMF and Löffler's endomyocardial disease are extremely serious conditions and usually prognosis is poor. While some patients in Africa may remain active though restricted for many years despite severe right-sided disease (Fig. 10.4), the condition can be rapidly fatal after a few months in the acute phase, or after a few years in the chronic phase [17]. In temperate climates earlier diagnosis improves medical treatment and encouraging surgical results have undoubtedly improved prognosis, but few patients are likely to live for more than 10 years after diagnosis, and significant numbers will die much sooner. Because of the rarity of the condition detailed evaluation of life span studies has not been possible. The poor prognosis in children is emphasised by a recent study in Abidjan [29]. Fifty-five of 98 children were treated surgically (usually with the use of a bioprosthesis). There were 10 operative deaths and 15 late postoperative deaths. Nevertheless, the surgical patients have a better prognosis than those treated medically.

References

1. Little WC, Downes TR, Applegate RJ (1990) Invasive evaluation of left ventricular diastolic performance. Herz 15: 362–376
2. Poole-Wilson PA (1990) Introduction to heart failure and diastolic dynsfunction: new insights. Eur Heart J 11 Suppl C:1
3. Goodwin JF (1985) Cardiomyopathies and specific heart muscle disease: definition, terminology and classification. In: Goodwin JF (ed) Heart muscle disease. MTP Press, Lancaster, pp 1–5
4. WHO Expert Committee (1984), Cardiomyopathies. WHO Tech Rep Ser 697
5. Wilmshurst PT, Katritsis D (1990) Editorial: restrictive cardiomyopathy. Br Heart J 63: 323–324
6. Chusid MJ, Dale DC, West BC, Wolff SM (1975) The hypereosinophilic syndrome: analysis of fourteen cases with review of the literature. Medicine (Baltimore) 54: 1–27
7. Olsen EGJ, Spry CJF (1979) The pathogenesis of Löffler's endomyocardial disease, and its relationship to endomyocardial fibrosis. In: Yu PN, Goodwin JF (eds) Lea and Febiger, Philadelphia, Progress in cardiology, vol 8 pp 281–303
8. Spry CJF, Davies J, Tai PC, Olsen EGJ, Oakley CM, Goodwin JF (1983) Clinical features of fifteen patients with the hypereosinophilic syndrome. Quart. J Med 52: 1–22
9. Parillo JE (1990) Heart disease and the eosinophil. N Engl J Med 323: 1560–1561
10. Ijaola O, Falase AO (1990) Distribution of antibodies against Coxsackie B viruses, arborvirus and *Toxoplasma gondii* among patients with endomyocardial fibrosis (EMF) compared with normal subjects form EMF endemic and non-endemic zones of Nigeria. Afr J Med Sci 19: 93–103
11. Olsen EGJ (1990) Morphological overview and pathogenetic mechanisms in endomyocardial fibrosis associated with eopsinophilia. In: Olsen EGJ, Sekiguchi M (eds) Restrictive cardiomyopathy and arrhythmias. University of Tokyo Press, Tokyo, pp 1–8 (Cardiomyopathy update 3)
12. Bedford DE, Konstam GLS (1946) Heart failure of unknown aetiology in Africans. Br Heart J 8: 216–237
13. Davies JNP (1948) Endocardial fibrosis in Africans. East Afr Med J 25: 10–14
14. Vijayaraghavan G, Sadanandan S, Cherian G (1990) Endomyocardial fibrosis in India: an overview. In: Cardiomyopathy update 3) Olsen EGJ, Sekiguchi M (eds) Restrictive cardiomyopathy and arrhythmias. University of Tokyo Press, Tokyo, pp 9–20
15. Brockington IF, Olsen EGJ (1973) Löffler's endocarditis and Davies endocardial fibrosis. Am Heart J 85: 308–322
16. WHO/ISFC (1980) Report of the Task Force on the definition and classification of cardiomyopathies. Br Heart J 44: 672–673
17. Parry EHO (1964) Endomyocardial fibrosis. Ciba Found Symp 322–352
18. Cohen J, Davies J, Goodwin JF, Spry CJ (1980) Arrhythmias in patients with hypereosinophilia: a comparison of patients with and without Löffler's endomyocardial disease. Post Grad Med J 56: 828–832
19. Spry CJF, Tai PC (1990) Clinical studies on endomyocardial fibrosis in patients with hypereosinophilia: an historical review. In: Olsen EGJ, Sekiguchi M (eds) Restrictive cardiomyopathy and Arrhythmias. University of Tokyo Press, Tokyo, pp 81–98 (Cardiomyopathy update 3)
20. Davies J, Spry CJ, Sapsford R, Olsen EGJ, de Perez G, Oakley CM, Goodwin JF (1983) Cardiovascular features of eleven patients with eosinophilic endomyocardial disease. Q J Med 52: 23–39

21. Chew C, Ziady GM, Raphael MJ, Oakley CM (1975) The functional defect in amyloid heart disease: the stiff heart syndrome. Am J Cardiol 36: 438–444
22. Parillo F, Fanci AS, Wolff SM (1978) Therapy of the hypereosinophilic syndrome. Ann Intern Med 89: 167
23. Zielinski RM, Lawrence WD (1990) Interferon alpha for the hypereosinophilic syndrome. Ann Intern Med 113: 716–718
24. Dubost C, Maurice P, Gerbaux A et al. (1977) L'endocardite fibreuse constrictive: Traitement chirugicale. Arch Mal Coeur 70: 155–162
25. Moraes CR, Buffolo E, Lime R et al. (1983) Surgical treatment of endomyocardial fibrosis. J Thorac Cardiovasc Surg 85: 738–745
26. John I, Mani GK, Muralidharans S, Krishnaswany Y, Cherian G (1980) Endomyocardial fibrosis from a surgical standpoint. J Thorac Cardiovasc Surg 80: 437–440
27. Davies J, Sapsford R, Brooksby I, Olsen EGJ, Spry CJ, Oakley CM, Goodwin JF (1981) Succcessful treatment of two patients with eosinophilic endomyocardial disease. Br Heart J 46: 438–445
28. De Oliveira SA, Barreto ACP, Mady C, Dallan LA de O, Lemos da Luz P, Jatene AD, Pileggi F (1990) Surgical treatment of endomyocardial fibrosis: a new approach. J Am Coll Cardiol 16: 1246–1251
29. Kakou-Gulkahue M, Chauvet J, Zabsome P, Tanank Y, Metros D, Ticolat R, Longechand A, Ekra A, Quezzin-Coulibaly A, Bexhaid ED (1991) Endocardite pariétale clinique Chez l'enfant: indications cliniques, résultat et évolution post-opération chez 98 enfants (ayant 55 opérés). Cardiol Trop 1: 71

CHAPTER 11

Pathology

E. G. J. Olsen and S. E. Trotter

According to the WHO/ISFC Task Force [1] recommendation endomyocardial fibrosis and Löffler's endocarditis parietialis fibroplastica have been included in the category of restrictive cardiomyopathy. It has been proposed that these conditions should be referred to as eosinophilic endomyocardial disease. Obliteration of the cavity is usually observed in advanced cases [1]. Excluded from the Task Force recommendation is amyloid disease; although presenting with restrictive signs and symptoms it is not included because it is an example of specific heart muscle disease, except in cases in which the amyloid disease is confined to the heart (see Chaps. 1 and 13).

At one time Löffler's endocarditis parietialis fibroplastica was believed to be confined to the temperate zones. Endomyocardial fibrosis was initially believed to be confined to Uganda, its range subsequently being extended to the tropical and subtropical region as reports from these areas appeared in the literature. Irrespective of geographical distribution the two conditions are new considered to be one entity [2,3]. Concurrently with another group of workers [4] Brockington and Olsen [5] examined retrospectively 91 autopsy-proven cases of endomyocardial disease associated with eosinophilia. Three major histological groups were identified dependent upon the length of history. If this had, on average, lasted for 5 weeks an initial necrotic stage was recognisable. This consisted of an intense eosinophilic cellular infiltrate with all the features of myocarditis (Fig. 11.1), together with vasculitis in the areas of inflammation; necrosis of myocytes was typical. When the length of history was on average 10 months, the thrombotic stage had been attained. The inflammatory cell infiltrate had largely abated, vascular connective tissue separating bundles of cardiac myocytes had made its appearance and endocardial thickening had become manifest. The striking histomorphological change was, however, thrombotic occlusion of some intramyocardial vessels and often severe superimposition of thrombus on the thickened endocardium. Finally, the fibrotic stage was reached, which was seen when the length of history was on average of $2\frac{1}{2}$ years. This was characterised by severe thickening of the endocardium (Fig. 11.2). Normally, ventricular endocardium is at its thickest in the left ventricular outflow tract, where it attains 20 μm. In endomyocardial disease thicknesses of 5 mm are regularly seen. This immensely thick endocardium is arranged in layers (Fig. 11.3). Superficially, a thin layer of thrombus of fibrin is identifiable over a layer of dense collagen tissue. This layer may also contain elastic fibres of varying

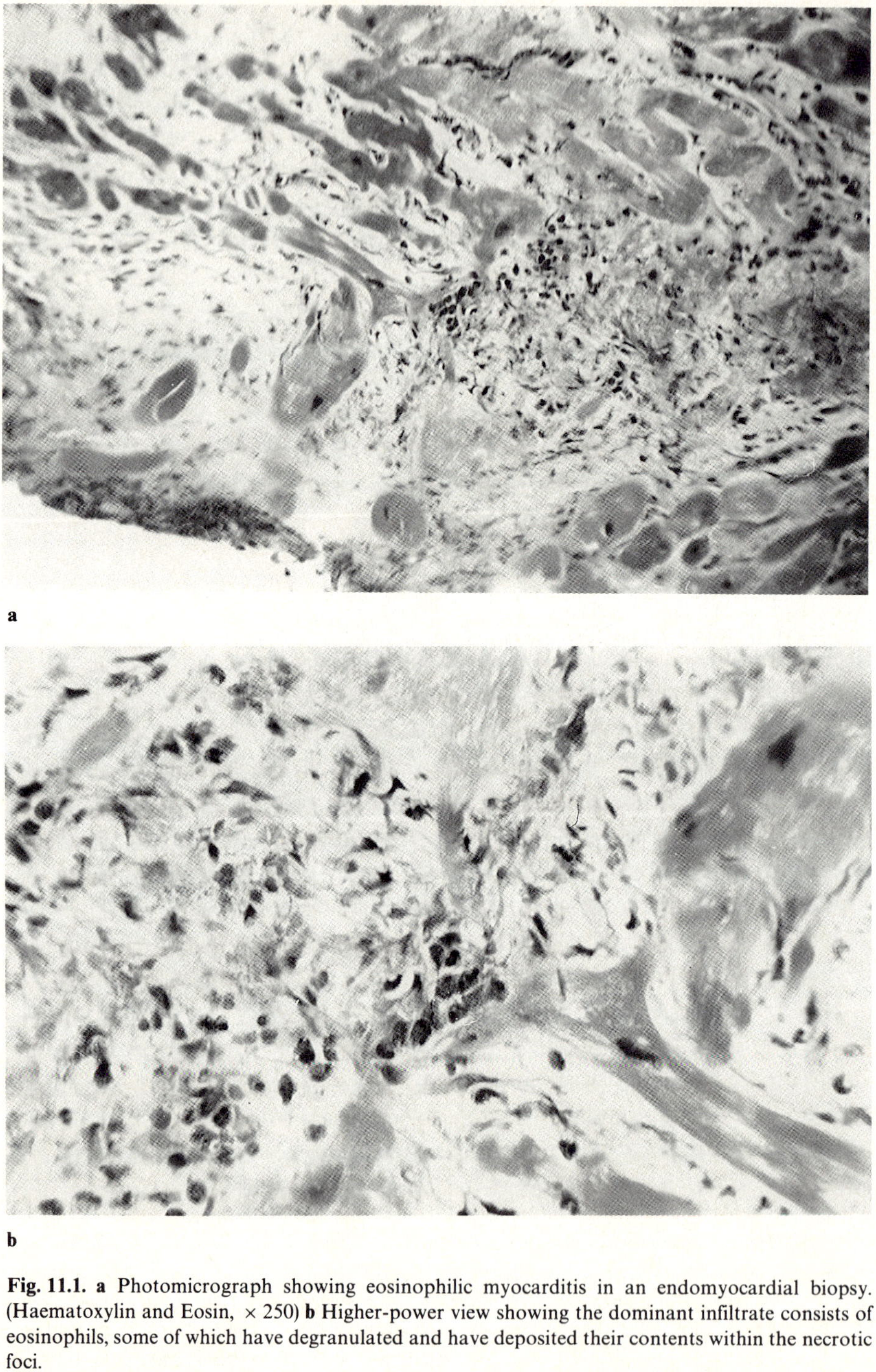

Fig. 11.1. a Photomicrograph showing eosinophilic myocarditis in an endomyocardial biopsy. (Haematoxylin and Eosin, × 250) **b** Higher-power view showing the dominant infiltrate consists of eosinophils, some of which have degranulated and have deposited their contents within the necrotic foci.

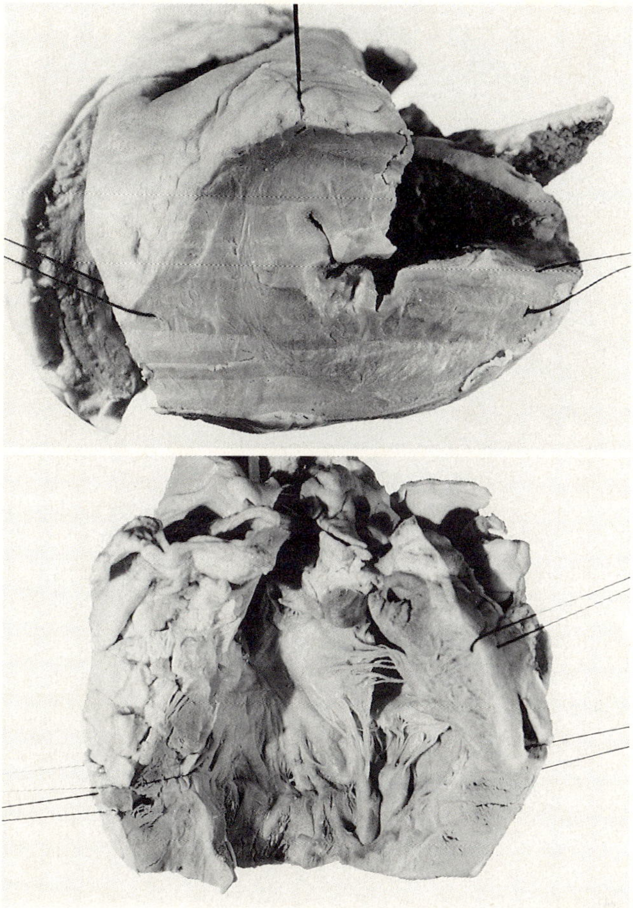

Fig. 11.2. **a** Cross section of a heart affected by endomyocardial fibrosis. Thickening of the endocardium is evident, with fibrous trabeculae extending into the myocardium. **b** The heart has been opened to expose the left ventricle. The thickened endocardium is seen apically and encroaches on the papillary muscles

distribution and sheet-like areas of calcification. The deepest layer, the granulation tissue layer, consists of loosely arranged connective tissue containing vascular and lymphatic channels and inflammatory cells including occasional eosinophils. From this deepest layer septa extend to varying degrees into the myocardium, occasionally reaching the sub-epicardium. The intramyocardial vessels, apart from occasional fibroelastic intimal changes, showed no specific morphological features.

As far as the macroscopic changes are concerned, serpiginous depressions haphazardly distributed in the ventricular myocardium are recognisable on the cut surface. Occasionally, haemorrhagic areas can also be identified. This is

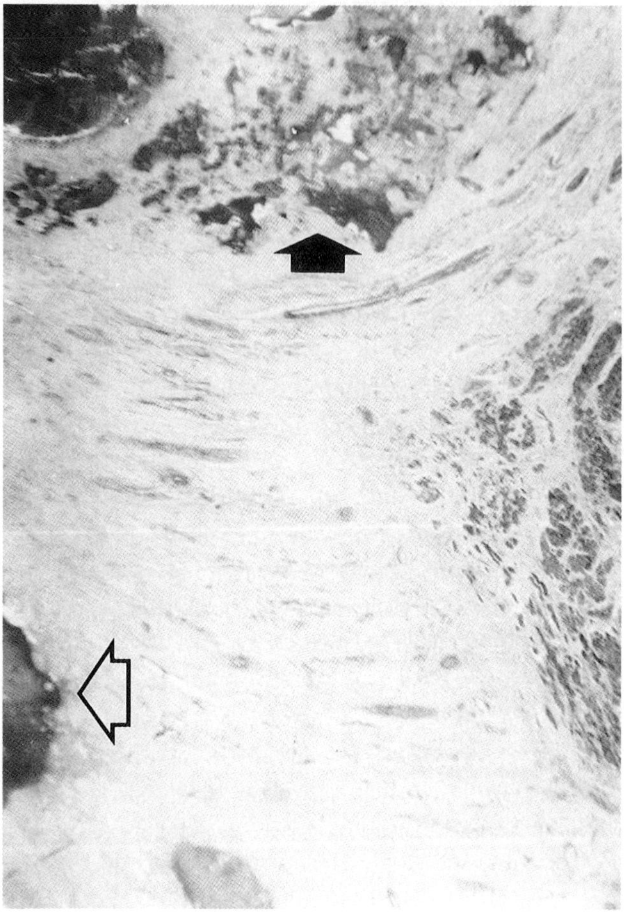

Fig. 11.3. Photomicrograph of the thickened endocardium. The tissue shows characteristic layering. Superficially there is thrombus (*black arrow*), and deeper fibrous tissue which shows an area of calcification (*open arrow*). Abutting onto the myocardium there is a vascular "granulation tissue" layer. Note the fibrous tissue extending into the myocardium. (Haematoxylin and eosin, × 250)

observed in the necrotic phase. In the thrombotic stage thrombus superimposition occasionally so severe as to obliterate the affected ventricular cavity is occasionally encountered. Typically, thrombus in the right ventricle is more prominent at the apex.

The fibrotic stage is characterised by an intense endocardial thickening. In left ventricular disease the inflow tract, the apex and part of the outflow tract are typically involved. When the region of the anterior mitral valve leaflet is reached the thick endocardium ceases abruptly, often ending in a thick rolled edge [6]. The posterior mitral valve leaflet, the papillary muscles and chordae tendineae are frequently involved by the disease process. Septa noted histologically can often clearly be seen macroscopically. The epicardium is unremarkable and the extra-mural coronary arteries are usually normal. In a study of 175 cases the thick endocardium was not invariably distributed as detailed above, but could involve on rare occasions the outflow tract or be haphazardly distributed [3].

In right ventricular involvement the apex is obliterated by thick endocardium and an area beneath the posterior (and part of the septal) leaflet also shows severe endocardial thickening. As the disease proceeds the apex becomes progressively drawn towards the tricuspid valve, giving externally the cardiac shadow of a W. In the retrospective study [5] 16 cases belonged to the fibrotic stage. When these were compared with 75 cases from Uganda, Nigeria and Brazil, no difference whatsoever could be observed in the fibrosis in terms of thickness, distribution, macroscopic appearances or histological arrangement, and it was concluded that Löffler's endocarditis and endomyocardial fibrosis belonged to the same disease spectrum, the origin of which could be traced back to the presence of abnormal eosinophils in the myocardium (see Chap. 10).

Subsequent examination of the eosinophils showed that these were abnormal. At the histological level, and observed in the blood stream, degranulation of the eosinophilic granular content were frequently observed [3, 7]. Decrease of granular content was sometimes so severe that electron microscopic examination had to be undertaken, which, in addition to degranulation of varying severity, also showed also mitochondrial changes [3]. These abnormal eosinophils also possessed receptors for rabbit IgG-coated erythrocytes and actively phagocytosed erythrocytes coated with rabbit IgG or human C3b [8]. It was found that if 20% of the circulating eosinophils showed vacuoles ($> 1.5 \times 10^9$/litre) and over 15%, i.e. $> 1 \times 10^9$/litre showed degranulation, endomyocardial disease was invariably present, proven by examination of endomyocardial biopsies even in the absence of clinical symptomatology. The cause of eosinophilia varied. In the retrospective study [5] in approximately 50% of patients the eosinophilia was idiopathic. In 25% of cases it was reactive consequent to polyarteritis nodosa, antituberculous therapy and parasitic infection. (This list has now been extended to include T cell lymphoma and others [3]). Twenty-two cases were considered to have eosinophillic leukaemia. Only 5 patients had a stem cell crisis, and it is therefore possible that most of these patients, thus labelled, had an intense eosinophilia.

The pathogenetic process of endomyocardial disease has been considered to take place as follows: As a result of stimulation causing an unmasking of Fc receptors for lgG (C3b) exocytosis of granular material cationic proteins resulted. By means of the microcirculation these stimulated granules reached the subendocardial region of the ventricular walls, together with substances such as peroxidase, resulting in intense myocarditis (the necrotic stage). The endocardium was often destroyed, resulting in superimposition of thrombus. It has further been shown that the cationic proteins are known to be thrombogenic [3, 9]. This explains the thrombotic stage. The fibrotic stage is the healed phase of the thrombotic stage. Studies with purified eosinophil granule basic proteins have been shown to act on the plasma membrane and pyruvic dehydrogenase and 2-oxygluterate dehydrogenase [10]. It has further been shown that the activated eosinophils, compared with normal eosinophils, have a surface charge activation of lysosomal acid phosphatase, membrane hexose transport and hexose transport monophosphate shunt activities [11]. Furthermore, the tissue-damaging effect of eosinophils is likely to be due to the granule and intracytoplasmic contents. Toxic substances have been identified, including neurotoxins [12] and eosinophil major basic proteins [13, 14], that are likely to result in induction of damage to epithelial cells [15] (see Chap. 10).

Furthermore, the incidence of the disease varies in different regions and also seasonal variations are encountered. These findings are unexplained, but the association of cardiac disease with abnormal eosinophils has become established. With this certainty in mind, it is therefore proposed that the condition should perhaps be re-classified under "specific heart muscle disease" rather than "cardiomyopathy". This suggestion is, however, controversial (see Chaps. 1 and 10).

An interesting theory has been reviewed by Gravanis [16]. It has been suggested that cardiotropic viral infection may be responsible for initial tissue damage, controlled by a mononuclear cell response, resulting in arrest of viraemia. Lymphocytes may make their appearance and there may be a release of eosinophilic haemotactic and eosinophilic differentiating factors, as well as substances such as lymphokines studied in long-term bone marrow cultures. Eosinophilic differentiating factors and other lymphokines may cause activation of eosinophils, resulting in unmasking of Fc receptors, and may have a cytolytic anti-viral and anticardiac tissue-specific (autoimmune) antibody on the cell surface. The presence of eosinophils activated by local eosinophilic haemotactic factors migrated to the heart, attack the damaged cardiac tissue, resulting in degranulation and induction of cytocidal effects leading to necrosis, thrombosis and finally, fibrosis. Much work remains to be done.

Endomyocardial Biopsies

Until about 1986 only 23 cases in which the principal diagnosis was eosinophilic heart disease were encountered in a total of nearly 2000 cases. Since the various publications [3, 5 and especially 7, 8], awareness of this entity has been stimulated and a total of 150 patients have now been obtained from these suspected cases (in a total of nearly 3000 patients). Personal examination by one of us (EGJO) of the tissue has revealed that in just over 50% of these cases a positive result has been found, especially in the early necrotic stage. In some cases biopsy had been performed in the absence of cardiac symptoms on the evidence of the blood film showing a significant number of degranulated eosinophils, irrespective of the severity of the eosinophilia. Even in the presence of a normal eosinophil count, if over 15% of these cells showed degranulation endomyocardial disease was observed.

Biopsies taken in the fibrotic stage have often resulted in negative samples. This can be explained on technical grounds as the bioptome may slip off the thick endocardium and sample unaffected regions.

In more recent years a group of patients has been recognised who have the signs and symptoms of restrictive haemodynamics without eosinophilia, affecting primarily the myocardium rather than the endocardium. An increase in interstitial fibrous tissue, focal or diffuse in distribution, has been interpreted as offering the likely explanation for the clinical manifestations. In other instances, mild endocardial thickening was all that was found. Occasionally, no morphological abnormalities have been detected, even though restrictive haemodynamics have been present. Personal observations have shown occasionally non-specific endocardial thickening and changes indistinguishable from dilated cardiomyopathy (see Chap. 10).

As far as classification is concerned, it is this group of cases for which no cause has, so far, been identified, nor any consistent morphological changes been established, that constitutes true restrictive cardiomyopathy.

Differential Diagnosis

A thick endocardium is found in several conditions, for example in infantile fibroelastosis where the thick endocardium has distinct histological features consisting of regularly arranged bundles of elastic tissue. Macroscopically the distribution of the thick endocardium which resembles candle grease, affects the outflow tract of the left or right ventricles and encases the trabeculae of the ventricular cavities, which are usually obliterated in all other types of endocardial thickening. Furthermore, the semilunar valves are frequently involved [17]. In myocardial infarction endocardial thickening overlying the infarcted area may also be extremely thick, but the histological changes do not include the characteristic layering seen in endomyocardial disease: instead they are haphazardly arranged and involve all endocardial components (collagen, elastic and smooth muscle fibres). In carcinoid heart disease the macroscopic distribution is typically in the right ventricular outflow tract beneath the pulmonary valve. Histologically, superimposition of mucoid-rich tissue overlying normal endocardium devoid of elastic tissue helps to distinguish this condition from endomyocardial disease [18].

Early recognition and timely treatment are essential, and in endomyocardial disease associated with eosinophilia estimation of the serum cationic proteins has also been shown to be of diagnostic value [3]. Examination of the blood film and the appearance of degranulated eosinophils in significant numbers clinch the diagnosis.

References

1. WHO/ISFC (1980) Task Force report on the definition and classification of cardiomyopathies. Br Heart J 44: 672–673
2. Oakley CM, Olsen EGJ (1977) Eosinophilia and heart disease (Editorial). Br Heart J 39: 233–237

3. Olsen EGJ, Spry CJF (1979) The pathogenesis of Löffler's endomyocardial disease, and its relationship to endomyocardial fibrosis. In: Yu PN, Goodwin JF (eds) Progress in cardiology, vol 8. Lea and Febiger, Philadelphia, pp 281–303
4. Roberts WC, Ferrans VJ (1975) Pathologic anatomy of the cardiomyopathies:idiopathic dilated and hypertrophic types, infiltrative types, and endomyocardial disease with and without eosinophilia. Hum Pathol 6: 287–342
5. Brokington IF, Olsen EGJ (1973) Löffler's endocarditis and Davies' endomyocardial fibrosis. Am Heart J 85: 308–322
6. Davies JNP (1968) The ridge in endomyocardial fibrosis. Lancet 1: 631–632
7. Spry CJF, Tai PC (1976) Studies on blood eosinophils. II. Patients with Löffler's cardiomyopathy. Clin Exp Immunol 24: 423–434
8. Tai PC, Spry CJF (1976) Studies on blood eosinophils. I. Patients with a transient eosinophilia. Clin Exp Immunol 24: 415–422
9. Venge P, Dahl R, Hollgren R et al. (1980) Cationic proteins of eosinophils and their role in the inflammatory reaction. In: Mahmoud AAF, Austin KF (eds) The eosinophil in health and disease. Grune and Stratton, New York, pp 131–144
10. Spry CJF, Tai PC, Davies J (1983) The cardiotoxicity of eosinophils. Postgrad Med J 59: 147–158
11. Bass DA, Grover WH, Lewis JC et al. (1980) Comparison of human eosinophils from normals and patients with eosinophilia. J Clin Invest 66: 1265–1273
12. Durack DT, Sumi SM, Klebanoff SJ (1979) Neurotoxicity of human eosinophils. Proc Natl Acad Sci USA 76: 1443–1447
13. Gleich GJ, Loegering DA, Frigas E et al. (1980) The major basic protein of the eosinophil granule: physicochemical properties, localization, and function. In: Mahmoud AAF, Austin KF (eds) The eosinophil in health and disease. Grune and Stratton, New York, pp 79–77
14. Gleich GJ, Loegering DA, Maldonado JE(1973)Identification of a major basic protein in guinea pig eosinophil granules. J Exp Med 137: 1459–1471
15. Gleich GJ, Frigas E, Loegering DA et al. (1979) Cytotoxic properties of the eosinophil major basic protein, J Immunol 123: 2925–2927
16. Gravanis MB (1987) Cardiovascular pathophysiology. McGraw-Hill, New York, pp 191–193
17. Olsen EGJ (1980) The pathology of the heart, 2nd edn. Macmillan, London, pp 327–329
18. Olsen EGJ (1980) The pathology of the heart, 2nd edn. Macmillan, London, pp 59–61

CHAPTER 12

Doppler Echocardiographic Investigations

H. Acquatella

Restrictive cardiomyopathy is characterised by abnormal filling of the ventricles, consisting of a disproportionate rise in ventricular pressure in early diastole for a given increase in volume. Pathological changes in endomyocardial disease (with or without hypereosinophilia) affect ventricular compliance by unknown mechanisms leading to a restrictive pattern of filling. This haemodynamic profile is usually documented by cardiac catheterisation but may be recognised non-invasively by pulsed Doppler echocardiography of mitral and tricuspid inflow velocities. This profile consists of a short isovolumic relaxation time, increased peak early inflow velocity, increased early deceleration time, decreased late atrial inflow peak velocity, and an increased ratio of early/late peak flow velocities. Vena cava and pulmonary venous blood flow velocities disclose predominant filling during early diastole and severe blunting of normal antegrade systolic flow. This restrictive profile is also presented by other endocardial or myocardial conditions. In pericardial constriction similar findings exist, but contrary to restriction these are greatly influenced by respiration. Endomyocardial biopsy is the diagnostic technique of choice during the early stages of endomyocardial disease. Two-dimensional echocardiography has increased the detection of endomyocardial fibrosis by showing a peculiar distribution of abnormal endocardium, obliteration of the ventricular apex, and the combination of near-normal-sized ventricles with dilated atria.

Restrictive cardiomyopathy is the least common of the three cardiomyopathies. By definition [1] it includes the classical tropical endomyocardial fibrosis (EMF) observed in Africa [2, 3], South America [4, 5] and India [6], and the hypereosinophilic endomyocardial disease of temperate countries [7–10]. As it has been demonstrated that the two entities are pathologically indistinguishable [11–13] the report of the WHO/ISFC Task Force [1] and a committee of the World Health Organization suggested that both clinical forms should be called "eosinophilic endomyocardial disease". With the exception of some regions of Africa [14] and India [15], endomyocardial disease is an infrequent cause of heart failure. Endomyocardial fibrosis (with and without hypereosinophilia) presents with the clinical and haemodynamic signs of a restrictive/constrictive physiology [16–22]. This consists in an abnormality of ventricular filling leading to severe venous congestion and manifested haemodynamically by an abrupt increase in ventricular pressure after early diastole in respone to small changes in volume [19, 23–28]. Systolic function may be normal or relatively spared. Restrictive physiology may be caused by other endocardial, endomyocardial or myocardial abnormalities [28], and therefore can be observed in various cardiac conditions. When extensive investigations in these patients do not unravel an aetiological factor the term "restrictive cardiomyopathy" is also used [27, 28]. Here the clinical and pathological findings of early endomyocardial disease and of endomyocardial fibrosis, and the usefulness of Doppler echocardiography in the recognition of restriction, are analysed (see Chaps. 10 and 13).

Acute/Necrotic and Thrombotic Stages of EMF

Most patients may display fever, rash, and a normal heart size and function at the onset of an acute hypereosinophilic syndrome [29, 30]. The initial acute/necrotic stage of eosinophilic myocarditis may be suspected on clinical grounds by the appearance of tachycardia and cardiomegaly with systemic and pulmonary venous congestion [30]. Degranulated eosinophils in peripheral blood smears should make one suspicious of eosinophilic myocarditis [21] and support the indication of endomyocardial biopsy [21, 22]. Cardiac hamodynamics may disclose a non-specific profile of florid congestive heart failure [30–32] with no evidence of restriction. In the few 2D echocardiographic reports from the literature obtained during this acute phase, non-specific ventricular dilatation with diminished cardiac contractility was found [30, 32, 33]. As the process advances to the thrombotic phase, subtle echocardiographic apical irregularities may be detected [29]. The most striking echographic finding in the acute hypereosinophilic stage is the demostration of apical thrombus superimposed on an akinetic or dyskinetic apex [34]. This is not specific, as up to 27% of cases of acute viral myocarditis may also present apical thrombus [37], and may have a similar echographic appearance. Electrocardiographic evidence of necrosis (QS wave) simulating myocardial infarction may be found [32] which may prompt coronary angiography to exclude coronary heart disease. A variety of cardiac manifestations other than endocardial restriction are shown by patients with hypereosinophilia, including congestive heart failure, arrhythmia, conduction disturbances and myopericarditis [32].

Fibrotic Stage of EMF

The scarring process leading to endomyocardial fibrosis is the origin of clinical restriction. Most echographic reports from the literature have focused on this late fibrotic stage of the disease [4, 6, 17, 29, 30a, 31, 34–36, 39–44]. The 2D echographic appearance is striking (Fig. 12.1), consisting in the combination of normal or slightly dilated ventricles with mildly dilated to huge atria and, most

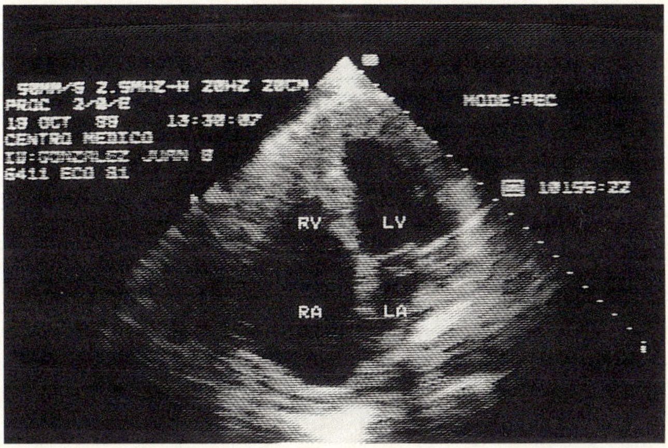

Fig. 12.1. Echographic four-chamber apical view from a patient with severe biventricular endomyocardial fibrosis, confirmed at autopsy. Note the apical obliteration by thick endocardium more pronounced in the right ventricle (*RV*) than in the left ventricle (*LV*), and the ventricular size contrast with the huge right atrium (*RA*). The left atrium (*LA*) appears tangentially obtained for technical reasons. The patient was in severe congestive heart failure

importantly, a peculiar distribution of fibrotic patches at the ventricular endocardial surface (Fig. 12. 2) [4, 41]. This pattern of localised fibrosis was described in detail in classic pathological work from Uganda [3]. Five preferential areas of ventricular endocardial fibrosis were observed at autopsy: in type 1 affecting only the apex with variable extension along the inflow tract; in type 2 extending from the apex to the mitral or tricuspid posterior valve along the inflow tract; in type 3 isolated valvar lesions; in type 4 at the apex and valvar regions

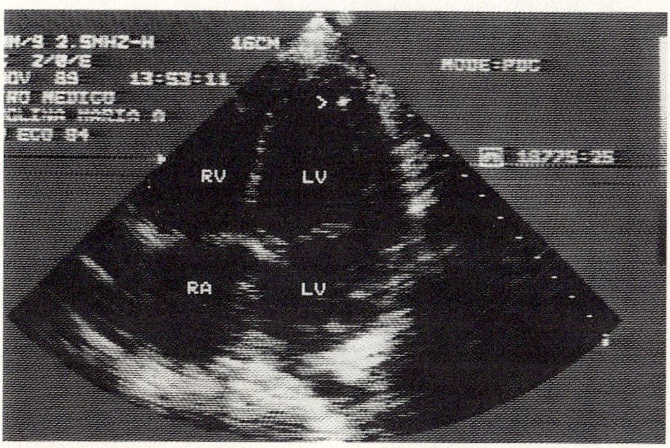

Fig. 12.2. Small echogenic fibrotic endocardial patch (>) overlying a partially obliterated left ventricular apex in a patient with mild symptoms. Abbreviations as in Fig. 12.1

without fibrosis of the intervening myocardium; and in type 5 in areas other than the apex or valves.

In those patients having left ventricular apical obliteration bright echoes of the endocardial surface are frequently seen moving inwards in systole [4]. The preservation of apical contraction in the majority of subjects with endomyocardial fibrosis contrasts with the dyskinetic apical thrombosis of myocardial infarction or of chronic Chagas' heart disease [4]. In these two conditions the apical myocardium, being ischaemic or fibrotic, will show an outward dyskinetic motion. Apical obliteration is found in most but not all patients [29, 41]. The thrombosed left ventricular apex may show a rounded appearance angiography while the right may have a "cut-off" shape [16–18]. Dilatation of the right ventricular infundibulum, greatly thickened tricuspid valves, severe tricuspid regurgitation, right ventricular volume overload and paradoxical septal motion are echo findings in the right heart [10, 31, 34, 36, 39].

An important echographic feature is fibrosis in patches filling the left ventricular cavity immediately below the mitral valve [34, 39, 41]. The posterobasal wall may only show diminished motion [41] as a subtle abnormality on M-mode tracings. The submitral and apical areas of fibrosis may constitute embolic sources which frequently complicate the clinical course of patients [41]. Left atrial thrombus of embolic potential (Fig. 12.3) can be detected also by transoesophageal echocardiography, which offers a unique posterior window on the area [4, 5]. Mild to severe mitral and/or tricuspid regurgitation is frequently present, and may in part be due to retraction and scarring of the posterior valve into the adjacent posterior ventricular wall [41]. Advances in instrumentation, including colour-coded amplitude-processing 2D echocardiographic imaging depicting regions of varying intensity, have demonstrated the distribution of

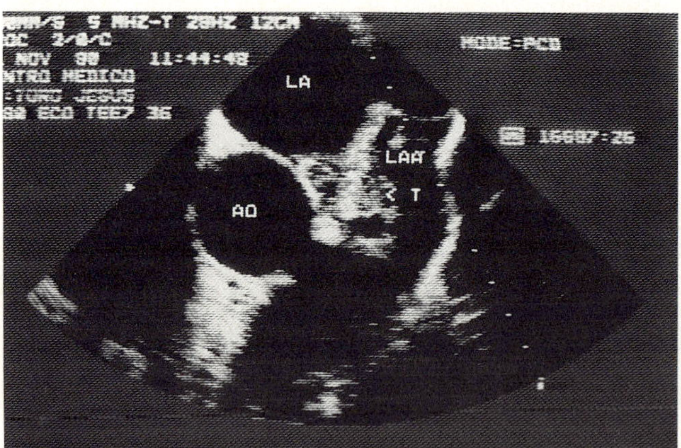

Fig. 12.3. Basal transoesophageal echocardiographic view of the left atrial appendage (*LAA*) from a patient with hypereosinophilic endomyocardial fibrosis shows a mobile thrombotic mass (< *T*) not seen with transthoracic echo. *AO*, aortic root

endocardial fibrotic areas, thus providing valuable information on the extent and severity of the disease [29].

M-mode echocardiographic findings of restrictive/constrictive physiology may be seen, such as a rapid early diastolic posterior motion of the left ventricular posterior wall [17, 29, 31, 46]. A rapid septal protodiastolic anterior "bounce" [34, 40], secondary to the abrupt early ventricular filling, may look on M-mode like an inverted dip and plateau [39]. This depends on the complex interplay between the two ventricular pressures, which might at a particular moment be greater in one chamber than the other [29].

Intraventricular pressure tracings display the square root pattern with unequal diastolic pressures between the ventricles [18, 29]. Digitised M-mode echocardiograms disclose two patterns of abnormal filling. When mitral regurgitation exists there is a decreased duration of rapid filling and increased peak rate of filling. When no mitral incompetence is present filling is normal or tracings show a reduced peak rate and prolonged duration of filling. No specific changes in eosinophilic myocardial disease were observed by digitised M-mode [29]. Other M-mode echocardiographic studies have shown increased left ventricular wall thickness and mass [47]. Small to large pericardial effusions are observed in some patients [4, 17, 43, 47] (see Chap. 10).

Ventricular and Atrial Filling: Usefulness of Doppler Echocardiography

Normal Findings

Diastole is a complex phenomenon, extensively studied by cardiac haemodynamics, in which for a given change in ventricular volume a change in intracardiac pressure occurs. It is divided (at a normal heart rate) [48–50] into an initial isovolumic relaxation period, a rapid-filling phase, a middle slow-filling phase or "diastasis", and a late atrial contraction period. Correlation studies between cineangiography and pulsed Doppler echocardiography have substantiated non-invasive estimation of ventricular filling dynamics [49–52]. These techniques nevertheless provide only partial information on diastolic function, as atrial and ventricular pressure are not measured. Changes in relaxation or filling observed by Doppler echocardiography should therefore be interpreted within the limitations imposed by the method.

Isovolumic relaxation begins with the closure of the aortic valves and lasts until the ventricular pressure falls below the atrial pressure [49, 50]. The monoexponential analysis of the left ventricular isovolumic pressure tracing or time constant of relaxation τ is used as an index. Non-invasive estimations of the isovolumic relaxation time include the phonocardiographic measurement from the aortic valve closure to the opening of the mitral valve [26, 49, 52], and the time recorded between valvar aortic closure and mitral opening, obtained by continuous wave Doppler intersection of the left ventricular outflow tract and mitral valve motion [26]. Rapid filling lasts from the opening of the mitral valves to peak ventricular filling. The pressure gradient between the left atrium and ventricle will influence peak filling rate. The initial rapid filling part of diastole will be influenced by abnormalities of ventricular relaxation, atrioventricular pressure gradient driving force, passive ventricular compliance, viscoelastic properties of the myocardium, and ventricular diastolic suction [48–50]. Active relaxation begins during the isovolumic period and extends further into the rapid filling phase; it takes one third of diastolic time for about 80% of ventricular filling to occur. During this time heart muscle fibres return to thier initial length and force, and active metabolic calcium extrusion takes place. As relaxation extends during rapid ventricular filling, other factors such as myocardial elastic recoil, viscoelastic forces, erectile effect of the coronary arteries, and passive ventricular compliance will influence the relation between pressures and volume. Loading conditions of the ventricle and of left atrial pressure will influence this ratio. After relaxation ceases a passive slow-filling phase ensues during which for a given ventricular volume increase a relatively small ventricular pressure change occurs. Approximately 5% filling occurs at a normal heart rate, but during tachycardia there is no time left for diastasis. Myocardial and chamber stiffness, and passive ventricular compliance might limit the increase in cavity size. At end-diastole, atrial contraction completes ventricular filling, contributing approximately 15% of the total volume. The late diastolic atrial-dependent ventricular filling might be influenced by the intrinsic atrial contractility, high end-diastolic ventricular pressure, and passive ventricular compliance or myocardial stiffness.

These three diastolic periods have previously been assessed clinically by high-fidelity pressure tracings and accurate time-consuming, angiographic volume measurements of the left ventricle [48–52], which it is not feasible to use on large groups of patients. The introduction of Doppler echocardiography to evaluate ventricular diastolic filling has created great interest because of its relative simplicity and repeatability in the same patient during changing conditions and at different times [26, 49–52]. Pulsed wave Doppler allows measurement of blood velocity within the cardiac chambers or across the mitral and tricuspid valves. Blood flow at the tip of the atrioventricular valve reflects the highest velocities produced by the driving forces. Good technical recording should demonstrate the opening clicks of the atrioventricular valve [26]. The beginning of mitral inflow reflects mitral opening. An initial high-velocity inflow rapidly peaks, representing filling in early (E) diastole. Acceleration time is measured from mitral valve opening to peak E velocity. This is followed by a decrease in velocities which is linear initially. Deceleration time is measured by linear extrapolation from Peak E velocity to the baseline of the Doppler tracing. During mid-diastole forward flow velocity is low, but might increase slightly because of venous (pulmonary or caval) flow. In late diastole normal atrial contraction increases blood velocity inflow again (A velocity). There is a normal range for mirtal and tricuspid Doppler measurements of peak E and A velocities

(E/A ratios), early inflow acceleration and deceleration velocities, and isovolumic relaxation time [19].

Late atrial filling can be assessed either by transthoracic pulsed Doppler of pulmonary veins with the sample volume positioned at their left atrial opening from a four-chamber apical window [53] or, more recently, from a transoesophageal window [54]. Pulminary flow velocities normally show a biphasic systolic and diastolic inflow pattern [53, 54]. The initial systolic component (while the mitral valve is normally closed) reflects the normal atrial filling when the left atrium is relaxed and the mitral annulus has an apical systolic descent. All these components contribute to a decreased left atrial pressure and optimise atrial filling. The second component of the biphasic inflow occurs in mid-diastole. After the conclusion of systole and opening of the mitral valve, the mitral annulus rapidly recoils in early diastole simultaneously with the rapid diastolic mitral inflow E wave and left ventricular filling: the rapid left atrial emptying decreases its pressure allowing a diastolic inflow from the pulmonary veins. Right atrial filling is commonly evaluated by pulsed Doppler of the inferior and hepatic veins from a subcostal window and of the superior vena cava from the suprasternal or right supraclavicular position [55]. Negative anterograde flows are observed in systole and diastole, corresponding to the x and y troughs of catheterisation venous tracings. Brief retrograde flows (positive) are observed at end-systole and at atrial contraction. Respiration profoundly influences the velocities and shapes of these wave forms [19, 26, 55].

Abnormal Filling in Restriction

Doppler echocardiography studies in endomyocardial fibrosis are scarce [56, 57]. Most recent publications on Doppler findings in a haemodynamically documented restrictive ventricular filling included various other conditions such as cardiac amyloidosis, myocarditis, idiopathic restriction, cardiac transplant, ventricular hypertrophy and infiltrative disorders [19, 26, 28, 50]. All showed a haemodynamics and Doppler profile indistinguishable from endomyocardial fibrosis.

The endocardial and myocardial pathological processes leading to the restriction [26–28, 49, 50] seen in endomyocardial fibrosis [17, 18, 29] affect ventricular compliance by poorly understood mechanisms. This results in a large abnormal increment in early diastolic ventricular pressures for a small increase in volume, halting ventricular filling in the initial third or half of diastole [19, 49–52]. As early diastolic filling is greatly increased, pulsed Doppler sample volume positioned at the tip of mitral or tricuspid valves [19, 25, 26, 49] shows normal or increased peak E wave velocity and velocity flow integrals, and, most importantly, a shortened deceleration time of the early filling E wave (Fig. 12.4). The rapid filling phase is greatly shortened. As a consequence, left ventricular isovolumic relaxation time [19] is also greatly diminished. This abnormality

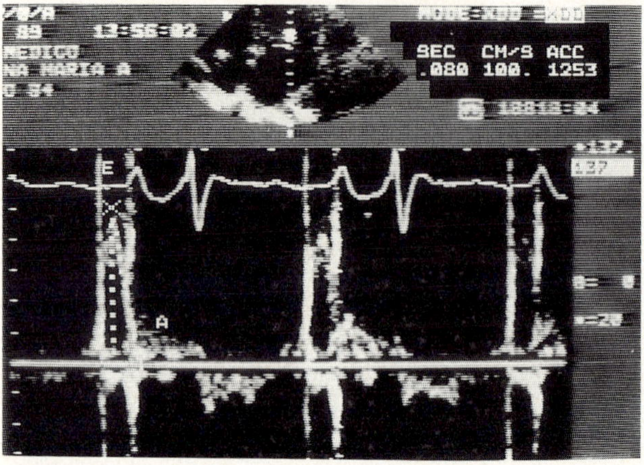

Fig. 12.4. Pulsed Doppler recording of mitral inflow velocities showing the restrictive pattern: high peak early (*E*) inflow velocity (100 cm/s), short deceleration time (80 ms) and small peak atrial (*A*) inflow velocity (25 cm/s). E/A ratio was increased to 4

occurs when a high atrial pressure and a rapid increase in ventricular pressure occur in early diastole due to the restrictive process, appearing at the early dip and plateau of the pressure curve. Subsequently in diastasis little or no apparent flow is seen, although in severe cases of restriction, if the ventricular pressure exceeds atrial pressure in mid-diastole, diastolic atrioventricular regurgitation might be seen as retrograde flow [19, 26]. At end-diastole peak velocity and flow velocity integrals of the atrial filling wave A are greatly decreased, expressing the remaining small atrioventricular pressure gradient. Therefore, the E/A ratio is significantly increased [19, 25, 26]. Abnormalities in tricuspid inflow velocities by pulsed Doppler similar to those observed in mitral inflow are seen. Tricuspid regurgitation or diminished right ventricular compliance will increase peak inflow E velocity and shorten deceleration time. These abnormalities are greatly influenced by inspiration. Some of the factors contributing to an increase in early abrupt diastolic filling [16, 17] may exist in endomyocardial fibrosis, such as increased left atrial pressure (or increased wedge pressure) [16, 18, 58] and normal end-systolic ventricular volume [16,18]. In chronic haemodynamically compensated patients whose initial hypereosinophilia responded favourably to steroid treatment a normal peak early E wave inflow velocity, normal to slightly decreased mitral deceleration time, and normal E/A ratio could be observed [56].

These abnormalities are, however, not confined to restrictive cardiomyopathy. Severe heart failure due to ischaemic heart disease or dilated cardiomyopathy, presenting high filling pressure in early diastole, might show similar Doppler findings: high peak E wave velocity, rapid deceleration time and small peak A wave velocity [26, 49, 52]. All have in common a stiffer less compliant ventricle in which, for a given end-diastolic volume, filling will occur at the expense of a much higher end-diastolic pressure. However, the usual Doppler profile in coronary heart disease, dilated cardiomyopathy, systemic hypertension or hypertrophic cardiomyopathy (see Chap. 8) is an abnormal relaxation pattern which is characteristically different to that of restriction [26, 50, 52]. This consists of a low initial peak E wave velocity, a greatly prolonged deceleration time, and an increased late filling peak A wave velocity E/A ratio <1). In these conditions a greatly prolonged relaxation and increased isovolumic relaxation time is characteristic (see Chap. 8). Right ventricular abnormal relaxation or hypertrophy may also prolong tricuspid early inflow deceleration time, increase peak A flow velocity and decrease the tricuspid E/A ratio [26]. Most importantly, clinical worsening leading to severe congestion with increasing left atrial and end-diastolic ventricular pressures will dramatically induce relatively rapid changes in the mitral and tricuspid Doppler inflows patterns, with change from that of abnormal, relaxation, through "pseudonormalisation" (E/A ratio close to 1) to a "worst" pattern indistinguishable from that of restriction (E/A ratio >2) [52].

Mitral and tricuspid regurgitation are common in endomyocardial fibrosis and in other restrictive disorders [10, 16–19, 27, 29, 41, 47, 56, 57]. Doppler echocardiography is most useful for estimating its detection and severity [59–61]. In one series of patients with restrictive physiology [19], almost all had mild to severe mitral and tricuspid regurgitation. Pulsed or continuous wave Doppler scanning from the apex [59, 60], and colour Doppler echocardiography, make this estimation rapid by allowing the shape, direction, width and extent of the regurgitant jet to be intracavitarily imaged [61]. The extension of the atrial systolic flow distortion will greatly depend on the systolic gradient between the ventricular and atrial chambers, its compliance, the gain setting of the instrument, the carrier frequency of the transducer, and the colour Doppler flow algorithm. As mentioned above, atrioventricular regurgitation by itself increases early inflow and thus may modify the Doppler pattern, increasing peak velocity of E wave and shortening of deceleration time.

Pulsed Doppler of the vena cava and hepatic veins in restriction may show a predominant diastolic forward flow, diminished or absent systolic forward flow, large and prolonged pre-systolic or atrial flow, diminished or absent systolic forward flow, and large and prolonged pre-systolic or atrial reversal which increases on inspiration [19, 49]. An increased reversal flow on inspiration is a sensitive index of restriction [19] because right ventricular filling is sharply reduced at end-diastole due to decreased ventricular compliance (Fig. 12.5). Severe tricuspid regurgitation may distort the analysis because it reverses all systolic flow and accentuates diastolic forward flow [19, 49]. When the tricuspid regurgitation is mild to moderate systolic reversal may not be apparent. Low atrial compliance, severe right ventricular dysfunction and atrial fibrillation will all accentuate the systolic reversal flow of tricuspid regurgitation. Since atrial fibrillation usually results in tricuspid regurgitation, the latter may show a diminished antegrade systolic flow, preserved diastolic flow and absence of the normal presystolic reversed flow. Right atrial compliance and size, atrial fibrillation, and right ventricular function will influence the venous velocity

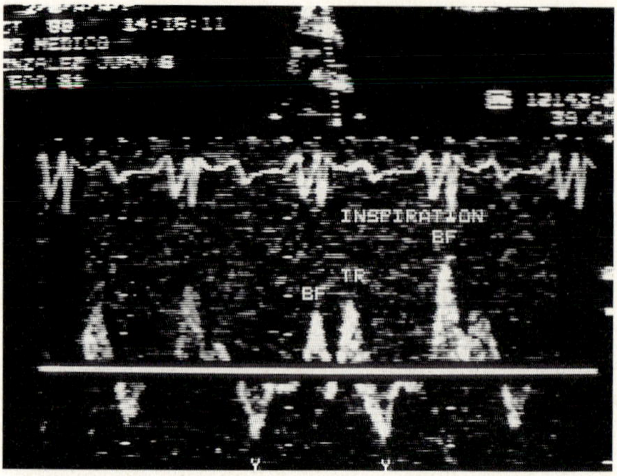

Fig. 12.5. Pulsed Doppler tracing of the suprahepatic vein from a patient with endomyocardial fibrosis displaying changes accentuated with inspiration: reversal of systolic antegrade flow due to tricuspid regurgitation (*TR*), increased early diastolic forward flow, and increased atrial backflow (*BF*)

flows. Increased right ventricular diastolic pressure, severe tricuspid regurgitation, diminished atrial contractility and depressed right ventricular systolic function will all make the venous inflow abnormalities more prominent. Right-sided congestion from restriction will make the inferior vena cava and intrahepatic vein look grossly plethoric.

Transoesophageal echocardiography permits the recording of strong Doppler signals from pulmonary veins. In a limited number of patients with endomyocardial fibrosis, abnormal filling of the left atria was noticed. Forward flow was mainly in diastole, while systolic filling was severely diminished (Fig. 12.6)

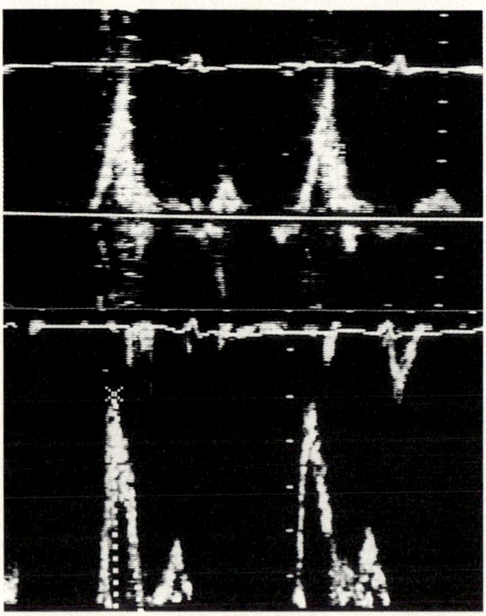

Fig. 12.6. Transoesophageal echocardiographic pulsed Doppler findings in a patient with hypereosinophilic endomyocardial fibrosis. *Upper panel*: tracing from the left upper pulmonary vein shows diminished forward systolic flow, greatly increased diastolic antegrade flow and absent atrial flow reversal. *Lower panel*: inverted tracing of mitral inflow obtained a few seconds later shows greatly increased early inflow with rapid deceleration, which coincides in time with the increased diastolic pulmonary vein flow. Tracings were make to coincide with the electrocardiogram.

Differential Diagnosis

Constrictive Pericarditis

The diagnosis of pericardial constriction is of the utmost importance. In an elegant Doppler echocardiographic study [25], differences in the respiratory responses were observed between restriction and constriction in early peak velocity flows of mitral and tricuspid valves and of isovolumic relaxation time. Simultaneous recording of respiration was important because changes occurred in the first beat after inspiration. In restriction there was little respiratory variation of diastolic pressure gradients between the pulmonary wedge and left ventricular diastolic pressures, as both pressures changed in a similar direction in inspiration or expiration. Therefore, little or no variation in mitral early peak E velocity flow occurs but shorter deceleration times are noted with inspiration. Tricuspid flow velocities, deceleration times and flow velocity integrals have similar changes to mitral. Tricuspid deceleration time further shortens with inspiration because of an abrupt increase in right ventricular filling [19, 25, 26].

In constriction, great respiratory variations occur because the rigid pericardium curtails ventricular filling as total cardiac volume is encased by the outer shell. On inspiration, right ventricular volume increases while the left decreases through septal displacement and ventricular interdependence [62]. There is an inspiratory decrease in pulmonary artery wedge pressure which diminishes the atrioventricular filling gradient. As a consequence, in pericardial constriction mitral early peak E velocity and deceleration time decrease and left ventricular isovolumic relaxation increases on inspiration [25]. On expiration opposite changes occur; there is an increase in left heart filling because the pressure gradient between pulmonary wedge and left ventricle increases in early diastole. Peak mitral inflow E velocity and deceleration time increase while left ventricular isovolumic relaxation time shortens [25]. Peak tricuspid flow velocity increases in inspiration in both restriction and constriction, but in pericardial constriction respiratory changes from expiration to inspiration were much larger, mainly because on expiration tricuspid flow velocity was markedly decreased. Comparison of the respiratory changes induced in early mitral and tricuspid flow velocities and in isovolumic relaxation time between restrictive and constrictive groups disclosed that in restriction no patient showed a difference greater than 15% between inspiratory and expiratory values, while in constriction respiratory variation was greater than 25% [25]. In obstructive pulmonary disease an inspiratory decrease in mitral peak early E velocity and increase in left ventricular isovolumic relaxation time may be observed but it was much less pronounced than in patients with constrictive pericarditis. In constriction inspiration induced a more pronounced decrease in aortic flow velocity and prolongation in left ventricular ejection time than in patients with restriction or normal controls.

Amyloid Heart Disease (see Chap. 13)

The echocardiographic findings [63–65] of cardiac amyloidosis show differences from endomyocardial fibrosis, but both may present a similar restrictive profile. A characteristic "granular sparkling" echographic texture of the ventricular walls is described in about half of cardiac amyloid patients. Increased thickness of papillary muscles, interatrial septum and valvar leaflets are observed. Biventricular normal dimensions with normal ejection fraction are seen early in the disease, but as the disease progresses impaired systolic function is common. Pulsed Doppler assessment of mitral and tricuspid inflow velocities and of pulmonary vein flow velocities has disclosed a spectrum of abnormal findings in biopsy-documented cardiac amyloidosis [66]. Patients were subdivided according to their left ventricular mean wall thickness as having early (12–15 mm) or advanced (> 15 mm) amyloid heart disease [65, 66]. In early cardiac amyloid and in amyloidosis without cardiac compromise findings suggestive of prolonged relaxation were found: the isovolumic relaxation time was prolonged, peak E velocity was decreased, peak A velocity was increased, and the E/A ratio was therefore decreased. Deceleration time was normal in most patients, but prolonged in some. By contrast, patients with advanced cardiac disease showed a restrictive pattern consisting in a markedly shortened deceleration time and a normal isovolumic relaxation time, a normal to increased peak E velocity and thus an increase in the E/A ratio. Pulmonary venous flow velocities were markedly abnormal, showing a decreased systolic flow velocity and an augmented diastolic flow velocity. It was noticed that when mitral peak E velocity was increased, there was also an increase in peak diastolic pulmonary venous velocity, as a consequence of the rapid left atrial emptying following the abrupt filling of the stiff amyloid left ventricle (increased E). In early amyloid most patients had a normal pulmonary venous flow. Interestingly, preservation of a prominent atrial reversal flow in pulmonary veins does not support the mechanism of impaired diastolic ventricular filling secondary to atrial systolic dysfunction [59]. Doppler follow-up of patients having early amyloidosis has proved useful in disclosing changes in the left ventricular filling pattern from one of abnormal relaxation, to "pseudonormalisation", and finally to restriction as the disease progresses in severity [66].

Other Conditions

Restrictive cardiomyopathy is clinically diagnosed after extensive investigations have carefully excluded other causes of restriction [23, 27, 28, 67, 68].

After 1 to 13 years of follow-up about 15% of a group of heart transplant recipients presented a restrictive physiology at cardiac catheterisation [69]. The diagnostic criteria for restriction were broader because the abnormal dip and plateau contour in some patients occured with normal diastolic pressure values and end-diastolic equalisation was not uniformly observed. On Doppler echocardiography the group with restriction had shorter left ventricular isovolumic relaxation time and pressure half-time (deceleration time), and the mitral E/A ratio was higher than in the non-restrictive allograft recipients. Similarly, right ventricular pressure half-time was shorter, and tricuspid peak early E inflow velocity and E/A ratio were higher in the restrictive group. This diastolic abnormality was invariably associated with and preceded systolic dysfunction. The patients with restriction were more symptomatic and had experienced more past episodes of rejection. There was a trend on biopsy to show a higher fibrosis score than the non-restriction group, but the difference did not reach statistical significance. Coronary artery disease of the graft found at autopsy may have contributed to the development of diastolic abnormalities in some patients [69].

Future Research

The contribution of invasive haemodynamics to the understanding of restrictive cardiomyopathy has been essential, but its expense and potential morbidity limits its role to selected patients. The extensive use of M-mode and 2D echocardiography [4, 6, 29, 31, 36, 39–44] and Doppler echocardiography [19, 25, 26, 49, 52] in patients with restrictive disorders has facilitated their non-invasive diagnosis. On the other hand, clinical electrocardiographic and haemodynamic predictors of mortality were found in a recent large series of endomyocardial fibrosis patients from India, but not echocardiographic predictors [70]. Other survival series including Doppler studies may be carried out. In endomyocardial disease Doppler investigation of an increasing number of patients may expand the spectrum of findings, especially during the acute/necrotic stage before restriction appears. The role of Doppler in helping to select candidates for surgical intervention or for monitoring therapy is unknown. Pulmonary venous flow velocities by transoesophageal echocardiography should help in the understanding of filling abnormalities in early and late restrictive cardiomyopathy [45, 53]. Recent developments in the technique of ultrasonic integrated backscatter myocardial pattern recognition [71, 72] as well as in amplitude-processed colour-coded imaging [29] may allow non-invasive investigation of the scarring process that leads to endomyocardial fibrosis.

References

1. WHO/ISFC (1980) Task Force report on the definition and classification of cardiomyopathies. Br Heart J 44: 672
2. Davies JNP, Ball JD (1955) The pathology of endomyocardial fibrosis in Uganda. Br Heart J 17: 337–359
3. Shaper AG, Hutt MSR, Coles RM (1968) Necropsy study of endomyocardial fibrosis and rheumatic heart disease in Uganda 1950–65. Br Heart J 30: 391–401

4. Acquatella H, Schiller NB, Puigbo JJ, Gomez-Mancebo JR, Suarez C, Acquatella G (1983) Value of two-dimensional echocardiography in endomyocardial disease with and without eosinophilia: a clinical and pathological study. Circulation 62:1219–1226
5. Andrade ZA, Guimaraes AC (1964) Endomyocardial fibrosis in Bahia, Brazil. Br Heart J 26:813–820
6. Vijayaraghavan G, Davies J, Sadanandan S, Spry CJ, Gibson DH, Goodwin JF (1983) Echocardiographic features of tropical endomyocardial disease in South India. Br Heart J 50:450–459
7. Löffler W (1936) Endocarditis parietalis fibroplastica mit Bluteosinophilie: ein eigenartiges Krankheitsbild. Schweiz Med Wochenschr 18:817–820
8. Roberts WC, Buja LM, Ferrans VJ (1970) Löffler's fibroplastic parietal endocarditis, eosinophilic leukemia, and Davies endomyocardial fibrosis: the same disease at different stages. Pathol Microbiol 35:90–95
9. Chusid MJ, Dale DC, West BC, Wolff SM (1975) The hypereosinophilic syndrome: analysis of fourteen cases with review of the literature. Medicine (Baltimore) 54:1–27
10. Goodwin JF (1983) Endomyocardial disease:clinical features. Postgrad Med J 59:154–156
11. Brockington IF, Olsen EGJ (1973) Löffler's endocarditis and Davies endomyocardial fibrosis. Am Heart J 85:308–322
12. Roberts WC, Buja LM, Ferrans VJ (1970) Löffler's fibroplastic parietal endocarditis, eosinophilic leukemia, and Davies' endomyocardial fibrosis: the same disease at different stages? Pathol Microbiol 35:90–95
13. Roberts WC, Liegler DG, Carbone PP (1969) Endomyocardial disease and eosinophilia: a clinical and pathologic spectrum. Am J Med 46:28–42.
14. Davies JNP (1948) Endomyocardial fibrosis in Africans. East Afr Med J 25:10–14
15. Kartha CC, Sandhyamani S (1985) An autopsy study of tropical endomyocardial fibrosis in Kerala. Indian J Med Res 82:439–446
16. Bell JA, Jenkins BS, Webb-Peploe MM (1976) Clinical, haemodynamic, and angiographic findings in Löffler's eosinophillic endocarditis. Br Heart J 38:541–548
17. Chew CYC, Ziady GM, Raphael MJ, Nellen M, Oackley CM 1 (1977) Primary restrictive cardiomyopathy: non-tropical endomyocardial fibrosis and hypereosinophilic heart disease. Br Heart J 39:399–413
18. Hess OM, Turina M, Senning A, Goebel NH, Scholer Y, Krayenbühl HP (1978) Pre- and postoperative findings in patients with endomyodardial fibrosis. Br Heart J 40:406–415
19. Appleton CP, Hatle LV, Popp RL (1988) Demonstration of restrictive ventricular physiology by Doppler echocardiography. J Am Coll Cardiol 11:757–768
20. Spry CJF (1987) Eosinophils and endomyocardial fibrosis: a review of clinical and experimental studies, 1980–86. In: Kawal C, Abelmann WM (eds) Pathogenesis of myocarditis and cardiomyopathy: recent experimental and clinical studies. University of Tokyo Press, Tokyo, pp 293–310
21. Olsen EGJ, Spry CJF (1979) The pathogenesis of Löffler's endomyocardial disease, and its relationship to endomyocardial fibrosis. In: Yu PN, Goodwin JF (eds) Progress in cardiology, vol 8. Lea and Febiger, Philadelphia, pp 281–303
22. Olsen EGJ, Spry CJF (1985) Relation between eosinophilia and endomyocardial disease. Prog Cardiovasc Dis 27:241–254
23. Benotti JR, Grossman W, Cohn PF (1980) Clinical profile of restrictive cardiomyopathy. Circulation 61:1206–1212
24. Goodwin JF (1985) Cardiomyopathies and specific heart muscle diseases: definition, terminology and classification. In: Goodwin JF (ed) Heart muscle disease. MTP Press, Lancaster, pp 1–5
25. Hatle LK, Appleton CP, Popp RL (1989) Differentiation of constrictive pericarditis and restrictive cardiomyopathy by Doppler echocardiography. Circulation 79:357–370
26. Nishimura RA, Abel MD, Hatle LK, Tajik AJ (1989) Assessment of diastolic function of the heart: background and current applications of Doppler echocardiography. II. Clinical studies. Mayo Clin Proc 64:181–204

27. Abelmann WH, Lorell BH (1989) The challenge of cardiomyopathy. J Am Coll Cardiol 13: 1219–1239
28. Child JS, Perloff JK (1988) The restrictive cardiomyopathies. Cardiol Clin 6: 289–316
29. Davies J, Gibson DG, Foale R, Herr K, Spry CJF, Oakley CM, Goodwin JF, (1982) Echocardiographic features of eosinophilic endomyocardial disease. Br Heart J 48: 434–440
30. Case Records of the Massachusets General Hospital (1980) Case no. 18. N Engl J Med 302: 1077–1083
30a. Andy JJ, Bishara FF, Soyinka OO (1981) Relation of severe eosinophilia and microfilariasis to chronic African endomyocardial fibrosis. Br Heart J 45: 672–680
31. Dienot B, Ekra A, Bertrand E (1979) L'echocardiographie dans 23 cas de fibroses endomyocardiques constrictives droites ou bilaterales. Arch Mal Coeur 72: 1101–1107
32. Take M, Sekiguchi M, Hiroe M, Hirosawa K, Mizoguchi H, Kijima M, Shirai T, Ishide T, Okubo S (1985) Clinical spectrum and endomyocardial biopsy findings in eosinophilic heart disease. In: Sekiguchi M, Olsen EGJ, Goodwin JF (eds) Myocarditis and related disorders. Springer, Berlin Heidelberg New York, pp 243–249
33. DePace NL, Nestico PF, Morganroth J, Ross J, Fox R, Kotler MN, Mintz GS, Vassallo R (1983) Dilated cardiomyopathy in the idiopathic hypereosinophilic syndrome. Am J Cardiol 52: 1359–1360
34. Acquatella H (1989) Echocardiographic overview of Chagas' disease and endomyocardial fibrosis: diagnostic implications for non-tropical countries. Echocardiography 6: 137–157
35. Hall SW, Theologides A, From AHL, Gobel FL, Fortuny IE, Lawrence CJ, Edwards JE (1977) Hypereosinophilic syndrome with biventricular involvement. Circulation 55: 217–222
36. George BO, Gaba FE, Talabi AI (1982) M-mode echocardiographic features of endomyocardial fibrosis. Br Heart J 48: 222–228
37. Richardson PJ, Daly K, Gishen P (1984) Hemodynamic findings in biopsy proven acute myocarditis. In: Bolte HD (ed) Viral heart disease. Springer, Berlin Heidelberg New York, pp 165–172
39. Pernod J, Gerbaux A, Vernin P, Terdjman M, Lelguen C, Droniou J (1980) Apport de l'echocardiographie dans le diagnostic des fibroses endomyocardiques. Arch Mal Coeur 73: 139–146
40. Candell-Riera J, Permanyer-Miralda G, Soler-Soler J (1982) Echocardiogrphic findings in endomyocardial fibrosis. Chest 82: 88–90
41. Gottdiener JS, Maron BJ, Schooley RT, Harley JB, Roberts WC, Fauci AS (1983) Two-dimensional echocardiographic assessment of the idiopathic hypereosinophilic syndrome: anatomical basis of mitral regurgitation and peripheral embolization. Circulation 67: 572–578
42. Puigbo JJ, Combellas I, Acquatella H, Marsiglia I, Tortoledo F, Casal H, Suarez JA (1983) Endomyocardial disease in South America: report on 23 cases in Venezuela. Postgrad Med J 59: 162–168
43. Bletry O, Scheuble C, Cereze P, Masquet P, Priollet P, Balafrej M, Godeau P (1984) Cardiac manifestations of the hypereosinophilic syndrome: the value of 2-dimensional echography (12 cases). Arch Mal Coeur 77: 633–641
44. Fawsy ME, Ziady G, Halim M, Guindy R, Mercer EN, Feteih N (1985) Endomyocardial fibrosis: report of eight cases. J Am Coll Cardiol 5: 983–988
45. Seward JB, Khandheria BK, Oh JK, Abel MD, Hughes RW Jr, Edwards WD, Nichols BA, Freeman WK, Tajik AJ (1988) Transesophageal echocardiography: technique, anatomic correlations, implementation, and clinical applications. Mayo Clin Proc 63: 649–680
46. Candell-Riera J, Garcia del Castillo H, Permanyer-Miralda G, Soler-Soler J (1978) Echocardiographic features of the interventricular septum in chronic constrictive pericarditis. Circulation 57: 1154–1158
47. Parrillo JE, Borer JS, Henry WL, Wolff SM, Fauci AS (1979) The cardiovascular manifestations of the hypereosinophilic syndrome: prospective study of 26 patients, with review of the literature. Am J Med 67: 572–582
48. Brutsaert DL, Rademakers Fe, Sys SU, Gillebert TC, Housmans PR (1985) Analysis of relaxation in the evaluation of ventricular function of the heart. Prog Cardiovasc Dis 28: 143–163

49. Nishimura RA, Housmans PR, Hatle LK, Tajik AJ (1989) Assessment of diastolic function of the heart: background and current applications of Doppler echocardiography. 1. Physiologic and pathophysiologic features. Mayo Clin Proc 64: 71–81
50. Harizi RC, Bianco JA, Alpert JS (1988) Diastolic function of the heart in clinical cardiology. Arch Intern Med 148: 99–109
51. Rokey R, Kuo LC, Zoghbi WA, Limacher MC, Quinones MA (1985) Determination of parameters of left ventricular diastolic filling with pulsed Doppler echocardiography: comparison with cineangiography. Circulation 71: 543–550
52. Appleton CP, Hatle LV, Popp RL (1988) Relation of transmitral flow velocity patterns to left ventricular diastolic function: new insights from a combined hemodynamic and Doppler echocardiographic study. J Am Coll Cardiol 12: 426–440
53. Keren G, Sherez J, Megidish R, Levitt B, Laniado S (1985) Pulmonary venous flow pattern: its relationship to cardiac dynamics. A pulsed Doppler echocardiographic study. Circulation 71: 1105–1112
54. Nishimura RA, Abel MD, Hatle LK, Tajik AJ (1990) Relation of pulmonary vein to mitral flow velocities by transesophageal Doppler echocardiography: effect of different loading conditions. Circulation 81: 1488–1497
55. Appleton CP, Hatle LK, Popp RL (1987) Superior vena cava and hepatic vein Doppler echocardiography in healthy adutls. J Am Coll Cardiol 10: 1032–1039
56. Acquatella H, Rodriguez L, Puigbo JJ, Gomez-Mancebo JR, Casanova M, Combellas I, Giordano H (1990) Echocardiographic recognition and Doppler abnormalities in eosinophilic endomyocardial disease and endomyocardial fibrosis. In: Sekiguchi M, Olsen EGJ (eds) Cardiomyopathy and myocarditis. University of Tokyo Press, Tokyo, pp 35–47 (Cardiomyopathy update 3).
57. Acquatella H, Rodriguez-Salas LA, Gomez-Mancebo JR (1990) Doppler echocardiography in dilated and restrictive cardiomyopathies. Cardiol Clin 8: 349–367
58. Moraes CR, Buffolo E, Lima R, Victor E, Lira V, Escobar M, Rodrigues J, Saralva L, Andrade JC (1983) Surgical treatment of endomyocardial fibrosis. J Thorac Cardiovasc Surg 85: 738–745
59. Miyatake K, Kinoshita N, Nagata S, Beppu S, Park YD, Sakakibara H, Nimura Y (1980) Intracardiac flow pattern in mitral regurgitation studied with combined use of the ultrasonic pulsed Doppler technique and cross-sectional echocardiography. Am J Cardiol 45: 155–162
60. Abbasi AS, Allen MW, DeCristofaro D, Ungar I (1980) Detection and estimation of the degree of mitral regurgitation by range-gated pulsed Doppler echocardiography. Circulation 61: 143–147
61. Helmcke F, Nanda NC, Hsiung MC, Soto B, Adey CK, Goyal RG, Gatewood RP (1987) Color Doppler assessment of mitral regurgitation with orthogonal planes. Circulation 75: 175–183
62. Santamore WP, Bartlet R, Van Buren SJ, Dowd MK, Kutcher MA (1986) Ventricular coupling in constrictive pericarditis. Circulation 74: 597–602
63. Falk RH, Plehn JF, Deering T, Schick EC, Boinay P, Rubinow A, Skinner M, Cohen AS (1987) Sensitivity and specificity of echocardiographic features of cardiac amyloidosis. Am J Cardiol 59: 418–422
64. Siqueira Filho AG, Cunha CLP, Tajik AJ, Seward JB, Schattenberg TT, Giuliani ER (1981) M-mode and two-dimentional echographic features in cardiac amyloidosis. Circulation 63: 188– 196
65. Cueto-Garcia L, Reeder GS, Kyle RA, Wood DL, Seward JB, Naessens J, Offord KP, Greipp PR, Edwards WD, Tajik AJ (1985) Echocardiographic findings in systemic amyloidosis: spectrum of cardiac involvement and relation to survival. J Am Coll Cardiol 6: 737–743
66. Klein AL, Hatle LK, Burstow DJ, Seward JB, Kyle RA, Bailey KR, Luscher TF, Gertz MA, Tajik AJ (1989) Doppler characterization of left ventricular diastolic function in cardiac amyloidosis. J Am Coll Cardiol 13: 1017–1026
67. Siegel RJ, Shah PK, Fishbein MC (1984) Idiopathic restrictive cardiomyopathy. Circulation 70: 165–169

68. Ortolani P, Rapezzi C, Binetti G, Baroni M, Mirri A, Alampi G, Benati A, Branzi A, Magnani B (1989) Idiopathic restrictive cardiomyopathy: clinical, hemodynamic, histologic and prognostic profile. Cardiologia 34: 759–768
69. Valantine HA, Appleton CP, Hatle LK, Hunt SA, Billingham ME, Shumway NE, Stinson EB, Popp RL, (1989) A hemodynamic and Doppler echocardiographic study of ventricular function in long-term cardiac allograft recipients: etiology and prognosis of restrictive–constrictive physiology. Circulation 79: 66–75
70. Gupta PN, Valiathan MS, Balakrishnan KG, Kartha CC, Ghosh MK (1989) Clinical course of endomyocardial fibrosis. Br Heart J 62: 450–454
71. Skorton DJ, Collins SM (1988) Clinical potential of ultrasound tissue characterization in cardiomyopathies. J Am Soc Echocardiogr 1: 69–77
72. Loomis JF, Waggoner AD, Schechtman KB, Miller JG, Sobel BE, Perez JE (1990) Ultrasonic integrated backscatter two-dimentional imaging: evaluation of M-mode guided acquisition and immediate analysis in 55 consecutive patients. J Am Soc Echocardiogr 3: 255– 265

Part V
Amyloid Heart Disease and Others

CHAPTER 13

Amyloid Heart Disease and Cardiomyopathies Difficult To Classify

C. M. Oakley

The development of increasingly precise and searching non-invasive techniques together with the experience of following some patients with cardiomyopathy for many years has shown that the three classical genres of dilated, hypertrophic and restrictive cardiomyopathy do not describe all the patients (see Chap. 1).

Some are seen with mild or moderate *systolic* impairment but major *restrictive* features who clearly do not have dilated cardiomyopathy in its typical form yet who are excluded from the designation of restrictive cardiomyopathy if that is defined by initial preservation of normal or near-normal systolic function.

We have been aware for years that surviving patients with *hypertrophic* cardiomyopathy may gradually lose systolic efficiency through the process of losing hypertrophied muscle and replacing it with fibrous tissue. They too develop restrictive features with high venous filling pressures, lack of dilatation but impaired systolic function often with little or no remaining increase in wall thickness. It is only if they have shown typical features years before that the disorder can be recognised for what it is. (see Chap. 10)

Whether or not eosinophilic heart disease and endomyocardial fibrosis are removed from the classification of restrictive cardiomyopathy or allowed to remain in it for historical reasons despite distinctive association and pathology, many patients with restrictive cardiomyopthay do not have endomyocardial fibrosis. Some with restrictive physiology show fine interstitial fibrosis quite different from the coarser patchy fibrosis seen in dilated cardiomyopathy or in hypertrophic cardiomyopathy. Others show widespread disarray, good systolic function but no increase in wall thickness (see Chaps. 6 and 9). These cases have recently been described as hypertrophic cardiomyopathy without hypertrophy, which is a contradiction in terms but accounts for occasional sudden deaths in previously asymptomatic young people with macroscopically normal hearts but who may have had family members with typical hypertrophic cardiomyopathy. Some restrictive cardiomyopathies including those with marked biatrial dilatation seen in childhood may show similar disarray with restrictive features but no increase in wall thickness. Some of these are familial, show progressive conduction system disorder and have been described under various titles including familial atrial cardiomyopathy.

Sudden cardiac death in young people is usually due to hypertrophic cardiomyopathy or to a long QT syndrome, but other causes may operate (Table 13.1).

Table 13.1. Causes of sudden death in young people including athletes

Hypertrophic cardiomyopathy
Right ventricular dysplasia
Aortic valve stenosis
Premature coronary artery disease
Congenital coronary artery anomalies
Long QT syndrome
Marfan's syndrome
Cerebrovascular accidents
Myocarditis
Pulmonary embolism

These "overlap" syndromes do not detract from the worth of describing the three major types of cardiomyopathy with their recognisably separate physiology and pathology. They are an inevitable product of increasing collective experience, the classification remaining valuable just as long as causes are still obscure. (see Chap. 1).

Other more discrete cardiomyopathies which do not fit include *endocardial fibroelastosis*—which can be regarded as a dilated cardiomyopathy with a temporal relationship to infancy, perhaps due to perinatal myocarditis. It may be associated with coarctation of the aorta, or with aortic atresia or variants of the hypoplastic left heart syndrome, when there may be ventricular restriction rather than dilatation.

Peripartum cardiomyopathy is a form of dilated cardiomyopathy with a temporal relationship to childbirth but which is now seen as a specific entity rather than the result of coincidental but very unfortunate timing.

Right ventricular dilated cardiomyopathy may represent a dilated cardiomyopathy which spares the left ventricle. If so, it is distinct from *arrhythmogenic right ventricular dysplasia*, which has a specific pathology, may be familial and displays arrhythmias and sudden death at a young age, rather than right ventricular failure.

Amyloid heart disease remains an important specific heart muscle disease in which knowledge of the pathogenesis and natural history has advanced in recent years. It is the great pretender, simulating hypertrophic, restrictive or even dilated cardiomyopathy in its different forms and at different stages of its course so that it cannot be omitted from a text on cardiomyopathies. Other specific toxic, infiltrative and storage diseases may be recognised by full investigation and especially by cardiac biopsy when they masquerade as cardiomyopathies (see Table 1.1).

Amyloid Heart Disease

Cardiac amyloidosis is an infiltrative myocardial disorder in which amyloid progressively accumulates in the interstitium between normal-looking myocardial cells. It may also be deposited in the walls of small coronary arteries. It is a disorder in which both the appearance and the functional disturbance of the heart change progressively and the study of patients with amyloid at differing stages of their relentless deterioration accounts for some apparent conflicts in previous descriptions of the amyloid heart [1]. It is through the freer use of early endomyocardial biopsy for diagnosis of mild but unexplained abnormality and serial echocardiography that the natural history of amyloid heart disease has become better known [2].

Amyloidosis is a disorder of protein metabolism in which the abnormal eosinophilic fibrillar protein, amyloid, is laid down intercellularly. Amyloid may be formed from a number of different precursor proteins but in all cases is bound to a non-fibriller glycoprotein that is a normal plasma constituent. The precursor protein determines the appearance of the amyloid fibrils, which can be identified by their distinct electron microscopic appearances [3].

Most clinically recognised amyloid heart disease results from the deposition of amyloid AL fibrils which are derived from monoclonal immunoglobulin light chains. It is associated either with myeloma, macroglobulinaemia or malignant B lymphocyte lymphomas or is of the so-called primary type in which the immunocyte dyscrasia cannot be identified. Primary type amyloid may either be limited to certain organs, sparing others, or generalised. In the localised type the heart, skeletal muscle, autonomic and peripheral nerves may be involved but there is wide variation. Less often it is the heart and gastrointestinal tract or the heart and the kidneys which are predominantly affected.

Although it used to be thought that deposition of amyloid in the hearts of elderly patients (senile amyloidosis) was a component of increasing age but unimportant, it is now apparent that not only does amyloid infiltration contribute to the functional abnormality of the senile heart but it may also be the cause of heart failure and death. In senile amyloidosis no monoclonal protein is to be found in the plasma or urine, the pre-albumin ACI fibrils being derived from a variant of plasma pre-albumin (now called thyretin). Senile cardiac amyloidosis is often clinically unrecognised in the very old but can also occur in some younger patients who show milder and more slowly advancing disease than is usual in AL amyloid [4–6].

In reactive amyloidosis associated with chronic inflammation or suppuration, the heart is not usually clinically involved but there are exceptions. The AA fibrils are derived from serum amyloid A protein. Massive cardiac infiltration is occasionally seen in patients with familial Mediterranean fever. In contrast to most patients with AL amyloid, these patients are usually young and they may be hypertensive from renal amyloid deposition.

Natural History (Figure 13.1)

Amyloid is generally known as a restrictive cardiac disease with an abnormality of diastolic filling resulting in a higher filling pressure for any increment of volume than in the normal heart.

The earliest abnormality is one of slight restriction to filling in an asymptomatic patient who shows normal systolic function on echocardiography and as yet no detectable increase in ventricular wall thickness. Such a patient will be asymptomatic but recognised perhaps by the chance finding of an atrial beat or of an electrocardiographic abnormality such as bundle branch block, even 1 or 2 years before the development of other evidence of heart disease. Left ventricular Doppler inflow recordings at this stage show abnormal relaxation with a reduced peak early velocity and increased peak late velocity and a prolonged deceleraton time [7] (see Chap. 12). Both isovolumic relaxation and passive filling are prolonged at this stage with the atrial contribution both to filling and to pressure being increased. Early on there is therefore reduced early and enhanced later filling, but as the amyloid deposition increases and the left ventricular wall thickens the heart becomes stiffer and late filling is diminished or abolished resulting in a changeover from enhanced late filling to a restrictive picture of early filling. In between may be detected a period of pseudonormalisation (see Chap. 10). This reflects the complexity of ventricular diastole, which is influenced by ventricular systole, pressure and ejection fraction, by filling pressure and therefore by diuretic status, by active myocardial relaxation, diastolic suction, the viscoelastic properties of the myocardium and atrial contractile force plus the PR interval. Pericardial restraint and ventricular interaction are probably less important in the amyloid heart (in which the total dimensions are often within normal limits), than in other forms of diastolic heart disease.

Eventually, although active relaxation is still prolonged, the isovolumic period is shortened if left atrial pressure is high and the amyloid heart is so stiff

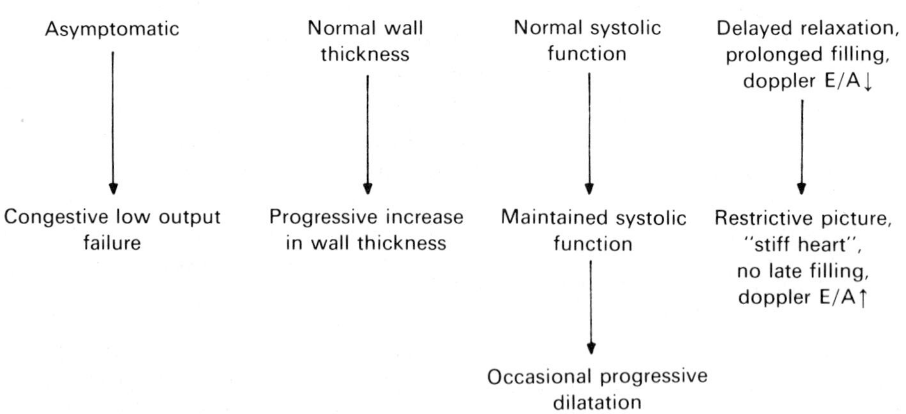

Fig. 13.1. Progression of amyloid heart disease

that filling is rapidly completed early on by diastolic suction during the period of shape change following the isovolumic period while the left ventricular diastolic pressure is still falling. There is no late filling and the plight of the patient is further worsened when the systolic function of this stiff but undilated ventricle begins to deteriorate without the means for compensatory dilatation (Fig. 13.1).

There is therefore a continuum of abnormality in the amyloid heart which reflects the extent of the amyloid deposition and whose rate of progression appears to be individually unpredictable. It varies from the fast rate of deposition reported in a young patient with primary cardiac amyloidosis during only a few months of close observation following cardiac transplantation [8], through the 1 or 2 years of progressive clinical difficulty usually seen [9], to the several years of slow deterioration now recognised in other patients, especially those with the senile form [6].

Serial echocardiography has been the means through which this process has been appreciated [10] and efforts have been made to enhance this by computerised quantitative texture analysis of the echo data [11, 12]. Imaging has shown a slow increase in left and in right ventricular wall thickness with a very characteristic thickening also of the atrial septum and valves which helps to differentiate the amyloid heart from the heart in advanced hypertrophic cardiomyopathy which may otherwise look very similar. Doppler echocardiography has enabled the filling characteristics of the ventricles to be examined serially in patients with amyloid heart disease and this has shown a wide range of mitral inflow velocity patterns representing a progressive spectrum of abnormality from the early prolongation of myocardial relaxation to the final highly restricted phase [13–15], by which time the prognosis has become very short and usually less than 1 year. Other imaging methods which have been used include radionuclide angiography to assess left ventricular diastolic function [16], magnetic resonance imaging [17] and technetium pyrophosphate scintigraphy [18]—none as readily available or repeatable as ultrasound (see Chap. 12)

Rarely, a predominance of amyloid infiltration in the walls of small coronary arteries rather than between myocardial cells may lead to progressive systolic failure with dilatation, but this is very rare though angina due to this cause is not uncommon in the early stages of amyloid heart disease. Patients with congestive features who have had chest pain may be thought to have suffered myocardial infarction [18].

Clinical Features

Primary cardiac amyloidosis is infrequent below the age of 50 but occasionally occurs in the thirties or forties. Except for patients who are detected at an early stage on account of a routine medical examination, patients with cardiac amyloidosis do not usually seek advice until there is evidence of heart failure [18]. They frequently look chronically sick having lost weight perhaps due to malabsorption from gastrointestinal involvement and from muscle wasting due to inanition from extreme fatigue and shortness of breath. Much less often the skeletal muscles may show increased bulk caused by amyloid infiltration. Patients may come to attention on account of a mono-neuritis or carpal tunnel syndrome before cardiac disability has been appreciated, or with gastrointestinal symptoms of diarrhoea or constipation, or with hepatomegaly.

Cardiovascular examination typically reveals a low output state with cool extremities, peripheral cyanosis and hypotension [9]. Conduction defects may lead to bradycardia due to sinoatrial disorder or atrioventricular block sometimes induced by digitalis [19]. Syncope may result either from this cause or from orthostatic hypotension caused by autonomic nerve involvement or diuretics given for treatment of the nephrotic syndrome. Diuretics given for oedema secondary to hypo-albuminaemia due to proteinuria may obscure cardiac involvement. Rarely, the jugular venous pressure may be normal even in the absence of diuretics and despite typical abnormality on echocardiographic examination. These may be patients who have been very inactive or failed to mount an adrenergic stimulation of the renin–angiotensin system to cause fluid retention.

A pericardial effusion is not uncommon but is often lax, removal of the fluid having no effect on raised intracardiac filling pressures. In one personal case with persistently normal venous filling pressures in the absence of diuretics, there was a pericardial effusion with echocardiographic features of tamponade, and diastolic collapse of the right atrium and right ventricular outflow tract walls. In this patient with normal intracardiac diastolic pressures the intrapericardial pressures must have been somewhat higher but aspiration of the effustion did not result in any improvement in cardiac output.

The amplitude of pulsation of the raised jugular venous pressure is usually small but there may be a predominant A wave or occasionally a regurgitant V wave. The cardiac impulse is quiet and usually impalpable. Murmurs and a left ventricular third heart sound are typically absent but occasionally a right ventricular third heart sound may be heard when the venous pressure is high, though this disappears when diuretics are given. Mitral regurgitation caused by papillary muscle infiltration is an occasional feature.

Investigations

Electrocardiography

The electrocardiogram typically shows low voltage and may indeed be the reason for first suspecting the diagnosis. Repolarisation abnormalities are not invariable, but q waves are common. An abnormal axis or fascicular block may be seen. There may be a marked discrepancy between a rather inconspicuous electrocardiographic abnormality and a very sick patient who is in severe clinical low output heart failure.

Chest Radiography

The chest radiograph may show little or no cardiac enlargement despite marked pulmonary venous congestion. Superior vena caval and azygous vein shadow may be prominent. If there is a pericardial effusion, this may give rise to considerable increase in the cardiac shadow radiographically, although echocardiography quickly reveals the reason for this.

Echocardiography

The role of echocardiography is described in Chap. 12.

Cardiac Catheterisation

Cardiac catheterisation usually reveals very high left ventricular diastolic and left atrial pressures in comparison to much less raised right atrial and right ventricular diastolic pressures. The pulmonary artery pressure may be moderately (or rarely considerably) raised. The large difference between left- sided and right-sided diastolic pressures distinguishes amyloid heart disease at all stages of its course from constrictive pericarditis [9, 18] (see Chap. 10).

Angiocardiography

Angiocardiography often shows deceptively normal appearances of the left and right ventricles. Typically the internal architecture of the ventricles is exaggerated due to amyloid infiltration of the subendocardial layers enhancing and coarsening trabeculation and increasing the size of papillary muscles. The cavities are usually small and the left ventricular ejection fraction preserved but there may be mitral regurgitation, though this is usually mild. The major coronary arteries are not affected by amyloid but they may show other sclerotic abnormalities common in middle-aged or elderly patients; if present, these should not deflect thoughts from the true diagnosis since coronary heart disease does not usually produce this pattern of global diastolic heart failure.

Endomyocardial Biopsy

Endomyocardial biopsy reveals the diagnosis because usually the infiltration is uniform, thus eliminating the possibility of sampling errors [18]. Only rarely does the amyloid deposition appear to be focal. One young patient aged only 15 showed marked tricuspid regurgitation with an akinetic though thickened right ventricular wall, normal left ventricle and valves and very thickened atrial septum. Right ventricular biopsies showed amyloid. Of course biopsies of the rectum or gingiva may be positive in patients with amyloid in these tissues, although in patients without evident amyloid outside the heart, cardiac biopsy is the preferred first biopsy (see Chap. 12).

Pathology

Characteristically, amyloid stains apple green with congo red when viewed by polarised light and gives a metachromatic reaction to methyl violet. Unfortunately the staining reactions of AL amyloid may be atypical, the iodine reaction first described by Virchow and even the histological stains being negative. It is very important, therefore, for the cardiac biopsy specimen to be examined by electron microscopy. The fibrillar amyloid masses can then be recognised (see Chap. 11).

Radioisotope Imaging

In the past, congo red injected intravenously was used as a diagnostic test for amyloid, the pigment having a physical affinity for the amyloid deposits and thereby being removed from the plasma, but false negatives were common since the test depended both on the amyloid deposits being fairly massive and on the amyloid having the usual physical affinity for the pigment. Moreover, allergic reactions sometimes occurred and the test was long ago abandoned. A recently developed technique involves labelling of purified serum amyloid P component (SAP) with iodine-123 [19]. Patients with amyloidosis show specific uptake of the label into the amyloid deposit. High-resolution scintigraphy then reveals even small deposits, but the specificity of the test acts to its own disadvantage when massive amyloid deposits in liver and spleen reduce the ability of the scan to detect amyloid elsewhere, and particularly in the heart where there is a relatively large blood pool containing the label. This technique shows promise for the detection and quantitation of amyloid deposition in the body and in following the rate of amyloid accumulation or regression should an effective treatment be found.

Treatment

No medical treatment yet exists which prevents progression of amyloid infiltration in primary cardiac amyloidosis, much less causes the amyloid material to be removed. Colchicine has been suggested for control of the clinical manifestations in familial Mediterranean fever [19a]. Cardiac transplantation therefore offers the only means of palliation and should not be refused on the grounds of likely involvement of the transplanted heart. Although this will occur, the rate of deposition in the transplanted organ is highly variable and may allow the patient many years of high-quality life. Patients with primary amyloidosis whose prognosis is limited by the cardiac involvement but whose amyloid deposition in other organs would otherwise have allowed a much longer outlook should be considered for cardiac transplantation.

Right Ventricular Dilated Cardiomyopathy and Arrhythmogenic Right Ventricular Dysplasia

Right ventricular cardiomyopathy and arrhythmogenic right ventricular dysplasia are now being seen as possibly separate conditions.

Dilated cardiomyopathy usually involves both ventricles globally and is recognised by ventricular dilatation and a low ejection fraction. Whilst in most patients the left ventricle is somewhat more severely affected than the right, in rare cases the right ventricle is predominantly or apparently solely involved—socalled *right ventricular cardiomyopathy*. The right ventricle is globally dilated, hypokinetic and thin-walled. The condition has been termed "partial Uhl's syndrome", but these patients present at any age, usually with congestive failure, and the right ventricular myocardium is not absent.

Arrhythmogenic right ventricular dysplasia is a primary disorder of the right ventricular myocardium characterised by minor or massive replacement of the right ventricular free wall by fibro-adipose tissue. The typical form is characterised by recurrent ventricular tachycardia of right ventricular origin with right ventricular enlargement detectable clinically or echocardiographically. Minor forms may be asymptomatic without overt right ventricular abnormality but with a risk of sudden death. Cases with massive replacement of the right ventricular myocardium may show right ventricular failure and simulate right ventricular dilated cardiomyopathy clinically, but this is exceptional and many points of differentiation are found on investigation.

The term "right ventricular dysplasia" was coined by Marcus et al. [20] in a description of 26 adult cases in 1982. Dalla Volta et al. [21] had previously described bizarrely severe cases of right ventricular cardiomyopathy under the title of "auricularisation of the right ventricular pressure curve" in 1961. These were cases with massive cardiomegaly, the right ventricle being dilated and functionally inefficient, the pulmonary artery being filled by right atrial drive. These authors also mentioned the replacement of the right ventricular myocardium with fibro-adipose tissue [22]. Gradually the evidence came to suggest two separate conditions: right ventricular cardiomyopathy with aetiology probably simillar to dilated cardiomyopathy, and arrhythmogenic right ventricular dysplasia, sometimes familial and showing a wide spectrum of severity. Differentiation may not necessarily always be clear-cut.

The term "arrhythmogenic right ventricular dysplasia" emphasises the tendency for serious arrhythmias in right ventricular dysplasia. It is most common in young adult males, the male to female ratio is 1.5:1, and the mean age at death was 24 years in a study which included 72 members of nine families. The age range was 8 to 77 years and included three generations in two families [23]. In Marcus et al.'s study [20] of 26 adult cases the age range was 17 to 65 with a male to female ratio of 2.7:1. The disorder has not been recognised in neonates or infants (in contrast to Uhl's syndrome) but has occasionally developed under observation.

In addition to the transformation of the musculature into fibrotic or adipose tissue in specific areas of the right ventricle, Thiene et al. [24] observed inflammatory changes with monocytic infiltration around necrotic myocytes in a quarter of the cases, but no viral or bacterial infection has been documented. A triangle of dysplasia develops in the free wall of the right ventricle, distal to the tricuspid valve, at the apex and below the pulmonary valve. The ventricular septum is unaffected and thus biopsies taken from the septum will not show diagnostic abnormalities. The left ventricle is usually normal but occasionally shows or develops focal wall motion abnormalities [25]. Unlike the right ventricle it does not dilate and some of the apparent left ventricular abnormality seen in severe cases may be consequent upon the right ventricular dilatation as has been described in other disorders of the right heart.

The Spectrum of Right Ventricular Dysplasia

As is usual the first descriptions were of the most florid cases, later of much less obvious ones, and now right ventricular dysplasia is recognised not to be nearly as rare as had originally been thought. Since the disease has been recognised to be familial, an autosomal dominant mode of inheritance with variable penetrance has been shown [23]. Affected families have shown a wide spectrum of severity from massive replacement of right ventricular myocardium, cardiomegaly and failure to the most localised forms. The true incidence and natural history of the disease are unknown. There is no evidence that it is regional or ethnic but this may be because it is still not widely recognised. It is of interest that no case has been observed in infancy and it is not known whether the disease is present at birth but with a gap between the anatomical and clinical onset, or whether it develops later. Asymptomatic members of afflicted families who have recognisable organic abnormality of the right ventricle have been observed and it is not yet known how many of these cases will go on to develop symptoms. As in hypertrophic cardiomyopathy, sporadic cases are also well known, but whether they are due to a new genetic mutation or are familial but with "low penetrance" is still not known. In family studies, apparently normal members may present with ventricular premature beats of right ventricular origin or even self-terminating runs of ventricular tachycardia with a left bundle branch block pattern. Indeed Waynberger et al. [26] described familial ventricular tachycardia of left bundle branch block type in 1974. These subjects may have a normal electrocardiogram and echocardiogram but it is not known whether they represent formes frustes or a pre-arrhythmic phase of the disease.

Arrhythmogenic right ventricular dysplasia is a cause of sudden death in asymptomatic young people [24] (Table 13.1) and more than 80% of cases present with arrhythmias. Ventricular arrhythmias dominate the disease, sometimes with syncope due to ventricular tachycardia provoked by exertion, but supraventricular arrhythmias also occur. Self-terminating ventricular tachycardia may be induced by treadmill exercise testing and provoked during electrophysiological study. The tachycardia is re-entrant, as shown by late QRS potentials implying fragmented conduction times on the signal-averaged electrocardiogram, the prime substrate for re-entry. Ventricular tachycardia of left bundle branch block type is usually readily inducible by timed extra stimuli. The electrocardiogram does not usually show a right ventricular conduction defect, suggesting that right ventricular dysplasia does not alter the sequence of ventricular activation, although this is invariably delayed as shown by the late potentials.

Clinical Features

The broad spectrum of severity of the dysplasia accounts for clinical features that vary from grossly abnormal to normal. Sustained ventricular tachycardia originating from the right ventricle which is dilated with regional bulges and akinesia in the presence of a normal left ventricle is diagnostic of right ventricular dysplasia. At the other extreme are asymptomatic patients in whom the right ventricular abnormality is only detected by echocardiography or indeed is only suspected because of right ventricular ectopic beats occurring in an asymptomatic member of an afflicted family.

Clinical features are usually much less impressive than echocardiographic and angiographic ones even when the ventricle is very abnormal. Eventually, right ventricular failure may occur in such cases or the development of supraventricular arrhythmias may be associated with progressive tricuspid regurgitation. Such patients may show right atrial dilatation on the chest radiograph but in most other cases the chest X-ray is normal. The electrocardiogram again is insensitive, but may show T wave inversion in the right chest leads or ventricular premature beats with a left bundle branch block morphology. The 24-h ambulatory Holter monitor may show bursts of ventricular tachycardia.

Other patients may have normal findings on examination and a normal electrocardiogram but experience disabling ventricular tachycardia provoked by exercise and have easily recognisable abnormalities on echocardiography or angiocardiography,

Echocardiography in the severe cases may show focal right ventricular dyskinesia with bulging in the inferobasal wall, apex and outflow tract with bizarre vermiform trabeculation as well as dilatation shown on angiography [27, 28]. Parallel deep fissuring of the anterior wall of the right ventricle resembling a "pile of plates" is typically recognised in diastole, with multisaccular bulging or hypokinesia of the inferior and anterior walls of the right ventricle seen during systole. The left ventricle only appears at all abnormal when the right ventricle is very abnormal. The dysplastic changes in the right and subsequently in the left ventricle appear to be progressive but the main concern is of a fatal ventricular arrhythmia at a stage when there may be little or no haemodynamic impairment [24, 29] and only small focal abnormalities on echocardiography [30].

Right ventricular biopsy taken from the septum may be quite normal but biopsy from the free wall may show the typical fibro-adipose changes, occasionally with some cellular infiltration. A negative biopsy does not exclude dysplasia but an adipose content of 20% in a young adult may be regarded as diagnostic.

Computed axial tomography or magnetic resonance imaging (MRI) will also allow recognition of right ventricular dysplasia in all but mild cases. These imaging modalities do not really add sufficiently to the information gained from echocardiography, angiocardiography and biopsy to justify their use, though MRI may make a biopsy redundant by allowing tissue recognition of adipose replacement. It is very expensive and not universally available.

Signal-averaged analysis of the QRS complex on surface electrocardiography has proved disappointing in predicting susceptibility to ventricular arrhythmia in right ventricular dysplasia, although delayed right ventricular free wall activity had been recognised by epicardial mapping and by endocavitary recordings before the development of signal averaging on the surface electrocardiogram [31]. Although it now appears that the dysplasia tends to be slowly progressive, serial recording of the signal-averaged QRS has not been useful in predicting ventricular tachycardia.

Treatment

Patients with symptomatic episodes of right ventricular tachycardia need treatment and amiodarone has shown itself to be effective in many of them. Unfortunately, a proportion of patients prove very resistant to therapy, needing a combination of amiodarone with a beta-adrenergic blocking drug or of amiodarone with a class IC agent such as flecainide. Electrode catheter ablation of resistant ventricular tachycardia has been tried. An attempt may be made to locate the site of origin of abnormal ventricular activation by endocardial mapping, but localisation of the area to be ablated is very difficult and these dysplastic ventricles may have many possible foci and re-entry circuits. Recognition of foci of maximal QRS dispersion is an easier target and electrical fulguration of such areas seems as good, although the success rate is not high. Combination of electrical fulguration with drug treatment may be helpful but recurrences of arrhythmias still tend to occur. For this reason surgical treatment has been attempted with a comprehensive disconnection of the right ventricular free wall which is then excluded from its left ventricular attachments by dissection. It is then re-sutured. The subsequent fibrous scar confines right ventricular tachycardias to that chamber [32]. The only other alternatives are an implanted defibrillator or cardiac transplantation.

Right ventricular dysplasia is a cause of sudden death in apparently healthy, young athletic people as well as older people. The propensity for this seems unrelated to the severity of the dysplastic change so that patients without haemodynamic disability may be faced with the possibility of needing such dramatic treatments if, despite all pharmacological and electrophysiological episodes, the risk of sudden death seems high. The efficiency of the implantable defibrillator has still to be evaluated in these patients.

Although the familial disorder is well documented, many patients with right ventricular dysplasia apparently have no family members affected. It has been suggested that in individuals with a genetic predisposition a number of different toxic, viral or bacterial agents may induce the typical histological alterations with adipose replacement of myocardial fibres. This might occur after infection with Mycoplasma or Coxsackie virus. In this connection MRI can be used to investigate the proportion of right ventricular myocardium that has been so replaced and would of course eliminate the small risks of taking a biopsy from the thinned right ventricular free wall. It is not yet known whether all forms of right ventricular dysplasia are progressive but certainly the familial forms seem to be and will eventually lead to right ventricular failure unless sudden death occurs earlier. The time course of this is not yet known and may be highly variable.

Right Ventricular Dilated Cardiomyopathy.

In patients with right ventricular dilated cardiomyopathy the right ventricle is dilated, thin walled and diffusely hypokinetic, and the first evidence of abnormality is usually right ventricular failure [33] with cardiomegaly on radiography, sometimes even simulating cardiac tamponade clinically although the true situation is quickly established by echocardiography [34]. Ventricular arrhythmias are not a feature but sudden death is likely. The left ventricle usually looks normal or only slightly abnormal, possibly due to the effect of the right ventricular abnormality or possibly because right ventricular dilated cardiomyopathy may result from previous virus infection which has incompletely spared the left ventricle. Tricuspid regurgitaion may be a feature and in older patients the clinical features may suggest advanced rheumatic heart disease until it is discovered that the mitral valve is normal. Sinoatrial disorders are a feature of some patients with atrial standstill more commonly than tachycardias. The possibility that the condition may be a variant of arrhythmogenic right ventricular dysplasia has to be considered.

Treatment is basically unhelpful except to correct the heart rate, and transplantation may be indicated.

Peripartum Cardiomyopathy

When myocardial failure develops late in pregnancy or within 6 months of delivery in a previously fit woman, the condition is known as "peripartum cardiomyopathy" [35, 36]. The term indicates our lack of understanding of the condition, the diagnosis usually being made by exclusion of other causes of heart failure.

Although it has been suggested that these patients may have had a previously undiagnosed mild cardiomyopathy with failure precipitated by the haemodynamic stress of pregnancy, this is unlikely because presentation is more frequent in the puerperium than in pregnancy.

Peripartum cardiomyopathy allegedly occurs approximately once every 2500 deliveries but the true incidence is unknown as mild cases may go undiagnosed. The relatively sudden development of often life-threatening heart failure at this time suggests that peripartum cardiomyopathy is a specific entity and caused by the pregnancy. Moreover, unlike patients with dilated cardiomyopathy, women with peripartum cardiomyopathy who survive often show dramatic improvement and cardiac function may return to normal [37].

Various suggested causes and associations have muddied the waters and made the incidence difficult to calculate. A high incidence reported in the West Indies and Africa has been related to the frequency of previous hypertension or pre-eclamptic toxaemia [38, 39]. Viral myocarditis in pregnancy has not been ruled out as a cause. My patients have not shown the low social class, high parity, previous hypertension, pre-eclamptic toxaemia or black skin which are supposed to contribute to the development of peripartum cardiomyopathy. An association with multiple births seems to be true.

In a recent study of 18 patients all of whom were submitted to endomyocardial biopsy, 14 showed evidence of myocarditis according to the Dallas criteria and 10 received immunosuppressive therapy [40]. Increased susceptibility to some bacterial infections in pregnancy may be due to diminished cell-mediated immunity for the protection of the child, but it seems possible that the "myocarditis" is of immunological origin rather than due to a virus or other infective agent—although two recent studies suggest an infective cause [40a]. This may have to do with a breakdown of the usual immune barrier between child and mother rather than that a healthy woman should succumb so disastrously to a virus just at this time.

Peripartum cardiomyopathy usually presents acutely in the puerperium, most often within a few days of the delivery of the child. Apart from the timing and the acute onset, there are no clinical distinctions from dilated cardiomyopathy. Both the left and the right ventricle are dilated and hypokinetic, the atria enlarged and the filling pressures raised, but the cardiac output may not be greatly reduced except in the most calamitous cases. Treatment of the heart failure therefore differs in no way from the treatment of dilated cardiomyopathy. Patients who are very ill may require pressure monitoring by a Swan–Ganz catheter during treatment with intravenous inotropes. Others, with less severe disease, may respond to oral treatment with digoxin, diuretics and angiotensin converting enzyme inhibitors. Patients who fail to improve may be treated with oral prednisolone (1 mg/kg per day) and azothioprine (1.5 mg/kg per day) for 6–8 weeks, tailing the drugs off gradually after this time. With the tendency even of seriously affected patients to improve if they do not die in the acute stages, and the widely varying severity of the myocardial failure together with the rarity of the condition, it is difficult to determine whether the immunosuppressive treatment is helpful or not. The results of a multicentre randomised trial of their treatment in myocarditis/dilated cardiomyopathy are awaited.

Prognosis

In the sparse literature it is suggested that the prognosis is good if the heart size has returned to normal within 6 months of delivery. This is clearly true but the converse is not. Improvement may begin considerably later than this. It may be delayed for as long as a year and then continue over a further year or more and the patient still recover normal myocardial function. Patients whose left ventricular function has returned to normal do not invariably suffer a recurrence of heart failure in subsequent pregnancies, though it seems wise to advise deferring further pregnancy for a few years. Patients with persisting impairment of left ventricular function should be strongly advised not to undertake further pregnancies.

The condition has a considerable mortality—allegedly up to 50%, but my own experience has been much happier than this. Fatalities tend to occur soon after onset, so facing the cardiologist with a desperate dilemma: to try to get the patient urgently transplanted lest she dies or to hang on in the hope of the considerable improvement that may still follow if the patient survives the acute phase. These patients have usually been rapidly transported from joy and elation at a safe delivery to the depths of despair and anguish about their likely fate and the welfare of the baby. They and their families need both skilled cardiological care and good doctoring.

Heart Failure in the Hausa Women of Northern Nigeria

A condition different from classical peripartum cardiomyopathy is found in the Hausa women of Northern Nigeria and is precipitated by heating of the body and excessive salt intake which is the custom for parturient women of that tribe [39]. The heart failure is due to excessive fluid retention, is of "high output" type and responds to salt restriction and diuretics. The prognosis is good.

Familial Cardiomyopathy

Apart from familial hypertrophic cardiomyopathy, there exist heterogeneous familial cardiomyopathies. Some of these have the features of dilated cardiomyopathy; others may have restrictive features.

Familial dilated cardiomyopathy exists in rare families with an apparently autosomal dominant mode of inheritance [41]. In other families exclusively males or exclusively females manifest the disease [42]. In some families the history of the development of congestive heart failure is long and the condition may remain stable for years. In other families the onset of heart failure tends to be explosive in young adults with early death unless cardiac transplantation can be arranged. Arrhythmias, embolism and sudden death occur.

It is now realised that a familial incidence in dilated cardiomyopathy is much commoner than previously realised. So dilated *familial* cardiomyopathy is likely to be identical with dilated cardiomyopathy (see Chap. 4).

In some families the condition shows varying severity, with some members dying in congestive heart failure and others asymptomatic but with electrocardiographic abnormalities.

At autopsy these hearts may look no different from the hearts of patients dying with the more usual sporadic form of dilated cardiomyopathy, but in other families there appears to have been progressive myocyte fall-out with replacement fibrosis and marked hypertophy of the remaining muscle fibres.

In yet other families the clinical picture is mainly restrictive with small, thin-walled active ventricles, raised filling pressures and biatrial dilatation sometimes with atrial standstill and with progressive atrioventricular conduction disease requiring pacing [43]. The pathology of the ventricular walls varies from seeming normality to marked disarray which may be generalised, so that some of these patients are designated as cases of hypertrophic cardiomyopathy and others as cases of restrictive cardiomyopathy. Two clinical syndromes are seen most frequently. Children or young adults with gradual onset of congestive failure in sinus rhythm are found to have normal-appearing left and right ventricles on echo cardiography and angiocardiography but raised filling pressures with a restrictive picture of rapid early fillng of the ventricles and high diastolic ventricular pressures. Some of these patients die from congestive failure in childhood. In others the picture simulates constrictive pericarditis, but usually marked atrial dilatation, disparity between the left- and right-sided diastolic pressuires of tricuspid regurgitation make a myocardial abnormality certain. Other patients are seen as young adults with sinoatrial disease, a tachybrady syndrome and high venous pressure but no other symptoms. They tend to develop progressively more restrictive physiology together with conduction system failure but may live for many years after pacemaker implantation. Ventricular arrhythmias are usually not a problem but symptoms of a low cardiac output such as weakness, lassitude, hepatomegaly, ascites and varicose veins may dominate the clinical scene. The condition has been seen in two generations as well as in siblings (see Chap. 4).

Endocardial Fibroelastosis

Endocardial fibroelastosis is characterised by thickening of the endocardium, especially of the left ventricle including the mitral and aortic valves. The fibrous thickening has been described as resembling porcelain and accounts for obliteration of the normal architecture on angiography. The primary form occurs in the absence of congenital heart disease but it may also occur in association with coarctation of the aorta. The condition causes heart failure in infancy which may be fatal, but survivors may reach early childhood or, in mild cases, may survive with stable although impaired left ventricular function into adult life. There is usually mild or moderate fixed mitral regurgitation caused by the involvement of the mitral valve.

The disorder is sometimes seen in siblings, suggesting an autosomal recessive inheritance [44], and an X-linked form has also been described [45]. However, the majority of cases are sporadic. The incidence of familial cases is sufficiently small to suggest that the sporadic cases do not have a genetic cause and that the aetiology is multifactorial. Myocarditis has been suggested as a likely cause. One form of recessively inherited endocardial fibroelastosis was attributed to deficiency of carnitine in a family with the cardiomyopathy in four out of five children [46]. Treatment of a surviving affected child with oral L-carnitine improved myocardial function.

References

1. Plehn JF, Friedman BJ (1989) Diastolic dysfunction in amyloid heart disease: restrictive cardiomyopathy or not? J Am Coll Cardiol 13(1): 54–56
2. Loire R (1989) Is myocardial biopsy necessary in the diagnosis of myocardial diseases? Arch Mal Coeur 82(11): 1887–1890
3. Isobe T, Osserman EF (1974) Patterns of amyloidosis and their association with plasma cell dyscrasia monoclonal immunoglobulins and Bence-Jones proteins. N Engl J Med 290: 473
4. Hodkinson M, Pomerance A (1977) The clinical significance of senile cardiac amyloidosis: a prospective clinico pathological study. Q J Med 46: 677
5. Pitkanen P, Westermark P, Cornwell GG (1984) Senile systemic amyloidosis. Am J Pathol 117: 391
6. Gertz MA, Kyle RA, Edwards WD (1989) Recognition of congestive heart failure due to senile cardiac amyloidosis. Biomed Pharmacother 43(2): 101–106
7. Klein AL, Hatle LK, Burstow DJ, Seward JB, Kyle RA, Bailey KR, Luscher TF, Gertz MA, Tajik LK (1989) Doppler characterization of left ventricular diastolic function in cardiac amyloidosis. J Am Coll Cardiol 13(5): 1017–1726
8. Valantine HA, Billingham ME (1989) Recurrence of amyloid in a cardiac allograft four months after transplantation. J Heart Transplant 8(4): 337–334
9. Chew C, Ziady GM, Raphael MJ, Oakley CM (1975) The functional defect in amyloid heart disease. Am J Cardiol 36: 438–444
10. Feigenbaum H (1989) Echocardiographic evaluation of left ventricular diastolic function. J Am Coll Cardiol 13(5): 1027–1029
11. Pinamonti B, Picano E, Ferdeghini EM, Lattanzi F, Slavich G, Lamdin L, Camerini F, Benassi A, Distante A, L'Abbate A (1989) Quantitative texture analysis in two-dimensional echocardiography: application to the diagnosis of myocardial amyloidosis. J Am Coll Cardiol 14(3): 666–671
12. Chandrasekarn K, Aylward PE, Fleagle SR, Burns TL, Seward JB, Tajik AJ, Collins SM, Skorton DJ (1989) Feasibility of identifying amyloid and hypertrophic cardiomyopathy with the use of computerized quantitative texture analysis of clinical echocardiographic data. J Am Coll Cardiol 13(4): 832–840

13. Kinoshita O, Hongo M, Yamada H, Misawa T, Kono J, Okubo S, Ikeda S (1989) Impaired left ventricular diastolic filling in patients with familial amyloid polyneuropathy: a pulsed Doppler echocardiographic study. Br Heart J 61(2): 198–203
14. Klein AL, Hatle LK, Taliercio CP, Taylor CL, Kyle RA, Bailey KR, Seward JB, Tajik AJ (1990) Serial Doppler echocardiographic follow-up of left ventricular diastolic function in cardiac amyloidosis. J. Am Coll Cardiol 16: 1135–1141
15. Hongo M, Fujii T, Hirayama J, Kinoshita O, Tanaka M, Okubo S (1989) Radionuclide angiographic assessment of left ventricular diastolic filling in amyloid heart disease: a study of patients with familial amyloid polyneuropathy. J Am Coll Cardiol 13(1): 48–53
16. Hawkins PN, Myers MJ, Lavender JP, Pepys MB (1988) Diagnostic radionuclide imaging of amyloid: biological targeting by circulating human serum amyloid P component. Lancet 1: 1413–1418
17. Von Kemp K, Beckers R, Vandenweghe J, Taeymans Y, Osteaux M, Block P (1989) Echocardiography and magnetic resonance imaging in cardiac amyloidosis. Acta Cardiol 44(1): 29–36
18. Goldstein SA, Lindsay J Jr, Chandeysson PL, Nolan NG (1989) Usefulness of technetium pyrophosphate scintigraphy in demonstrating cardiac amyloidosis in persons aged 85 years and older. Am J Cardiol 63(11): 752–753
19. Ridolfi RL, Bulkley SH, Hutchins GM (1977) The conduction system in cardiac amyloidosis: clinical and pathological features of 23 patients. Am J Med 62: 677
19a. Goldfinger WE (1972) Colchicine for familial Mediterranean fever. N Engl J Med 287: 1302
20. Marcus FI, Fontaine GH, Guiraudon G et al. (1982) Right ventricular dysplasia: a report of 26 adult cases. Circulation 65: 384–398
21. Dalla Volta S, Battaglia G, Zerbini E (1961) Auricularization of right ventricular pressure curve. Am Heart J 61: 25–33
22. Dalla Volta S (1990) Right ventricular arrhythmogenic cardiomyopathy: the clinical point of view. In: Boraldi G, Camerini F, Goodwin JF (eds) Advances in cardiomyopathies. Springer, Berlin Heidelberg New York, p 104
23. Nava A, Thiene G, Canciani B et al. (1988) Familial occurrence of right ventricular dysplasia: a study involving nine families. J Am Coll Cardiol 12: 1222–1228
24. Thiene G, Nava A, Corrado D, Ross L, Pennelli N (1988) Right ventricular cardiomyopathy and sudden death in young people. N Engl J Med 138: 129–133
25. Webb JG, Kerr CR, Huckell VF, Mizgala HF, Ricci DR (1986) Left ventricular abnormalities in arrhythmogenic right ventricular dysplasia. Am J Cardiol 58: 568–570
26. Waynberger M, Courtadon M, Peltier JM et al. (1974) Tachycardies ventriculaires familiales: à propos de 7 observations. Nouv Presse Med 30: 1857–1860
27. Robertson JH, Bardy GH, German LD, Gallagher JJ, Kisslo J (1985) Comparison of two-dimensional echocardiographic and angiographic findings in arrhythmogenic right ventricular dysplasia. Am J Cardiol 55: 1506–1508
28. Chiddo A, Locuratolo N, Gaglione A, Bortone A, Trotto G, Musli S, Grimaldi N, Rizzon P (1989) Right ventricular dysplasia: an angiographic study. Eur Heart J 10 Suppl D: 42–45
29. Maron BJ (1988) Right ventricular cardiomyopathy: another cause of sudden death in the young. N Engl J Med 318: 178–180
30. Scognamiglio R, Fasoli G, Nava A, Miraglia G, della Valentina, Thiene G (1989) Relevance of subtle echocardiographic findings in the early diagnosis of the concealed from of right ventricular dysplasia. Eur Heart J 10 Suppl D: 27–28
31. Blomstrom-Lundqvist C, Hirsch I, Olsson SB, Edvardsson N (1988) Quantitative analysis of the signal-averaged QRS patients with arrhythmogenic right ventricular dysplasia. Eur Heart J 9: 301–312
32. Guiraudon GM, Klein GJ, Gulamhusein SS et al. (1983) Total disconnection of the right ventricular free wall in surgical treatment of right ventricular tachycardia associated with right ventricular dysplasia. Circulation 67: 463–470
33. Fitchett DJ, Sugrue DD, McArthur CG, Oakley CM (1984) Right ventricular dilated cardiomyopathy. Br Heart J 51: 25–29

34. Ribeiro PA, Shapiro LM, Foale RA, Crean P, Oakley CM (1987) Echocardiographic features of right ventricular dilated cardiomyopathy and Uhl's anomaly. Eur Heart J 8:65–71
35. Homans DC (1985) Peripartum cardiomyopathy. N Engl J Med 312: 1432
36. Julian DG, Szekeley P (1985) Peripartum cardiomyopathy. Prog Cardiovasc Dis 27:223
37. Gilchrist AR (1963) Cardiological problems in young women, including those of pregnancy and the puerperium. Br Med J 1: 209
38. Stuart KL (1968) Cardiomyopathy of pregnancy in the puerperium. Q J Med 37:463–478
39. Sanderson JE, Adesanya CO, Anjorin FI, Parry E (1979) Postpartum cardiac failure: heart failure due to volume overload? Am Heart J 97:613
40. Midei MG, Dement SH, Feldman AM et al. (1990) Peripartum myocarditis and cardiomyopathy. Circulation 81: 922–928
40a. Falase AO (1985) Peripartum heart disease In: Sebiqueli M, Olsen EGJ, Goodwin JF (eds) Myocarditis and related disorders. Springer, Berlin Heidelberg New York, p 232
41. Ross RS, Bulkley BH, Hutchins GM et al. (1978) Idiopathic familial myocardiopathy in three generations: a clinical and pathologic study. Am Heart J 97:170
42. Berko BA, Swift M (1987) X-linked dilated cardiomyopathy. N Engl J Med 316:1186
43. Stables RH, Bailey C, Ormerod DJM (1989) Idiopathic familial atrial cardiomyopathy with diffuse conduction block. Q J Med 71: 325–332
44. Vestermark S (1962) Primary endocardial fibroelastosis in siblings. Acta Paediatr 51: 94
45. Westwood M, Harris R, Burn JL, Barson AJ (1975) Heredity in primary endocardial fibroelastosis. Br Heart J 37: 1077
46. Trip ME, Katcher ML, Deters HA et al. (1981) Systemic carnitine deficiency presenting as familial endocardial fibroelastosis. N Engl J Med 305:385

Part VI
Experimental, Clinical, Immunological and Molecular Biological Research

CHAPTER 14

The Significance of Autoantibodies and the Role of the ADP/ATP Carrier in the Pathogenesis of Viral Heart Disease, Myocarditis and Dilated Cardiomyopathy

H.-P. Schultheiss

Introduction

Current concepts of autoimmunity emphasise the role of antibodies in the development and maintenance of autoimmune disorders. The problem concerning the role of autoantibodies in mediating disease is to show that a given autoantibody is an essential component of a pathological mechanism which leads to tissue damage and organ dysfunction. As well as contributing to an understanding of the pathogenesis, the precise characterisation of the antibodies involved in an autoimmune process may have diagnostic and prognostic value.

In this chapter we discuss the role of autoantibodies against a mitochondrial membrane protein—the ADP/ATP carrier—in the pathogenesis of myocarditis and dilated cardiomyopathy. To elucidate the role of autoantibodies against the ADP/ATP carrier in the pathogenesis of heart muscle diseases, we studied the hearts of guinea pigs immunised with the isolated carrier protein. The subcellular distribution of the adenine nucleotides was measured, as an inhibition of the carrier should change the intracellular energy balance by diminishing the ATP efflux from the mitochondiria into the cytosol. On the basis of these results we discuss our working hypothesis that autoimmunity to intracellular proteins, such as the ADP/ATP carrier, may contribute to the pathophysiology of viral heart disease, dilated cardiomyopathy and suspected autoimmune diseases (see Chap. 4).

Characterisation of the ADP/ATP Carrier as an Organ-Specific Autoantigen

The ADP/ATP carrier is an intrinsic hydrophobic protein located in the inner mitochondrial membrane [1]. The protein has a relative molecular mass of around 30 000 kDa and exists in the native form as a dimer. The carrier exists in two major states, alternating in the translocation process: the "c-state", where the single binding site is facing the cytosolic side of the membrane and can bind carboxyatractylate (CAT), and the "m-state", where it faces the matrix side and can bind bongkrekate (BKA) [2]. Since the inner mitochondrial membrane is *a priori* impermeable to hydrophilic metabolites, the transfer of ATP to the cytosol with its energy-consuming processes and the return of ADP to the inner mitochondrial space for regeneration by oxidative phosphorylation requires a particular transport catalysis. The ADP/ATP shuttle, the only active nucleotide transport system in mitochondria, is highly specific for ATP and ADP. Of great metabolic significance is the differentiation between ADP and ATP in the transport by the energisation of the inner mitochondrial membrane, which makes the exchange strongly asymmetric [3]. By preferential uptake of ADP and release of ATP this energisation of the membrane modulates the ADP/ATP carrier activity so as to correspond exactly to the requirement of ATP production in the cell [2].

To characterise the targets of the antibodies specific for the CAT–protein complex, different methods such as radioimmunoassay (RIA), immunoprecipitation and Western blotting have been used [4]. To test the possible effect of the antibodies on nucleotide transport in vitro, the exchange rate of mitochondria was determined by the inhibitor-stop method combined with back-exchange [4].

For the interpretation of antigen–antibody systems it is very important that the antigen is intact. Once proteins are solubilised from the membrane with a non-ionic detergent such as Triton X-100, they are labile and rapidly lose their ability to bind specific ligands. The ADP/ATP carrier was isolated as a ligand–protein complex. The non-covalent ligant (CAT) protects the protein against denaturation and gives a quantitative assay for the proportion of intact protein [1]. Given this protection of the translocator against proteolytic

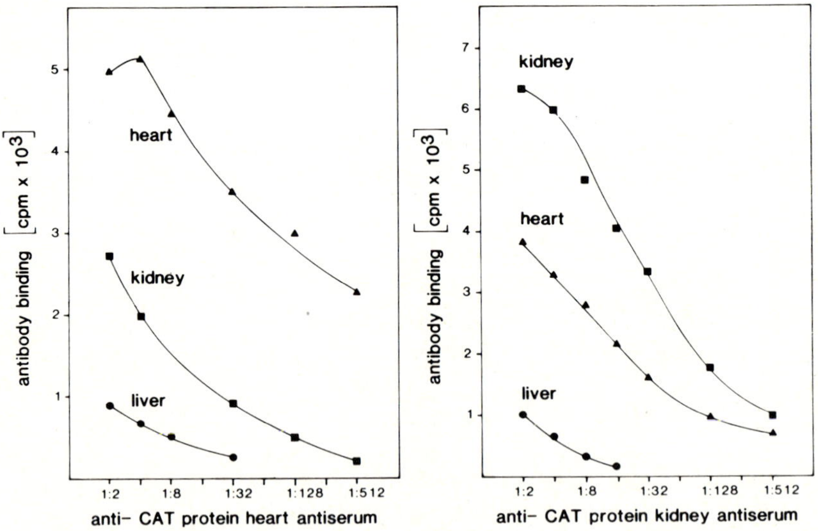

Fig. 14.1. Organ specificity of the ADP/ATP carrier

degradation, once can assume that the protein's structure and antigenicity are not destroyed by the isolation procedure [5]. Antibodies specific for the CAT–protein complex from heart or kidney were elicited in rabbits.

In indirect solid-phase radioimmunoassay the anti-heart protein antibody showed the highest bindnig activity with the heart protein (Fig. 14.1a). The maximum binding of the anti-heart antibody to the kidney protein was about 50% and to the liver protein about 20% of the binding to the heart protein. Anti-kidney antibody showed the highest binding activity with the kidney protein, but cross-reacting antibodies with the heart and liver protein were seen (Fig. 14.1b). Although a partial cross-reactivity was observed these results enlarged earlier observations on the existence of organ-specific antigenic determinants.

Immunoadsorption studies were performed to differentiate the observed cross-reactivity into heterogeneity with respect to determinants recognised on the antigen, and heterogeneity of affinity within the antibody subpopulation reacting with each determinant. As shown representatively for the anti-heart protein antiserum in Fig. 14.2, the adenine nucleotide translocator from heart absorbed most of the antibodies, while the residual activity of the antiserum after immunoabsorption on liver or kidney protein was about 80% or 50%, respectively. These results, indicating the existence of organ-specific non-cross-reacting antibodies, were confirmed by immunoadsorption studies on intact mitochondria. The fact that organ specificity is observed both with the solubilised and with the membrane-bound carrier protein shows that some organ-specific antibodies are directed against exposed regions of the carrier which are then preserved during solubilisation. The inability of the protein from kidney and liver to displace all of the anti-heart protein antibodies excludes the possibility that the organ

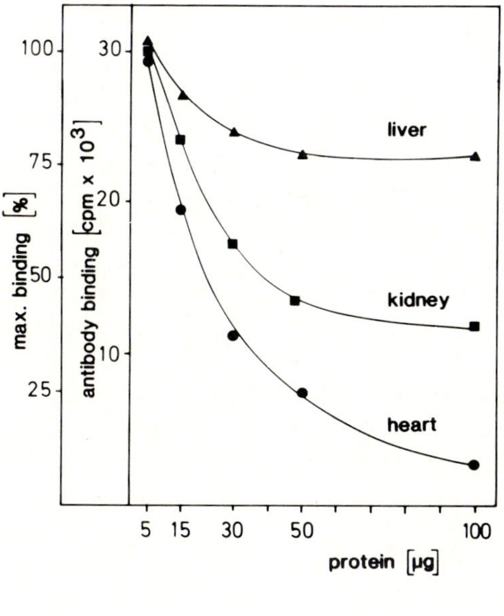

Fig. 14.2. After immunoadsorption

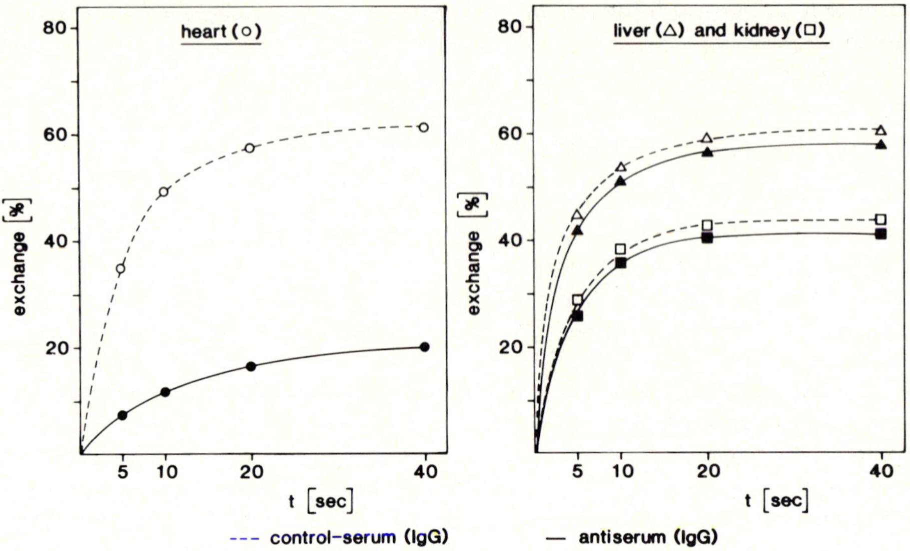

Fig. 14.3. Organ-specific inhibition of the ADP/ATp carrier

specificity is only the result of a lower affinity of the anti-heart protein antibody for the antigenic determinants of the liver and kidney proteins. Instead, the determinants appeared to be sufficiently different to exclude binding, indicating only a partial cross-reactivity between the carrier proteins from the three organs.

In an attempt to gain further evidence for the organ specificity of the ADP/ATP carrier, we determined whether the antibodies against the ADP/ATP carrier from heart inhibit mitochondrial nucleotide transport in heart, liver and kidney mitochondria. The ADP/ATP exchange rate was measured by the inhibitor-stop method combined with back-exchange. Figure 14.3 shows the immunoinactivation of the ADP/ATP carrier of heart mitochondria by the anti-heart protein antiserum. Serial dilution of the antiserum resulted in a progressive decrease of the blocking effect of the antibody. In support of organ-specific binding of antibodies to the carrier protein, it is of interest to note that the anti-heart protein antiserum showed no inhibition of adenine nucleotide transport in kidney and liver mitochondria (Fig. 14.3). Furthermore, the inhibitory activity of the anti-heart protein antiserum was not abolished by adsorption to kidney or liver mitochondria, while preadsorption of the antiserum to heart mitochondria did abolish its inhibitory activity.

This remarkable organ specificity of the ADP/ATP carrier was previously interpreted as reflecting isoenzyme distribution of the carrier in various organs. Although the concept of isoenzymes seemed at first bold and premature, it has since been extended to several other situations [6, 7]. The organ specificity of the ADP/ATP carrier, which was confirmed by peptide maps and studies of the cDNA sequence, may reflect tissue-specific regulation of nucleotide transport.

This regulation may be adapted to the specific requirements in different tissues by the expression of specific isoenzymes.

Characterisation of the Autoantibodies

Sera of 49 patients with proven dilated cardiomyopathy and 66 patients with clinically suspected myocarditis were tested. The diagnosis of dilated cardiomyopathy was established according to the WHO/ISFC task force as a chronic disorder of heart muscle of unknown cause or association. Cases of specific heart muscle diseases or secondary cardiomyopathies were excluded. Diagnosis was principally based on cardiac catheterisation data and the morphological analysis of endomyocardial biopsies, which were compatible with dilated cardiomyopathy. The diagnosis of myocarditis was established on the basis of anamnestic data, especially with regard to a common cold infection, an accompanying change in viral neutralisation titre on follow-up, clinical features and morphological evidence of myocarditis in myocardial biopsy samples. The biopsy specimens were classified into three major groups according to Olsen: active myocarditis, healing myocarditis and healed myocarditis [8,9]. Sera from

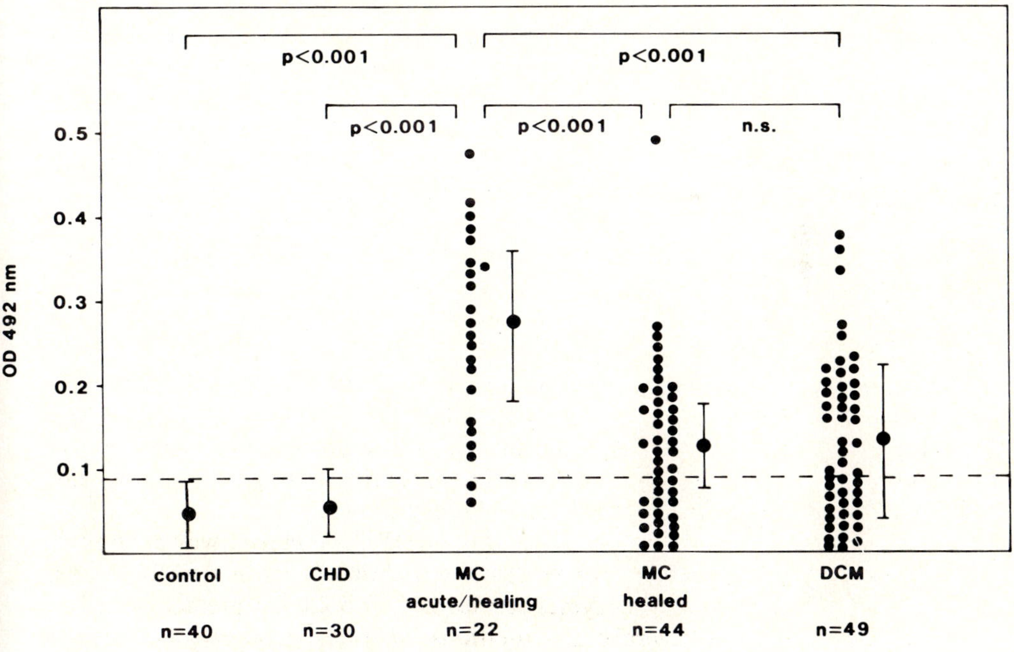

Fig. 14.4. Autoantibodies against the ADP/ATP carrier in patients with myocarditis (*MC*) and dilated cardiomyopathy (*DCM*). *CHD*, coronary heart disease

patients with proven coronary heart disease ($n = 30$) and from healthy blood donors (controls) ($n = 40$) were used for comparison.

When the sera of patients with myocarditis were tested in the enzyme-linked immunosorbent assay (ELISA) against the ADP/ATP carrier from heart, a significant antibody titre was seen in 20 of 22 patients with acute/healing myocarditis and in 26 of 44 patients with the histological diagnosis "healed myocarditis" (Fig. 14.4). In comparison to the controls, the sera from patients with coronary heart disease did not contain autoantibodies against the ADP/ATP carrier. If the positive sera from patients with suspected myocarditis reacting with the heart protein were tested against the ADP/ATP carrier from kidney or liver, the binding to the kidney and liver protein was significantly lower than the binding to the heart protein. The organ specificity of the auto antibodies was also confirmed by immunoadsorption studies on intact mitochondria or on the isolated protein from heart and lever (data not shown).

To test a possible inhibitory activity of the autoantibodies on the nucleotide exchange rate of mitochondria, we measured nucleotide transport in vitro. After preincubation of the mitochondria with isolated IgG from myocarditis sera, the exchange rate was determined by the inhibitor-stop method combined with back-exchange [4]. None of the control sera produced a significant inhibition of

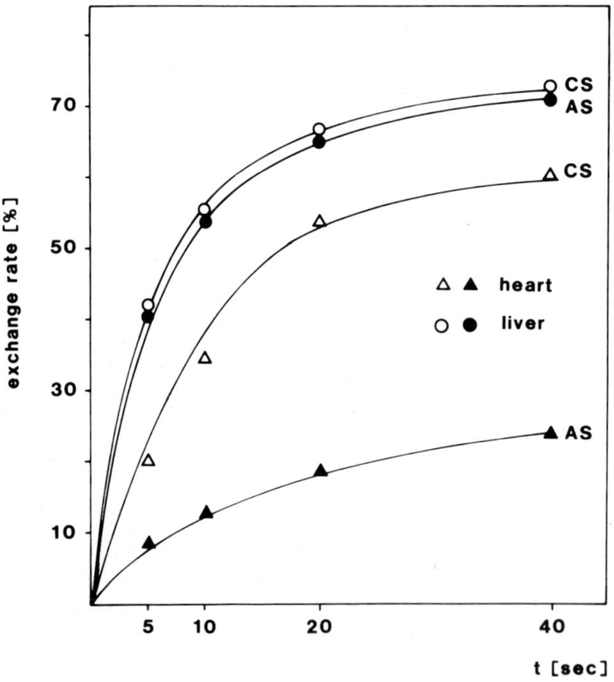

Fig. 14.5. Antibody-mediated organ-specific inhibition of the nucleotide transport. *CS*, control serum (lgG); *AS*, antiserum (lgG)

nucleotide transport. However, about 60% of the positive sera from patients with acute or healing myocarditis and 45% of the dilated cardiomyopathy sera immunoinactivated the ADP/ATP carrier from heart.

None of the sera which inhibited the nucleotide transport of heart mitochondria inhibited the transport of liver mitochondria. Again, these results demonstrate the organ specificity not only of the autoantibodies but also of the ADP/ATP carrier itself (Fig. 14.5).

The results described here demonstrate the existence of organ-specific autoantibodies against the ADP/ATP carrier, an immunochemically well-characterised constituent of the inner mitochondrial membrane, in myocarditis and dilated cardiomyopathy. Besides the importance of organ specificity for understanding the basic regulatory mechanisms in differentiated organisms, it has become particularly significant as regards autoimmune processes. In relation to the pathogenetic aetiology of these diseases, it is certain that the factors causing production of the highly specific autoantibodies are limited to the local milieu. If the autoantibodies directed against the ADP/ATP carrier play a fundamental role in the pathogenesis of myocarditis and dilated cardiomyopathy, one would suspect a correlation between the concentration of these antibodies and the clinical severity of the disease. However, the antibody titres correspond poorly with haemodynamic function, suggesting that factors other than the anitbody titre may be important in determining clinical severity. One possible explanation is that the functional activity of the antibodies, i. e. their ability to inhibit nucleotide transport across the inner mitochondrial membrane, may be clinically relevant in the pathogenesis of these diseases.

The principal ability of the antibodies to inhibit nucleotide exchange activity was shown in vitro, and regression analysis revealed a significant relationship between the immunoinactivating autoantibodies and clinical class [10].

Characterisation of Myocardial Energy Metabolism in Patients with Dilated Cardiomyopathy

In suggesting a pathogenetic role for the antibodies, it has to be asked whether nucleotide transport across the inner mitochondrial membrane is decreased not only in vitro but also in vivo. This should lead to an imbalance between energy production and energy use in the failing heart. There is substantial evidence that the failing heart in dilated cardiomyopathy is in an energy-depleted state [11, 12]. However, the cause for the disturbed myocardial energy metabolism in dilated cardiomyopathy is not yet clear. On one hand, the changes in myocardial energy metabolism might be a direct result of the underlying compensating mechanisms during the failing process. On the other hand, the imbalance between energy need and supply could be the result of an antibody-mediated disturbance of the energy-producing mechanisms.

Recently we were able to show a significant increase in LDH_5 concomitant with a decrease in LDH_1 in myocardial biopsy samples from patients with severe chronic heart failure resulting from dilated cardiomyopathy [12]. Concomitant with the shift in the LDH (lactate dehydrogenase) isoenzyme pattern, a decrease in myocardial ATP content and a significant increase in ADP/ATP carrier concentration were observed. These findings support the hypothesis of metabolic changes in chronic heart failure. The shift of the isoenzyme pattern toward LDH_5 indicates enhanced anaerobic glycolysis in the myocardium. Whether the increase in ADP/ATP carrier concentration represents an upregulation of the carrier as a consequence of an insufficient energy supply to the energy-consuming processes in the cytosol, or whether it is a disease-specific alteration (e.g. the expression of a distinct ADP/ATP carrier), is as yet unknown. However, the data show that the carrier concentration is not elevated in ischaemic heart disease, although the haemodynamic data were in the same range [13]. From this it can be surmised that the elevated carrier concentration in dilated cardiomyopathy is not simply an upregultion secondary to a disturbed energy metabolism. This assumption is also supported by the fact that nucleotide transport across the

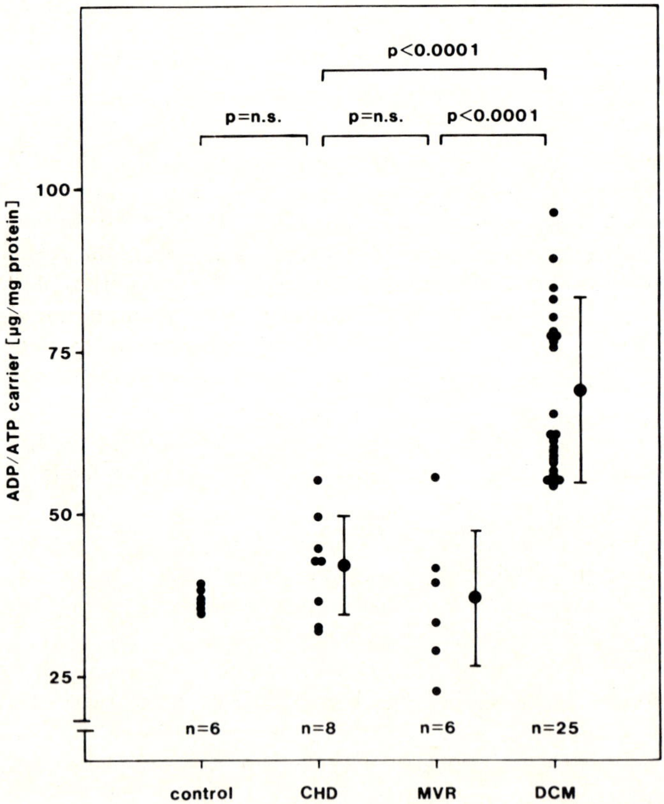

Fig. 14.6. ADP/ATP carrier content in human cardiac tissue. *CHD*, coronary heart disease; *MVR*, mitral valve replacement; *DCM*, dilated cardiomyopathy

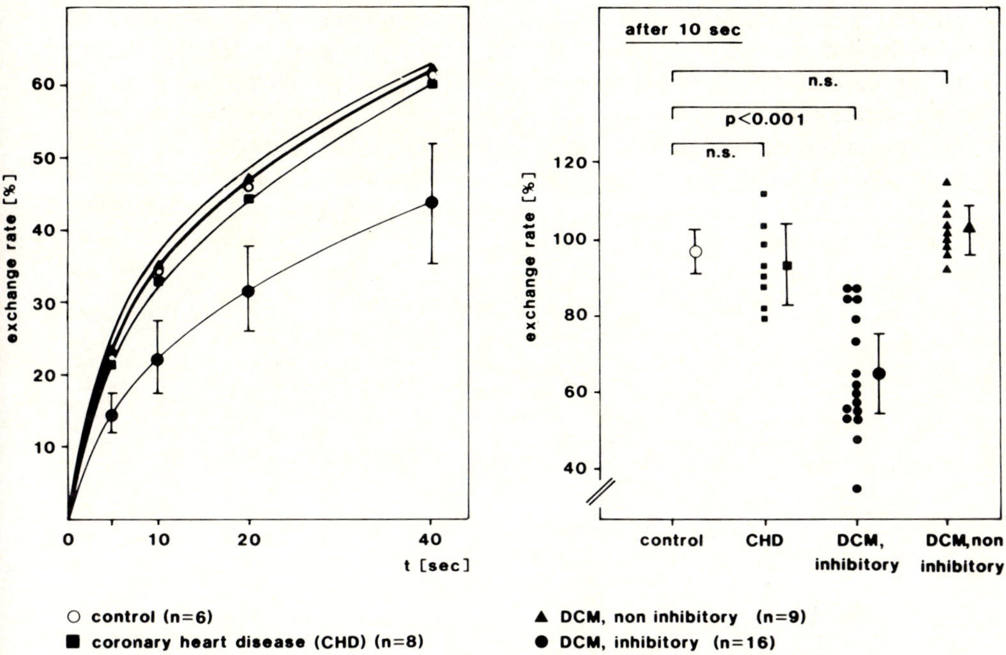

Fig. 14.7. Nucleotide exchange rate in mitochondria from explanted hearts

mitochondrial membrane is decreased in dilated cardiomyopathy. To do these measurements we isolated mitochondria from explanted hearts of patients with dilated cardiomyopathy undergoing heart transplantation. After isolation of the mitochondria, the nucleotide exchange rate was measured without adding antibodies to the mitochondria. In comparison with controls or with patients with coronary heart disease, the nucleotide exchange rate was significantly lowered in 16 of 25 patients with dilated cardiomyopathy [14]. These data indicate that the total transport capacity for ATP is decreased in these patients, again implicating a diminished energy supply to the cytosol (Fig. 14.6, 14.7).

Characterisation of Myocardial Energy Metabolism and Function in Immunised Animals

The ability of antibodies against the ADP/ATP carrier to inhibit nucleotide exchange activity from heart mitochondria was demonstarted in vitro. Regression analysis revealed a significant relationship between the immunoinactivating autoantibodies and clinical class. In postulating a pathophysiological role for these autoantibodies it has to be shown that they are an essential component of the pathological mechanism leading to organ dysfunction. To determine this we immunised guinea pigs with the isolated carrier protein and measured on one hand the subcellular distribution of the adenine nucleotides and on the other the haemodynamic parameters of the immunised animals in comparison with the control animals.

Analysis of the subcellular distribution of ATP and ADP provides a sensitive marker for defining the transport acitivity of the carrier protein. According to Klingenberg and Heldt [2] this is given by the characteristics of the ADP/ATP transport:

1) Nucleotide exchange is strongly asymmetric in energised mitochondria.
2) Nucleotide exchange is membrane-potential driven (outside positive, inside negative).
3) As a result, ATP and ADP are highly asymmetrically distributed across the mitochondrial membrane: the concentration ratio ATP/ADP is significantly higher in the extra than in the intramitochondrial space.

On the basis of these characteristics it was shown by Klingenberg [3] that the force for the regulation of adenine nucleotide exchange is derived from the potential difference between the cytosolic and motochondrial ATP. As the energisation of the mitochondrial membrane, which is expressed by the cytosolic-mitochondrial difference of the phosphorylation potential of ATP, G (cyt − mit), modulates ADP/ATP carrier activity so as it operates in the manner required for the energy needs of the cell, a decreased phosphorylation potential difference of ATP can be taken as an indicator of a reduced transport capacity of the carrier protein.

To evaluate the cytosolic and motochondrial adenine nucleotide concentrations, the hearts of the immunised and non-immunised guinea pigs were isolated and perfused as working heart preparations. Perfusion experiments were terminated by stop-freezing the myocardium between aluminium blocks precooled in liquid nitrogen. The cytosolic and mitochondrial adenine nucleotide concentrations were then measured in the haemoglobin-free perfused working

Table 14.1. Subcellular distribution of myocardiac high-energy phosphates in isolated perfused guinea pig hearts. Ratios for free cytosolic ATP/ADP were calculated from the mass action ratio of the creative kinase reaction

	Control ($n = 5$)		After immunization ($n = 6$)	
	Cytosol	Mitochondria	Cytosol	Mitochondria
ATP (mmol/l)	13.2 ± 2.0	8.1 ± 2.3	11.3 ± 2.9	18.3 ± 5.9**
ADP (mmol/l)	1.9 ± 0.4	1.6 ± 0.3	2.5 ± 0.5*	1.1 ± 0.2*
ATP/ADP (overall)	6.7 ± 0.4	5.1 ± 0.5	4.5 ± 1.1**	17.1 ± 4.9**
ATP/ADP (free)	61.8 ± 7.9	—	50.2 ± 8.8*	—
(ATP)/(ADP) × (P_i)	5487 ± 644	926 ± 215	4105 ± 624**	3349 ± 1445**
ΔG (cyt − mit) (kJ/mol)	4.6 ± 0.5		0.7 ± 1.2**	

ΔG (cyt − mit), difference in phosphorylation potential between cytosol and mitochondria
*f < 0.01, **f < 0.001 vs control

guinea pig hearts using density gradient centrifugation of the myocardial homogenates in non-aqueous media [15].

The hearts of the control animals exhibited a normal intracellular distribution of ATP (13.2 mol/l in cytosol, 8.1 mol/l in the matrix). These values are in agreement with those reported in the literature. In the hearts of the guinea pigs which showed immunoinactivating antibodies against the ADP/ATP carrier, however, the concentration of ATP was slightly lower in the cytosol (11.3 mol/l) but tremendously increased in the mitochondria (18.3 mol/l) (Table 14.1). Consequently, the ATP/ADP ratio as well as the phosphorylation state of ATP—expressed as the ratio (ATP)/(ADP) × (P_1)—were significantly lower in the cytosol, while in the mitochondrial a substantial increase was observed. Whereas in the hearts of the immunised animals G (cyt − mit) was only 0.7 kJ/mol, the difference was significantly higher in the controls (4.6 kJ/mol, $p < 0.001$).

As discussed previously, under physiological conditions the asymmetric transport of ATP creates a high cytosolic and low mitochondrial ATP/ADP ratio. A decrease in the cytosolic-mitochondrial difference of the phosphorylation potential of ATP indicates an imbalance between energy delivery and demand in the cell. Thus, the data demonstrated that the total transport capacity for ATP is decreased in the immunised animals, indicating an inadequate delivery of high-energy phosphates to the cytosol [15].

This raises the question of whether the disturbance of cellular energy balance caused by diminishing the ATP efflux from mitochondria into cytosol alters myocardial function. To evalute this hypothesis we measured the haemodynamic data from immunised guinea pig hearts which were stimulated by high calcium and maximum elevation of the afterload. The hearts were isolated and perfused as working heart preparations as described previously. The preload of 12 cmH_2O and the mean developed afterload determined the pressure–volume work of the left ventricle. External heart work was calcuated as the sum of pressure–volume work and acceleration work [$\frac{1}{2}$ × ejected volume × (mean velocity of flow)^2] during ejection.

Beating heart preparations from guinea pigs immunised with the ADP/ATP carrier showed a marked decrease in cardiac function compared with controls hearts from non-immunised animals [16]. Mean aortic pressure, stroke volume, stroke work and external heart work of the left ventricle were 40%–80% lower, external heart work being diminished from 375 to 62 mJ/g per minute (Fig. 14.8). In parallel, myocardial oxygen extraction was found to be lowered while myocardial lactate production was significantly increased.

These functional data support the hypothesis that the antibodies reacting with the ADP/ATP carrier alter myocardial function by means of an antibody-mediated dysfunction of the carrier protein which causes an imbalance between energy demand and energy supply. Thus, the experimental data suggest that the autoantibodies against the ADP/ATP carrier found in patients with myocarditis and dilated cardiomyopathy might be an essential component of the pathological mechanisms involved in post-myocarditic cardiomyopathy. This is confirmed by recent data demonstrating a direct relation between the impairment of energy

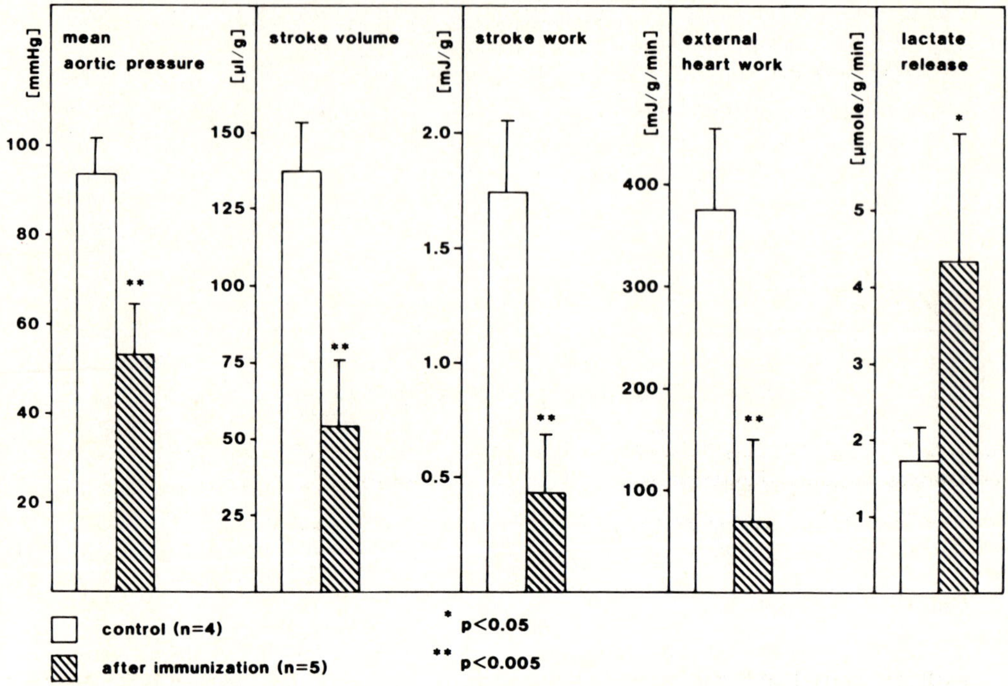

Fig. 14.8. Haemodynamic parameters of immunized vs control animals

metabolism and myocardial function. It was shown that the magnitude of the reduction in G(cyt – mit) correlates directly with the maximum work guinea pig hearts perform after being immunised with the ADP/ATP carrier.

Molecular Mimicry: The Cause of Autoimmunity (see Chap. 15)

A relationship between infectious agents (viruses) and the development of outoimmune disease has been suggested many times. Several theories have been proposed to explain the connection. One mechanism by which a virus could trigger an autoimmune response is by molecular mimicry, defined as the sharing of antigenic determinants by the virus and host cell [17]. Structural similarities have frequently been noted between a number of RNA and DNA viruses and "self" proteins. Since Coxsackie B3 virus (CB3) has been shown to induce myocarditis, we searched for homologous determinants between the recently determined sequence of CB3 and that of the ADP/ATP carrier. For the identification of antigenic epitopes we used the "pepplot" of the University of Wisconsin Genetics Computer Group. This is an amalgam of different methods for predicting the secondary structure of amino acid sequences on the basis of

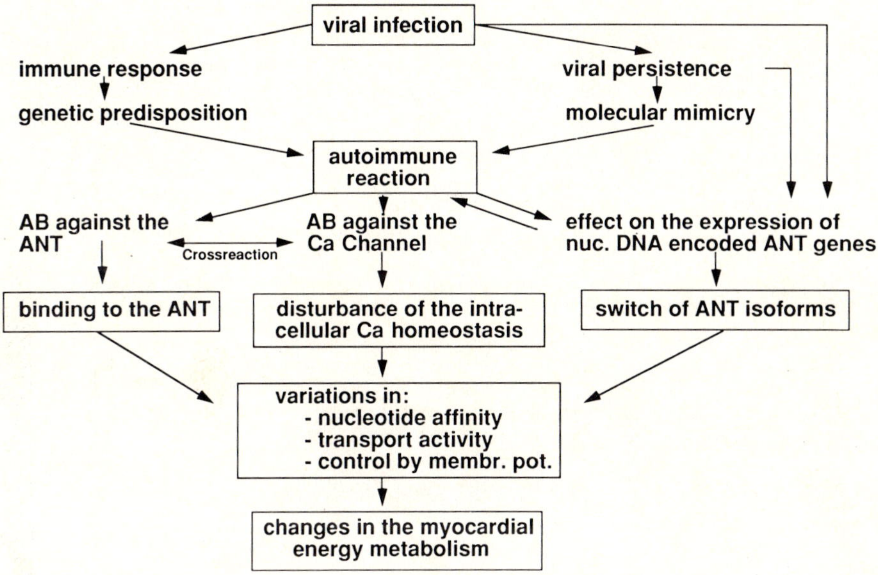

Fig. 14.9. Possible pathomechanism of dilated cardiomyopathy

hydrophilicity/hydrophobicity, acidity, basophilicity, charge, molecular size, structure and empirical data about the presence of sequences in defined proteins. Based on this analysis, a region of homology was found between the ADP/ATP carrier (amino acide 27–36) and CB3 (amino acids 1218–1228) [18]. Further experiments demonstrated that this homology translated into immunological cross-reactivity [19]. These results show that the sharing of cross-reacting antigenic determinants between the ADP/ATP carrier and CB3 may play a role in the induction of an autoimmune process following viral myocarditis. This assumption is confirmed by the fact that more than 60% of sera from patients with dilated cardiomyopathy or myocarditis bind to this sequence, while only 5% of control sera showed a positive binding on ELISA [20]. Thus, molecular mimicry may account for the enigma of persistent immunity in the absence of continued exposure to the virus (Fig. 14.9).

Characterisation of Myocardial Energy Metabolism In CB_3 Infected Mice

On the basis of the possible link between viral infection and the induction of autoimmunity we investigated whether an immunological reaction against the ADP/ATP carrier could be incited by viral infection (Fig. 14.10). After infection of H-2 congenic mice (A. SW/Sn-J mice) with CB3 viruses, circulating heart-reactive antibodies were found. A further characterisation of the antibodies

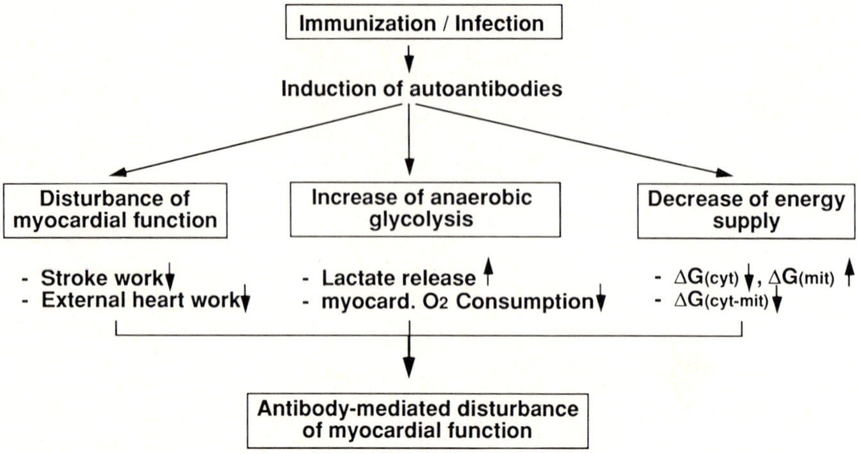

Fig. 14.10. Possible link between viral infection and induction of autoimmunity

using Western blotting showed that the antibodies stained a 30 kDa protein in the mitochondrial extract. Absorption studies revealed that the antigen was the ADP/ATP carrier. In a next step we measured—in parallel to the experiments described above—the cytosolic-mitochondrial differences of the phosphorylation potential of ATP, G(cyt – mit), by non-aqueous fractionation of the myocardium. Similar to the data seen in guinea pigs immunised with the ADP/ATP carrier, in mice infected with CB3 a decreased virus-induced immunoreaction against the ADP/ATP carrier leads to a disturbance of cellular energy metabolism. Together with the molecular mimicry between Coxsackie B3 virus and the ADP/ATP carrier, the virus-induced antibody-mediated disturbance of nucleotide transport can be taken as a further indication for the role of the ADP/ATP carrier in the pathogenicity of viral heart disease.

Conclusion

A number of investigations have suggested that immunopathological mechanisms, both humoral and cellular, may contribute, at least in part, to the pathogenesis of myocarditis and dilated cardiomyopathy [21–23]. Recent data demonstrating persistence of viral RNA in the myocardium of patients with myocarditis and dilated cardiomyopathy make a persistent viral infection in the latter quite likely [15, 24–26] (Fig. 14.11). Interest is now focused on the link between persistent viral infection, the induction of autoimmunity and the alteration of differentiated functions of the myocardium in myocarditis and dilated cardiomyopathy.

One hypothesis to explain virus-induced autoimmunity is that immunogenic determinants of a virus can induce the formation of antibodies during an

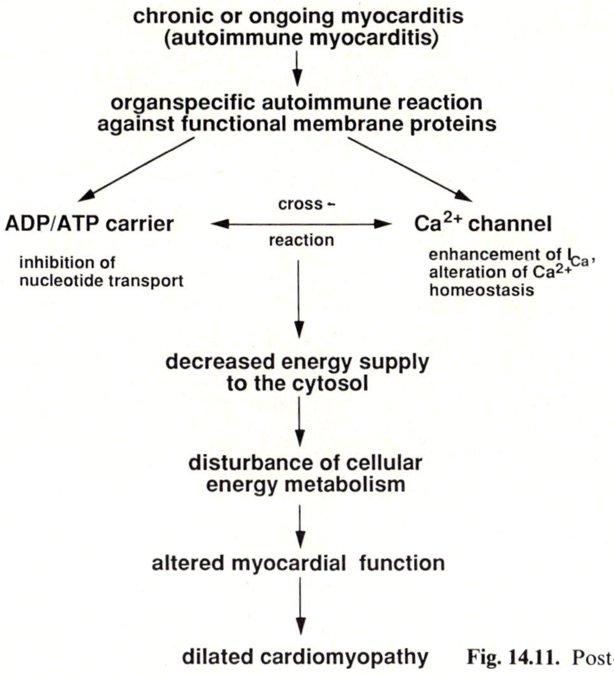

Fig. 14.11. Post-infection cardiac autoimmunity

infection which in turn may react with homologous but not identical epitopes on a host protein.

The immune response initiated against the foreign virus material may therefore react not only with the virus but also with the "self" protein. Depending on the biological function of the host protein that is recognised, the outcome of the interaction may be disease. The data presented here show, for the first time, molecular mimicry between Coxsackie B3 virus and the adenine nucleotide translocator (an autoantigen in myocarditis and dilated cardiomyopathy) as a possible mechanism for the development of autoimmunity in viral heart disease.

However, it has to be emphasised that the induction of cross-reactivity does not require a replicating agent. The immunologically mediated injury can occur also after removal of the immunogen. This means that the viral infection initiates the autoimmune phenomenon but does not need to be present at the time overt disease develops. The autoimmune response itself leads to tissue injury that, in turn, releases more self-antigen, thereby inducing more autoantibodies, and so on.

The specificity of the autoantibodies against the ADP/ATP carrier and their ability to inhibit nucleotide exchange acitivity in vitro suggests that they might be mediators of the disease at the molecular level [27–29]. Since there are no methods available for measuring the function of the ADP/ATP carrier in living organs, we measured the cytosolic-mitochondrial difference of the phosphorylation potential of ATP in guinea pigs. The ratio of the subcellular concentrations of ATP and ADP is particular suitable for evaluating the balance between mitochondrial ADP phosphorylation, ATP transport and the consumption of ATP in the cytosol. On the basis of these functional characteristics of the carrier protein, the data provide strong experimental evidence for a diminished total activity of nucleotide transport in vivo in the immunised animals [15].

In parallel with to the disturbed energy metabolism, the functional data of the isolated perfused hearts from the immunised guinea pigs performing maximum pressure-volume work showed a significantly altered myocardial function [16, 29]. Stroke, volume, stroke work and external heart work calculated as the sum of pressure-volume work and acceleration work during ejections were greatly reduced. Thus, the biochemical and functional data clearly support the hypothesis that the antibodies against the ADP/ATP carrier cause a dysfunction of the heart by an antibody-mediated disturbance of cellular energy metabolism.

Clinical findings support the experimental results from the animal model. First, sera from patients with myocarditis and dilated cardiomyopathy inhibit nucleotide exchange in isolated mitrochondria. Second, isolated mitochondria of explanted hearts from patients with dilated cardiomyopathy show a reduced carrier function. Third, carrier protein concentration is increased in endomyocardial biopsy samples from patients with cardiomyopathy and in explanted cardiomyopathic hearts. Fourth, a relationship exists between the presence of immunoinactivating antibodies against the ADP/ATP carrier in the sera of patients with myocarditis and the prognosis of the disease.

Nevertheless, the mechanism by which the antibodies are enabled to exert their deleterious effect on energy metabolism and myocardial function needs to be elucidated. Using immunofluorescence techniques and peroxidase-antiperoxidase staining we found immunoglobulin deposits in mitochondrial membranes in cryosections of the myocardium of immunised animals. In isolated cardiac myocytes, the formation and cytosolic internalisation of immunoglobulin-containing membrane-coated vesicles could be shown [30]. These results might support the hypothesis of a direct binding of the cytosolically internalised antibodies to the ADP/ATP carrier. Cytosolic uptake of the plasma-membrane-bound antibodies could result from receptor-mediated endocytosis. The connexon and the calcium channel have been identified as cross-reacting structures at the cell surface, such as would needed for receptor-mediated endocytosis. To bind to the carrier protein the antibody does not need to penetrate the outer mitochondrial membrane, for the carrier is synthesised in the cytosol and imported post-translationally into the inner mitochondrial membrane. Thus the binding of antibodies to the pre-mature carrier protein could result in hindering carrier uptake into the inner mitochondrial membrane or carrier dysfunction after membrane incorporation.

A second possibility is that antibody binding to the cell surface influences carrier function indirectly by activating a messenger system. This is supported by the observation of cross-reactivity between the ADP/ATP carrier and the calcium channel [31, 32]. By electrophysiological and functional studies it was demonstrated that anti-ADP/ATP carrier antibodies bind specifically at the calcium channel of the cell surface and enchance calcium influx into the cell.

A raised intracellular calcium concentration could cause an intramitochondrial calcium overload and lower the mitochondrial transmembrane potential, which seems to be dependent on the intra-mitochondrial calcium concentration and on calcium fluxes through the mitochondrial membrane. Any lowered mitochondrial transmembrane potential would downregulate the activity of the electrogenic nucleotide exchange via the ADP/ATP carrier, finally decreasing the cytosolic–mitochondrial phosphorylation potential difference of ATP. Thus, an antibody-mediated change in cellular calcium homeostasis would initiate cellular metabolic impairment via calcium as a "second messenger". In principle, abnormalities in calcium metabolism of the myocardium are thought to be involved in the pathogenesis of cardiomyopathies.

Regardless of the mechanism of action of the antibodies—either directly through antibody-mediated inhibition of the carrier protein or indirectly through antibody-mediated disturbance of intracellular calcium homeostasis—our data indicate a new role for an antibody-mediated dysfunction of the myocardium. These results may be of major importance for understanding the pathogenesis of myocarditis and dilated cardiomyopathy and, subsequently, may result in new therapeutic regimes for these diseases.

References

1. Klingenberg M (1985) The ADP/ATP carrier in mitochondrial membranes. In: Martonosi AN (ed) The enzymes of biological membranes, vol 4. Plenum, New York, pp 511–553
2. Klingenberg M, Heldt HW (1982) The ADP/ATP translocation in mitochondria and its role in intracellular compartmentation. In: Sies H (ed) Metabolic compartmentation. Academic, London, pp 101–122
3. Klingenberg M (1980) The ADP/ATP carrier translocation in mitchondria: a membrane potential controlled transport. J Membr Biol 56: 97
4. Schultheiss H-P, Klingenberg M (1984) Immunochemical characterization of the adenine nucleotide translocator: organ specificity and conformation specificity. Eur J Biochem 143: 599–605
5. Schultheiss H-P, Schulze K, Kühl U, Ulrich G, Klingenberg M (1987) The ADP/ATP carrier as a mitochondrial autoantigen: facts and perspectives. Ann NY Acad Sci 488: 44–64
6. Neckelmann N, Li K, Wade RP, Shuster R, Wallace DC (1987) cDNA sequence of a human skeletal muscle ADP/ATP translocator: lack of a leader peptide, divergence from a fibroblast translocator cDNA, and coevolution with mitochondrial DNA genes. Proc Natl Acad Sci USA 84: 7580
7. Rasmussen UB, Wohlrab H (1986) Conserved structural domains among species and tissues-specific differences in the mitochondrial phosphate-transport protein and the ADP/ATP carrier. Biochim Biophys Acta 852: 306–314
8. Olsen EGJ (1983) Myocarditis: a case of mistaken identity? Br Heart J 50: 303–311
9. Aretz HT, Billingham ME, Edwards WD, Factors S, Fallon JT, Fenoglio JJ Jr, Olsen EGJ, Schoen F (1986) Myocarditis: a histopathologic definition and classification. J Cardiovasc Pathol 1: 3–14
10. Schultheiss H-P, Schwimmbeck P (1986) Autoantibodies to the adenine nucleotide translocator (ANT) in myocarditis (MC): prevalence, clinical correlates and diagnostic value. Circulation 74 Suppl 2: 142
11. Schultheiss H-P, Witzenbichler B, Strauer BE (1991) Disturbed myocardial energy metabolism in dilated cardiomyopathy. Circulation 82: 2257

12. Schultheiss H-P (1990) Effect on the myocardial energy metabolism of angiotensin-converting enzyme inhibition in chronic heart failure. Am J Cardiol 65: 74G–81G
13. Schultheiss H-P (1989) The significance of autoantibodies against the ADP/ATP carrier for the pathogenesis of myocarditis and dilated cardiomyopathy: clinical and experimental data. Springer Semin Immunopathol 11: 15–30
14. Schultheiss HP, Kühl U, Schauer R, Schulze K, Kemkes B, Becker BF (1988) Antibodies against the ADP/ATP carrier alter myocardial function by disturbing cellular energy metabolism. In: Schultheiss HP (ed) New concepts in viral heart disease. Springer, Berlin Heidelberg New York, pp 243–258
15. Schulze K, Becker BF, Schultheiss H-P (1989) Antibodies to the ADP/ATP carrier—an autoantigen in myocarditis and dilated cardiomyopathy-penetrate into myocardial cells and disturb energy metabolism in vivo. Circ Res 64: 179–192
16. Schulze K, Becker BF, Schauer R, Schultheiss H-P (1990) Antibodies to ADP-ATP carrier—an autoantigen in myocarditis and dilated cardiomyopathy—impair cardiac function. Circulation 81: 959–969
17. Oldstone MBA, Schwimmbeck P, Dyrberg TI, Fujinami R (1986) Mimicry by virus of host molecules: implications for autoimmune disease. Prog Immunol 6: 787–795
18. Schwimmbeck PL, Schultheiss H-P, Strauer BE (1989) Identification of a main autoimmunogenic epitope of the adenine nucleotide translocator which cross-reacts with Coxsackie B3 virus: use in the diagnosis of myocarditis and dilative cardiomyopahty. Circulation 80 Suppl: II-665
19. Schwimmbeck PL, Schultheiss H-P, Strauer BE, Oldstone MBA (1989) Sharing of antigenic determinants between Coxsackie B3 virus and autoantigens in viral myocarditis and dilative cardiomyopathy. J Am Coll Cardiol 13: 253-A
20. Schwimmbeck PL, Schultheiss H-P, Strauer BE (1990) Isolation of myocardial autoantibodies using immunadsorption with synthetic peptides as antigens. Eur Heart J 11 Suppl: 280
21. Witzenbichler B, Christmann C, Schulze K, Schultheiss H-P, Strauer BE (1991) Disturbance of the myocardial energy metabolism in A. SW/SNJ mice after viral infection (Coxsackie virus B3). J Am Coll Cardiol 17: 264-A
22. Zanetti M (1986) New concepts in autoimmunity. Immunol Invest 15: 287
23. Rose NR, Herskowitz A, Neumann DA, Neu N (1988) Autoimmune myocarditis: a paradigm of post-infection autoimmune disease. Immunol Today 9: 117–119
24. Archard LC, Freeke AC, Richardson PJ, Meany B, Olson EGJ, Morgan-Capner P, Rose ML, Taylor P, Banner NR, Yacoub MH, Bowles NE (1988) Persistence of enterovirus RNA in dilated cardiomyopahty: a progression from myocarditis. In: Schulthei H-P (ed) New concepts in viral heart disease. Springer, Berlin Heidelberg New York, pp 349–362
25. Kandolf A, Kirschner P, Ameis D, Canu A, Erdmann E. Schultheiss H-P, Kemkes B, Hofschneider P (1988) Enteroviral heart disease: diagnosis by in-situ hybridization. In: Schultheiss HP (ed) New concepts in viral heart disease. Springer, Berlin Heidelberg New York, pp 337–348
26. Editorial (1990) Dilated cardiomyopathy and enteroviruses. Lancet 336: 971–973
27. Schultheiss H-P, Bolte HD (1985) Immunological analysis of autoantibodies against the adenine nucleotide translocator in dilated cardiomyopathy. J Mol Cell Cardiol 17: 603–617
28. Schultheiss H-P (1987) The mitochondrion as antigen in inflammatory heart disease. Eur Heart J 8: 203–210
29. Schultheiss HP, Kuhl U, Schauer R, Schulze K, Kemkes B, Becker BF (1988) Antibodies against adenosine di-/triphosphate carrier alter myocardial function by disturbing cellular energy metabolism. In: Schultheiss H-P (ed) New concepts in viral heart disease. Springer, Berlin Heidelberg New York, pp 243–258
30. Janda I, Herzog V, Kühl U, Schultheiss H-P (1990) Biochemical and immunocytochemical evidence for endocytosis of antibodies against the ADP/ATP carrier—an autoantigen in dilated cardiomyopathy. Circulation 82: III–268
31. Schultheiss H-P, Kühl U, Janda I, Melzner B, Ulrich G, Morad M (1988) Antibody-mediated enhancement of calcium permeability in cardiac myocytes. J Exp Med 168: 2105–2116
32. Morad M, Davies NW, Ulrich G, Schultheiss H-P (1988) Antibodies against ADP–ATP carrier enhance Ca^{2+} current in isolated cardiac myocytes. Am J Physiol 255: H960–H964

CHAPTER 15

Experimental Studies of Humoral and Cellular Immunological Parameters of Viral Heart Disease

B. Maisch and M. Herzum

Human Studies

Retrospective

Realisation and expectation, hopes and frustration in the diagnosis, the pathogenetic understanding and the treatment of viral heart disease in general and viral myocarditis in particular can be appreciated best from a historical retrospective, from which current perspectives will become clearer.

In 1772 J. B. Senac (quoted in [219]), private physician of the ordinary to Louis XV, the emperor of France, in *Traité de la structure du coeur, de son action et de ses maladies*, characterised the "state of the art" in myocarditis in a fashion that could also have been done some 200 years previously: "We have examined the course and sequelae of inflammatory processes and abscesses of the heart. But what is the fruit of our investigations? The inflammation of the heart is difficult to diagnose and if we have diagnosed it, can we then treat it better?" In the eighteenth century inflammation was a common cause of disease. Cardiotropic viruses and bacteria, however, were not yet known as causes of disease.

In 1899, more than 100 years later, von Schroetter [240] postulated that "the most important role in aetiology of heart failure is played by inflammatory processes of myocardium". This happened in a century which underestimated the incidence of coronary heart disease and attributed diseased organs mostly to inflammation. At this stage bacterial aetiology was suspected in some diseases of the heart. Rheumatic fever was later associated with a disease process following streptococcal attack; infective endocarditis was known to be caused mostly by infective bacterial agents. Comparable hypotheses were applied to myocardial and pericardial inflammation. As reviewed by Christian [34] the disease that we know today as viral myocarditis, pericarditis or myopericarditis had been described as a clinical syndrome as early as 1854, long before virus isolation, viral serology, dot blot techniques or in situ hybridisation were available. Descriptions of cardiac involvement in mumps [17], in influenza, in cytomegalovirus and Epstein-Barr virus myocarditis followed a century later (Table 15.1). Even more important, enteroviral pleuropericarditis in the course of Bornholm's disease or pleurodynia [233] was described long before its viral origin could be ascertained (Table 15.1).

Table 15.1. Viral heart disease in humans [updated from 272]

Classification	Virus	Selectecd references
1.0 RNA virus		
1.1 Picorna virus (Enterovirus)	Coxsackie A	Bell and Grist [16], Grist and Bell [71, 72];
	Coxsackie B	Javett et al. [105], Kibrick and Benirschke [115], Fletcher and Brennan [55], Fletcher et al. [56], Sainani et al. [209], Hirschmann and Hammer [91], Jennings [106] Bowles et al. [23], Kandolf et al. [109], Maisch et al. [186], Longson et al. [142];
	Echo	Russel and Bell, quoted from [158]; Bell and Grist [16]; Monif et al. [192];
	Polio	Ludden and Edwards [147], Dolgopol and Cragen [48], Kipkie and McAuley [116], Laake [129], Weinstein and Shelokov [245];
1.2 Orthomyxovirus	Influenza ASB	Lucke et al. 1919, quoted from [158]; Hamburger [76], Finland et al. [54], Giles and Shuttleworth [65], Adams [3], Oceasohn et al. [199], Coltman [35];
1.3 Paramyxovirus	Mumps	Rosenberg 1945, quoted from [158];
	Rubeola (measles)	Giustra and Nilsson [66];
1.4 Togavirus	Chikunguna	Obeyeserke and Hermon 1972, quoted from [158]; Cannell [33];
	Dengue	
	Yellow fever	Cannell [33], Bugher [26];
	Rubella	Ainger et al. [55];
1.5 Rhabdovirus	Rabies	Ross and Armentrout [207a]; Cheetham et al. [33a];
1.6 Arenavirus	Lymphocytic choriomeningitis	Thiede [226a];
2.0 DNA virus		
2.1 Herpesvirus	Cytomegalovirus	Ahvenainen [4], Bodey et al. [21], Maisch et al. [161, 168, 183], Schönian et al. [218];
	Epstein-Barr virus	Hoagland [92];
	Varicella zoster	Hackel [74], Sampson [210], Tatter et al. [235], Moore et al. [193];
	Herpes simplex	Lowry et al. [145]; Maisch et al. [186];
2.2 Adenovirus	Adeno	Berkovich et al. [18], Henson and Mufson [84], Gardiner and Short [62];
2.3 Poxvirus	Variola	Gore and Saphir, [70], Anderson et al. [8];
	Vaccinia	Dalgaard [40], Caldera et al. [30], Maut [189];
3.0 Unclassified	Hepatitis	Abelmann et al. [1], Saphir et al. [214];
4.0 HTLV	AIDS	Besterri [19], Grody et al. [73], Lewis [137]

Gore and Saphir [70] classified a large cohort of probably fairly heterogeneous forms of myocarditis cases in 1947 and Gore and Kline [69] reviewed it some 20 years later. But even recently, James [103] adapted Churchill's saying to inflammatory heart disease in stating that "myocarditis has become the medical equivalent of a riddle wrapped in a mystery inside an enigma." In the second half of the twentieth century the central role of viruses in originating and in some cases in perpetuating heart disease with its facets of myocardial, pericardial and endocardial involvement, and the effects on the vascular endothelium and the conduction system, have been elucidated. In an attempt to characterise the central haemodynamics and aetiology the WHO/ISFC task force defined cardiomyopathy [205] as "heart muscle disease of unknown cause" and classified cardiomyopathies into hypertrophic, dilated and restrictive forms. A more diverse pathogenetic distinction was not yet possible by this rough definition, however. Since then we have reached a new understanding and better concept of myocarditis and viral heart disease and it interrelationship with virus myocardiopathy [134] by means of new techniques in molecular biology, experimental and clinical immunology, virology and biochemistry:

1. While a humoral immune response to the virus in myocarditis and dilated cardiomyopathy by antibodies of different istotypes has been known for some time [11, 12, 31] viral persistence has now been demonstrated in patients who have been clinically classified as having either dilated cardiomyopathy or myocarditis. This has been done using a positive probe of Coxsackie virus RNA with in situ hybridisation [108, 109] or dot blot techniques [23] or by finding persistent cytomegalovirus in the myocytes, endothelial cells and interstitial cells of the heart [183, 185, 218] even when the overt inflammatory process has subsided.

2. Both cellular and humoral autoreactivity have been clearly demonstrated in myocarditis [6, 14, 22, 28, 50, 63, 93–96, 122, 123, 140, 149–158, 162–172, 174–186] and dilated heart muscle disease [7, 32, 42, 43, 57, 58, 102, 145, 146, 149–156, 158, 162–172, 174–186, 254]. In addition mediators and soluble factors of inflammation have been found, as has de novo expression of major histocompatibility antigens [83, 86, 97, 206, 207]. Immunocardiology has answered many questions on the pathogenesis and aetiology of myocarditis and dilated heart muscle disease, but has also posed new questions:

1. Is myocarditis, as seen by the pathologist and defined according to the Dallas criteria [9] or similar definitions [20, 47, 124, 154, 157, 184, 188, 191, 194] (Baughman 1991, personal communication), identical with or just a minor part of the newly evolving entity of immune-mediated heart disease [155, 156, 190]? How should we define the latter clinically, since it is still more characterised by in vitro assays?
2. Is the murine model of myocarditis truly a model of the human disease or are we in search of a human equivalent to the murine model and often unable to find it?
3. Are our animal models of myocarditis [27, 67, 90, 93, 94, 96, 140, 181, 195, 196, 206, 207, 248, 248–254] truly models leading to dilated cardiomyopathy?

This chapter deals with our knowledge on humoral and cellular immune mechanisms in viral heart disease in man and is followed by an overview on experimental enteroviral heart disease in mice, since our current understanding of the human disease has received numerous inputs from animal work.

Definition of Terms

Histologically validated myocarditis is defined here as active, healing or healed myocarditis according to Daly et al. [41]or the almost identical Dallas criteria [9] (Table 15.2a). It has been suggested recently by others that myocarditis be subdivided clinically and histologically into fulminant forms with severe acute complications (cardiogenic shock) and either acute death or almost complete recovery, and chronic forms with incomplete recovery or a worse long-term prognosis [53, 113] (Baughman 1991, personal communication). Japanese authors have suggested separating acute from chronic forms by different criteria which are not identical even when similar words are employed.

Chronic myocarditis in a purely histological sense remains controversial in international histopathology although features of chronicity have been known

Table 15.2. Criteria for myocarditis and perimyocarditis, cardiomyopathy and post-myocarditic heart-muscle disease

(a) Criteria for myocarditis and perimyocarditis
Essential criteria:
Inflammation of the myocardium determined by biopsy/necropsy with infiltrate, focal necrosis, interstitial oedema) with or without fibrosis. According to Daly et al. [41] and Aretz et al. [9] one can distinguish different forms of *myocarditis*:
- active myocarditis (prominent infiltrate close to myofibres, necrosis $\pm$ fibrosis)
- healing myocarditis (scarce (interstitial) infiltrate, fibrosis, no or very little necrosis)
- healed myocarditis (second biopsy: focal fibrosis, no infiltrate; but in first biopsy: active inflammation)

or
Pericardial rub or pericardial effusion with segmental wall motion abnormality and dysrhythmia after exclusion of coronary artery disease by coronary angiography (= *perimyocarditis*)
Additional criteria:
Positive RNA or DNA probe for cardiotropic viruses
A more then threefold alteration of titer in complement-fixation or neutralisation test against cardiotrophic viruses

(b) Criteria for dilated cardiomyopathy
Essential criteria
Clinical examination (see Chaps. 2–5)
Cardiomegaly (left ventricular end-diastolic volume index > 100 ml/m^2 and reduced ejection fraction (< 55%)
Exclusion or coronary artery disease, valvar heart disease, hypertension and other forms of secondary heart muscle diseases (e.g. diabetes mellitus, neuroendocrine disorder, alcohol consumption)
Additional criterion:
Indicative histomorphology with hypertrophy and branching of myocytes, diffuse or focal fibrosis

(c) Criteria for post-myocarditic heart muscle disease
Biopsy-proven cellular infiltrate in first biopsy and missing infiltrate in second biopsy
or
Perimyocarditis proven by clinical criteria (Table 15.2a) at first examination; no infiltrate in second biopsy but cardiomegaly with reduced ejection fraction at the second examination

for a long time [47]. Our recent studies on the secondary immunopathogenesis in protracted forms of (peri)myocarditis and in enteroviral heart disease with viral persistence suggest that an effort to reintroduce this term in a clinical context may be worth while [158]. There have been attempts to further subclassify these forms histologically, and partly clinically, into chronic and chronic persistent types [53, 57] (Baughman 1991, personal communication).

Perimyocarditis is defined here as pericardial effusion and cardiomegaly or segmental wall motion abnormality (Table 15.2a). Demonstration of pericardial effusion (in the absence of neoplastic, post-radiation or post-injury syndromes or uraemea) denotes the inflammatory epicardial or pericardial process, while cardiac dilatation or wall motion abnormality defines the myocardial involvement in such inflammatory heart disease [173–182, 184, 185]. As Woodruff already pointed out [252] viral pericarditis is nearly always associated with underlying epicardial and myocardial lesions which led to the use of the term myopericarditis or more precisely perimyocarditis [173]. Since in turn myocarditis is not always associated with pericardial effusion, the two clinical entities overlap but are not identical. For these patients a biopsy with demonstration of active inflammation is helpful.

Inflammatory heart muscle disease therefore includes both myocarditis and perimyocarditis and, in addition, rejection episodes (which are not dealt with in this review). The terms chronic and acute as used here are not derived from histology but used in a clinical fashion and are applied to both myocarditis and perimyocarditis.

Dilated cardiomyopathy (Table 15.2b) may be secondary to myocarditis [45], perimyocarditis or a secondary immunopathogenesis (Table 15.2c). The diagnostic criteria for (peri)myocarditis or dilated heart muscle disease have been summarised in Table 15.2a–c. Most specific heart muscle diseases produce a dilated form of ventricular disease (see Chaps. 1, 4 and 5).

Viral heart disease is defined as structural abnormalities in inflammatory or dilated heart disease with the demonstration of virus, viral RNA or DNA in the myocardium. The association of electrical, haemodynamic or structural abnormalities in the heart in the context of an apparent viral illness is only suggestive of viral heart disease as is the demonstration of increased viral titres.

Immune-mediated heart disease or secondary immunopathogenesis refers to the large number of patients having either inflammatory heart disease or dilated heart muscle disease with signs of autoimmunity [174–180, 190]. We recently distinguished several forms of this disorder by immunohistopathology and in vitro assays of humoral and cellular autoreactivity (Table 15.3).

Histological Diagnosis in Viral or Autoimmune Heart Disease

The Dallas criteria for myocarditis [9, 41] are now widely accepted as a histopathological working definition. They were primarily designed as a diagnostic tool for the American Myocarditis Trial, and are not necessarily the best

Table 15.3. Immunological classification of dilated heart muscle diseases

	Endomyocardial biopsy			Peripheral blood						
	Lymphocytic infiltrate	IgG,M,A,C3 binding	Class II expr. on myocyctes	Cardio-LC[a]	NK cell activity[b]	AMLAs[c]	anti-ANT	AFAs[d]	Matrix ab	AEAs[e]
Myocarditis	++	++	+	+	Reduced	++	++	–	++	+
Perimyocarditis	++	++	+	+	Reduced	++	n.d.	+	+	+
Pericarditis	–	+	+/–	–[f]	=	+	n.d.	–	++	+
Post-myocarditic heart muscle disease	–	++	–	+	Reduced	++/+	+	–	+	+
Dilated cardiomyopathy	–	+/–	–	+/–	Reduced	+	+	(+)	+	+

=, unchanged; –, negative or less than 25% of patients positive; +, positive finding in more than 50% of patients; ++, positive finding in more than 80% of patients.

[a] Lymphocytotoxicity to isolated rat heart cells by peripheral blood lymphocytes (non-MHC-controlled lymphocytotoxicity.

[b] Natural killer cell activity to K562 erythroblast cell line [203].

[c] Antimyolemmal antibodies.

[d] Antifibrillary antibodies mostly from the antimyosin type.

[e] antiendothelial antibodies.

[f] No cardiocytotoxicity of peripheral blood lymphocytes but strong lymphocytotoxicity from lymphocytes of the pericardial fluid (unpublished data).

or most comprehensive definition of myocarditis or viral heart disease. Problems with the Dallas classification and other histopathological definitions centre around three issues [133, 232]: The first is interobserver variability. Even when the same histopathological criteria were applied by all pathologists, Shanes et al. [232] demonstrated extraordinary variation in the interpretation of the Dallas criteria by the pathologists involved.

The second issue is that "myocarditis" in one patient, centre or publication does not equal myocarditis in another. The criteria that Parillo et al. [201] used in their therapeutic trial demonstrate this impressively: although they preclassified their "reactive patient group" as being either positive for lymphocytic infiltrations ($n=2$), having grade 1 (mild), 2 (moderate), or 3 (severe) fibroblastic infiltrations ($n=36$), having immunoglobulin deposition ($n=16$), or having positive findings in a gallium scan ($n=7$) or an elevated erythrocyte sedimentation rate ($n=18$), only 2 patients of this cohort would have been admitted to the American Myocarditis Trial because they were positive for lymphocytic infiltration, not to mention the second obligatory requirement, which is necrosis. Thus the criteria used by Parillo et al. [201] are too heterogeneous and non-specific for myocarditis, which is never mentioned in their paper. They may, however, become of interest when one looks for viral persistence in heart muscle disease. Their small group of patients who tested positive for lymphocytic infiltration, however, corresponds closely to data from other authors who demonstrated lymphocytic infiltrations in dilated heart muscle diseases only in 4.4%–8.0% in adults [157] and up to 25% in children [133, 137a].

Lie, comparing findings from 13 reports on the incidence of myocarditis over 6 years, gives figures ranging from less than 25% to 67% and concludes that myocarditis in acute heart failure is as predictable as Russian roulette. The vagueness of the histological diagnosis of myocarditis is not new, however. The German pathologist Doerr [47] claimed already in 1971 that every pathologist has his own view of myocarditis. The Dallas criteria may have changed some if this vagary, but not all of it. This dilemma, by no means one that applies to this study alone, thus results from the bias of individual pathologists and the sampling error.

The latter is substantiated by Hauck et al. [80] who, from post-mortem studies of patients with active perimyocarditis at necropsy, evaluated the insensitivity of endomyocardial biopsy for the diagnosis of myocarditis. Even when 10 biopsy specimens were evaluated, the frequency of false-negative findings was 45% for the left and 37% for the right ventricle. This finding was even more prominent in patients who died of focal myocarditis, which points to at least two conclusions: (1) a negative biopsy does not rule out myocarditis, and (2) other methods are needed to demonstrate inflammation or immunological activation.

The need for better methods is, therefore, the third issue in enteroviral heart disease. This issue contrasts with "the need to find a diagnosis for myocarditis in dilated cardiomyopathy", as Lie [137a] has put it. Since molecular and immunological methods are now available they should be employed in routine diagnosis. They include major histocompatibility complex classes I and II expression, the deposition of IgM, IgA and complement C3 as known from the Wuerzburg Multicenter Study, and probes to define viral persistence and altered protein biosynthesis.

New Diagnostic Approaches in Viral Heart Disease

The diagnosis of viral heart disease cannot be made from clinical features with sufficient accuracy. Assessing serum antibody titres in suspected cases also proved to be of limited diagnostic value, except in an epidemic or endemic situation, although an increased incidence of positive microneutralisation tests in dilated cardiomyopathy has been reported [31]. Molecular genetic techniques are the most powerful tools for defining the role of enteroviruses and cytomegaloviruses [183, 218] in the induction of myocarditis and in the further pathogenetic process. Using in situ hybridisation of enterovirus RNA in infected cells in endomyocardial biopsies, Kandolf and Hofschneider [108] demonstrated a positive finding in 19 of 81 patients with suspected myocarditis, and in 8 of 27 patients with dilated cardiomyopathy. This is about half the percentage that Bowles et al. [23] demonstrated with a blot technique. The latter does not allow histological attribution of this finding to different cells in the biopsy. Their data indicate that viral persistence may be one important feature of dilated cardiomyopathy.

Whether the virus induces an autoreactive cellular and humoral response or is itself responsible for myocardial necrosis remains unresolved [29]. Preliminary data, including those from experimental work in myocarditis, show that even in mice this issue is controversial. Necrosis can be attributed either to virus cytopathology [96] or to the immunocompetent cells [96]. As will be discussed later this difference of opinion may arise at least partly from the use of different strains of animals with different genetic backgrounds or different batches of viruses.

Other cardiopathic agents have been defined in the past few years. These are cytomegalovirus (CMV), human T -cell lymphotropic virus (HTLV), and a bacterial agent that can be treated with antibiotics, i.e. *Borrelia burgdorferi*, the agent responsible for borreliosis or Lyme disease, which may be associated in up to 20% of cases with myocarditis [121].

Immune Response and Structural Alterations

Virus induction of myocardial inflammation was demonstrated in many patients with myocarditis and dilated cardiomyopathy. Viral persistence, however, does not prove that myocardial inflammation and destruction or the induction of reparative processes are mediated or caused by the virus that may have just left its fingerprints. Some of the reparative features, e.g. hypertrophy, may be controlled by proto-oncogenes, such as c-*myc* and c-*fos*, or by collagen genes [44, 51, 52], which have been expressed de novo in different forms of heart disease and were first described in rejection [128]. For the induction of fibrosis in inflammatory heart disease mediators such as the platelet-derived growth factors (A and B) are likely to be an early competence signal, which is followed by a progression signal, e.g. insulin-derived growth factor. Platelet-derived growth factor and insulin-derived growth factor reside in macrophages, a cell population the role of which has just begun to be understood and that has also been demonstrated in myocarditis. Activated macrophages produce fibronectin, fibroblast growth factor, and interleukin-1, which stimulates collagen synthesis. The role of cytokines is just emerging in inflammation and is still mostly speculative in myocarditis. Samsonov et al. [211] and Klappacher et al. [119, 120] have demonstrated that in dilated cardiomyopathy as in any other form of congestive failure neopterin is increased. Neopterin is released by monocytes under control of activated T lymphocytes via interferon-γ thus reflecting T cell activation (since it was associated with an increase of β_2-microglobulin) and monocyte activation. Tumour necrosis factor alpha (TNF_α) was found to be increased in advanced stages of heart failure independent of their cause. TNF_α appeared to be closely associated to increased right atrial pressure and a concomitant increase in atrial natriuretic peptide (ANP). In addition β_2-microglobulin levels were found to be increased in sera of patients with dilated cardiomyopathy due either to impairment of renal function in advanced heart failure or to T cell activation. These first data on mediators in dilated heart muscle disease domonstrate similar trends as are found in rejection after heart transplantation.

Function and structure of the heart muscle are maintained both by the contractile filaments actin, myosin [212] and tropomyosin [130] and by the often neglected cytoskeleton [79, 204], the intermediate filaments [61, 132, 200] and the extracellular matrix [81, 82, 135]. The adhesion of the myocytes to the components of the extracellular matrix has been clearly documented [148]. So have the anchorage sites of the microfilaments in the cytoskeleton by specific autoantibodies [231]. This may explain in part the close interrelation between systolic and diastolic function on a microscopic level. Structural alterations of the cytoskeleton in diseased human myocardium, particularly in dilated cardiomyopathy, were preliminary described by Schaper et al. [215, 216] and may be secondary to myocarditis:

1. Desmin, normally located at the Z band [64, 131], may be formed irregularly, as found when probed for with a monoclonal antidesmin antibody.
2. Tubulin [68, 213] may be diffusely increased or altered.
3. Vinculin, which is incorporated into the sarcolemmal membrane and the intercalated discs, may be increased or have an irregular shape.
4. Laminin, a 220 kDa protein closely associated with the basement membrane [114], has been demonstrated to be irregularly shaped and increased in content.

5. Fibronectin, another basement protein that binds cells to collagen [99, 100], may also appear in irregular forms.
6. Vimentin, which is found in endothelial cells and in fibroblasts, may be increased due to increased fibrosis.

An increase in interstitial collagen has been obvious to pathologists after viral infection [112], myocarditis or in dilated cardiomyopathy [113] for years and was also shown in an experimental situation [136, 265] even in areas without an inflammatory infiltrate. It has been demonstrated to occur not only in reparative processes but also in cardiac hypertrophy [243] with a distinct impact on diastolic function.

Viral Antigens in Viral Heart Disease

Until the demonstration of the genetic code in cells was possible the demonstration of viral infection relied primarily on the humoral antiviral response by the complement fixation test or microneutralisation test to cardiotropic viruses. These circulating antiviral antibodies, however, never permitted diagnosis of viral heart disease, only the confirmation of viral infection in an individual. In animal experiments it has also become clear that the antiviral response is not restricted to B cells but also includes T cells that appear at an even earlier stage of infection. Antigenic mimicry has evolved as an important pathomechanism in sensitised T cells and autoantibodies that could cause cardiac damage independent of any viral infection of the myocardium.

Immunological Regulator and Effector Mechanisms in Viral Heart Disease

Lymphocyte Subpopulations in Myocarditis and Dilated Heart Disease

Peripheral Blood Cells. In our own patients [166–168, 173, 183] blood white cell counts did not show significant differences between patients with myocarditis, perimyocarditis, pericardial effusion, dilated cardiomyopathy, post-myocarditic heart diasease and non-cardiac controls. Although in one fourth of patients with acute carditis lymphocytosis was observed this was not a consistent finding. By the enumeration of circulating T-lymphocyte subpopulations in patients with carditis a significant difference in pan-T (OKT3-positive, OKT11-positive) and T helper (OKT4-positive) cells was not demonstrated. In perimyocarditis the OKlal-positive B cells and activated T lymphocytes were significantly increased, and in post- myocarditic heart disease a tendency for a decrease in T suppressor cells was demonstrated (Table 15.4). In contrast in primary dilated cardiomyopathy circulating OKMI-positive monocytes were increased [154]. The T4/T8 ratio did not differ from that of age- and sex-matched controls. These findings correspond to those from studies by other investigators.

Table 15.4. Lymphocyte subsets in the peripheral blood of patients with (peri)myocarditis ($n = 62$), post-myocarditic cardiomegaly ($n = 19$), primary dilated cardiomyopathy ($n = 49$) and healthy controls ($n = 56$)

	(Peri) myocarditic	Post-myocarditic cardiomegaly	Primary dilated cardiomyopathy	Healthy and non- –cardiac controls
Pan-T cells (OKT3)	74.3 ± 6.1	75.6 ± 3.5	71.1 ± 1.4	72.6 ± 7.0
Helper/inducer (OKT4)	48.6 ± 4.7	50.0 ± 2.8	50.4 ± 1.9	48.7 ± 7.3
Suppressor/ cytotoxic (OKT8)	23.2 ± 5.3	17.8 ± 2.8*	21.2 ± 1.8	22.9 ± 5.7
B lymphocyte (+ activated T cells) (OKIal)	28.3 ± 8.5*	19.8 ± 3.2	22.7 ± 1.7	23.6 ± 7.6
Monocytes + NK cells (OKMI)	14.5 ± 4.3	10.8 ± 2.4	19.1 ± 1.9*	13.2 ± 5.6

*$p < 0.05$ by chi-squared analysis, when compared with controls.

Lymphocytes from Endomyocardial Biopsies. Lymphocytes can also be grown from the biopsies of patients with suspected myocarditis (Fig. 15.1) or dilated cardiomyopathy [127] and cultured and expanded in the presence of human recombinant interleukin-2 (rIL2). This is possible in about every third to fourth patient with myocarditis both in our own experience and that of others [127] (Schultheiss personal communication). CD4+ cell populations prevailed in two thirds of patients when compared with CD8+ cells or a mixed population. They may exert natural killer cell activity and produce lymphokines such as IL2, whereby phenotypic appearance does not correlate with lymphokine production or cardiocytotoxicity. Attempts have also been made target to culture specific T cells, e.g.to defined cardiac antigens such as the ADP/ATP carrier (Schultheiss, personal communication) and sarcolemmal proteins (own unpublished data); only a few patients have proved positive in established culture systems.

T Suppressor Cell Activity. In contrast to the findings of others [50, 57] in our patients spontaneous (assessed according to [25] in vivo and Con-A-generated T suppressor cell activity (assessed according to [75]) did not differ from that in sex- and age-matched controls without heart disease. In post-myocarditic dilated heart disease, however, in selected indicator systems such as the autologous irradiated mixed lymphocyte reaction and the allogeneic mitogen stimulation system a significant reduction in T suppressor cell activity was seen when compared with patients with acute myocarditis, who themselves demonstrated a significantly enhanced, but not a decreased suppressor cell activity when compared with non-cardiac controls. It should be pointed out, however, that

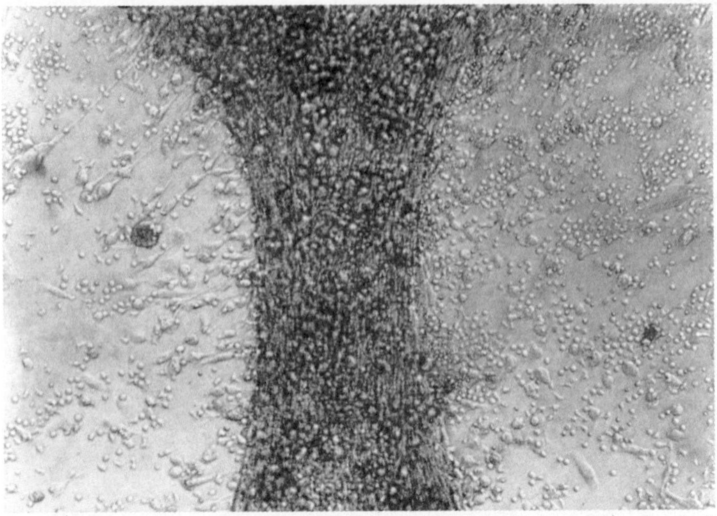
a

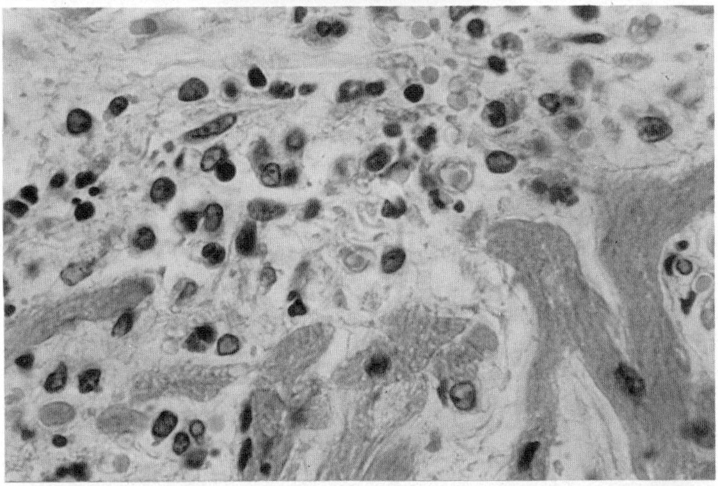
b

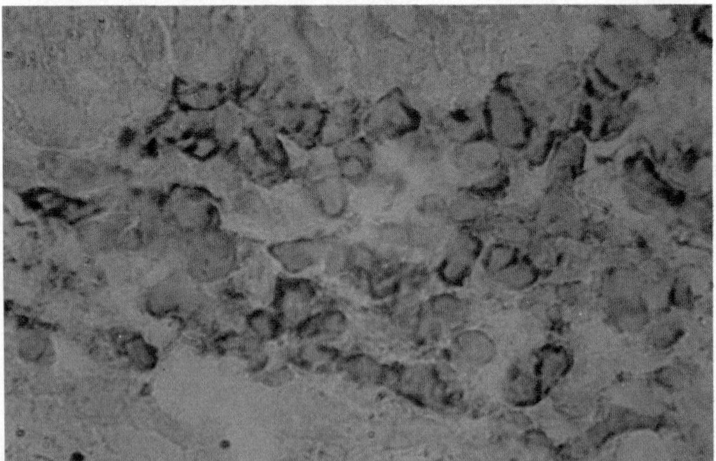
c

there is broad variance in T suppressor cell activity, both in controls and in patients with acute inflammatory heart disease, and that while the different indicator systems for the assessment of T suppressor cell activity may be particularly sensitive in expressing changes in some of the T suppressor cell subpopulations, most are not altered in myocarditis and dilated cardiomyopathy. Even though a global reduction of T suppressor cell activity is not evident from our data, it cannot be ruled out that the antigen-specific T suppressor cell activity may have been changed. The assessment of antigen-specific T suppressor cell activity would need cloned T cell subpopulations elicited by specific cardiac membrane antigens (or other molecules), a prerequisite which is not yet available.

Assessment of Cellular Effector Mechanisms in Man. In patients with perimyocarditis peripheral blood analysis of lymphocyte subpopulations demonstrated an increase in the OKlal-positive cells whilch may be either B and/or activated T lymphocytes. An increase in B lymphocytes would explain the increased antibody response found in carditis; an increase in activated T cells would explain the strong activity of cytolytic T cells as demonstrated in mice, for which no adequate assay system in man is yet available.

Natural Killer Cell Activity. Natural killer (NK) cell activity in patients with carditis was markedly decreased in the acute state in all three lymphocyte/target cell ratios examined (Fig. 15.2a). In post-myocarditic dilated heart muscle disease, NK cell activity had almost returned to normal (Fig. 15.2b). In primary dilated cardiomyopathy, however, a significantly decreased NK cell activity was observed again (Fig. 15.2c) [154]. This confirms previous investigations in dilated cardiomyopathy by Anderson et al. [7].

Target-Cell-Specific Non-MHC-Restricted Lymphocytotoxicity. In contrast in myocarditis target-cell-specific non-MHC-restricted lysis against living adult allogeneic rat myocytes is sustained or slightly enhanced. This also applies to postmyocarditic dilated heart disease and primary dilated cardiomyopathy in which one third of patients demonstrated an increase of target cell, specific cytotoxicity. Other than a sporadic increase in cell lysis, analysis of antibody-dependent cellular cytotoxicity (ADCC) showed little variation from normal in perimyocarditis or primary and secondary post-myocarditic heart muscle disease [166–168, 173]. In the myocardial biopsy, the infiltrating cell populations operating at the site of the lesion were mostly round cells, particularly lymphocytes.

◄

Fig. 15.1. a Lymphocytes isolated and expanded with interleukin-2 from the endomyocardial biopsy of a patient with active myocarditis. **b** the majority of the lymphocytes belonged to the T helper subpopulation **c** As evidenced by labelling with a monoclonal anti-CD4 antibody (peroxide staining)

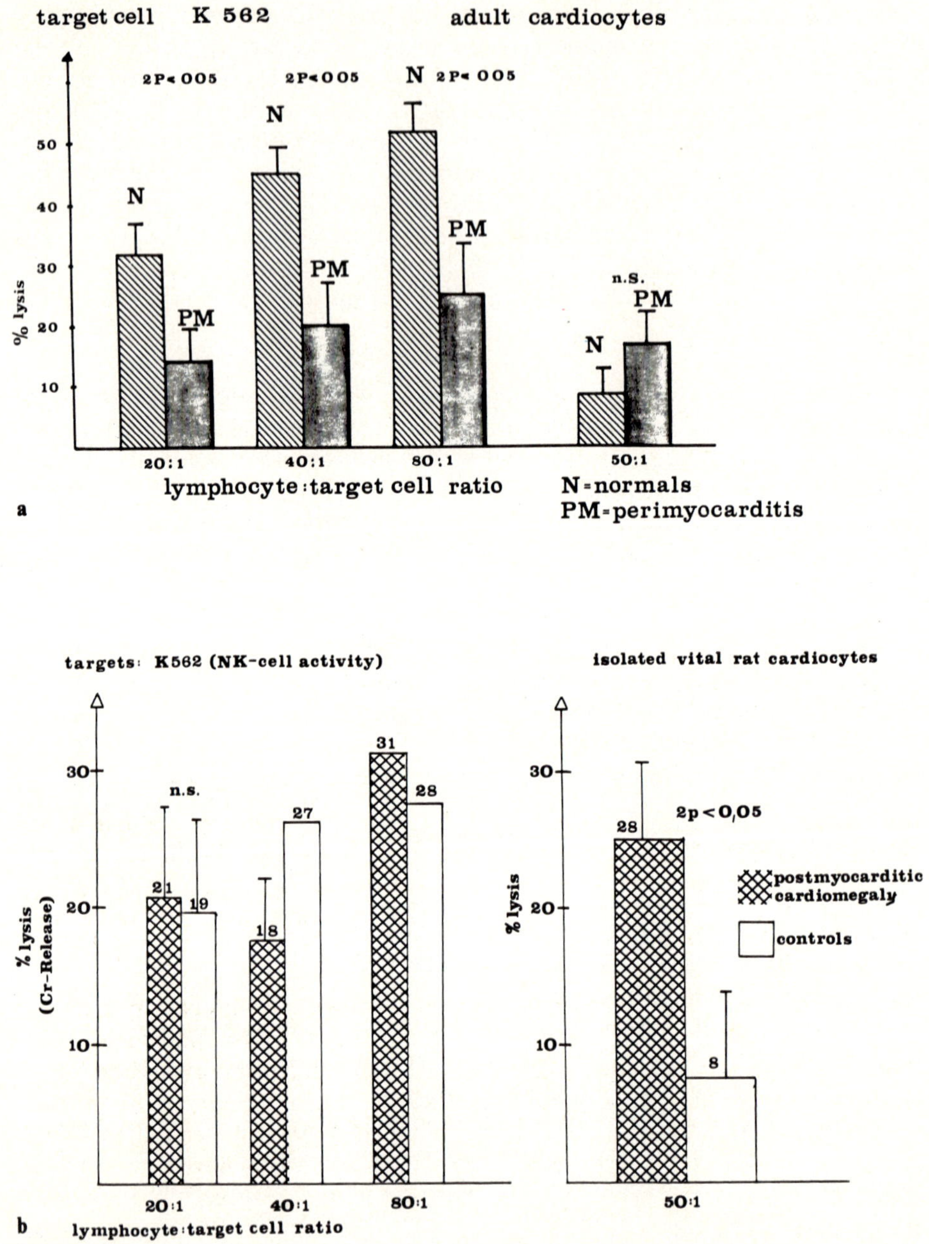

Fig. 15.2 a–c. Natural killer (NK) cell activity to K 562 [203] and cardiospecific non-MHC-restricted lymphocytotoxicity (LC) in active myocarditis (**a**), post-myocarditic heart disease (**b**) and primary dilated cardiomyopathy (**c**). NK cell activity is decreased in myocarditis (**a**) and dilated cardiomyopathy (**c**) whereas LC is sustained or slightly enhanced [155]. In post-myocarditic heart disease NK-cell activity normal but cardiospecific non-MHC-restricted lymphocytotoxicity (LC) with isolated vital resting rat cardiocytes is significantly ($2p < 0.05$) increased

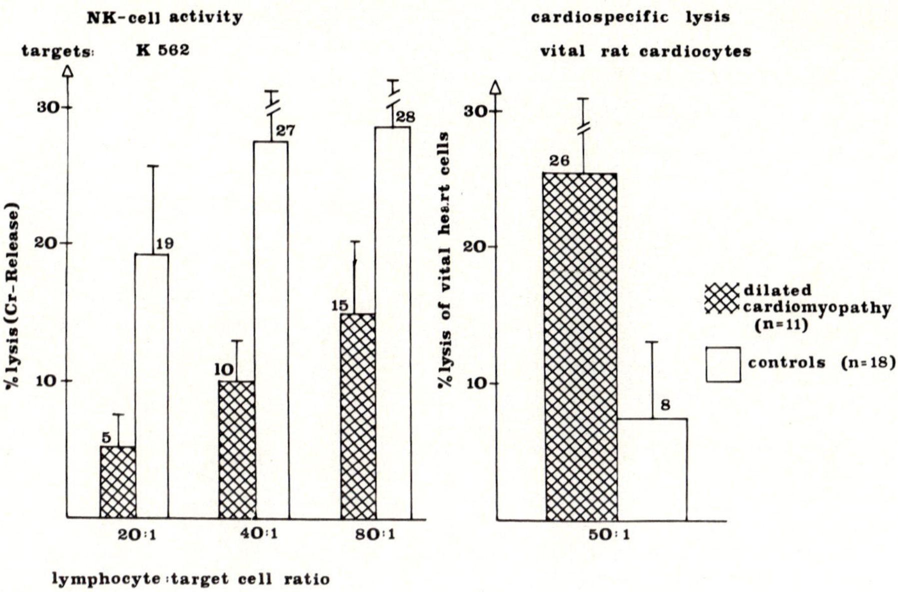

Fig. 15.2c

Myocardial Antigens in Autoreactive Heart Disease

Autoantigens of the Myocyte

Cardiac antigens can be identified as targets of humoral and cellular autoreactivity. These include all components that can be identified with light microscopy on cryostat sections (Fig. 15.3). Some antigens have been characterised further biochemically or defined by monoclonal antibodies. The most important antigens so far described are:

Antibodies to the Cardiac Membrane and its Constituents. It has been postulated that there is membrane damage of the myocardium in the pathogenesis of cardiomyopathies independent of the demonstrated autoreactivity to the cardiac membrane [111]. Of particular interest are circulating and bound antibodies to the membrane of the cardiomyocyte, the sarcolemma and myolemma, to which cytolytic complement-fixing antibodies (AMLAs; Fig. 15.4a) have been demonstrated in Coxsackie virus B, mumps, and influenza myocarditis [88]. They have been elucidated further in human [117, 149, 150, 154, 168, 186], and murine myocarditis [155–160, 162–167, 170–175]. Recent evidence suggests that antigenic mimicry may play an important role: epitopes on the sarcolemmal surface [186] and to the ANT-carrier [228], which in turn shares antigenic properties with the membrane-bound calcium channel, were found to cross-react with Coxsackie B viruses. In classic absorption experiments it was conclusively shown that in viral myocarditis the sarcolemmal fluorescence was greatly

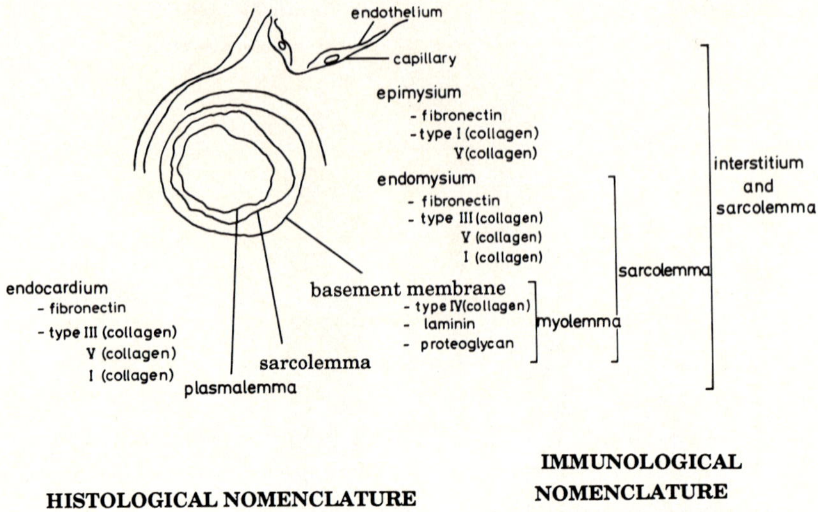

Fig. 15.3. Autoantigens of the heart: comparison of the classic histological and the immunological nomenclature. The myolemma, which can be identified clearly in isolated human heart cells, consists of the plasmalemma, the sarcolemma and basement membrane and is made up of laminin, proteoglycans, membrane-bound receptors and membrane-specific epitopes. The sarcolemma as identified by immunofluorescence techniques includes the endomysium containing fibronectin and types. I, III and V collagen. The interstitium comprises the epimysium with its biochemically defined components

diminished, and the cytolytic serum activity could be absorbed by the virus [154, 156, 181].

The correlation of antibody titre (AMLAs) and cytolytic serum activity clearly demonstrates the presence of a complement-fixing cytolytic anti-membrane antibody which can be shown to be cross-reactive with enteroviral core proteins by Western blot analysis [186], in which viral and sarcolemmal membranes [202] have been used both for identification and absorption, or by defining cross-reactive epitopes by using monoclonal antibodies [229]. In diseases induced by streptococci, such as rheumatic fever [110] or infective endocarditis [237], cross-reactive relationships between antigens of streptococci and mammalian cardiac tissue (sarcolemmal membranes in particular) have also been demonstrated.

It is remarkable but understandable from cell anatomy that antibodies directed against fibronectin, laminin, desmin and vinculin, which are proteins of the extracellular matrix, also stain the "myolemma" in isolated heart cells and that monoclonal antibodies to actin, a-actinin and myosin stain both fibrils and the membrane (Table 15.5). The incidence of circulating AMLAs and antisarcolemmal antibodies in inflammatory and dilated heart muscle disease as compared with controls is given in Table 15.6a–d.

Antibodies to the beta-adrenoceptor have recently been shown to exist in patients with dilated cardiomyopathy [138, 139]. Whether these antireceptor

Table 15.5. Antibody pattern derived from nonoclonal or "monospecific" antibodies to components of the interstitial tissue and extracellular matrix [from 158]

Antibody type[a]	Human or rat myocytes					Heart tissue (human)			Endothelial fibroblasts human cell BHK-21				Hep-2
	AMLA	Zb	AFA	ID	ASA	Zb	AFA	ID	net	cap	net	pc	net
a-collagen I	−	−	−	−	+	−	−	−	nd	nd	nd	nd	nd
a-collagen III	−	−	−	−	+	−	−	−	nd	nd	nd	nd	nd
a-fibronectin	+	(+)	−	+	+	+	−	+	−	−	−	−	−
a-laminin	+	−[c]	−	+	+	−	−	−	+	−	+	−	+
a-desmin	+	++	−	+	+	+	−	(+)	+	+	+	+	+
a-vimentin	−	−	−	−	−	+	−	−/+	−/+	+	+	+	+
a-keratin	−	−	−	−	−	−	−	−	−	−	−	−	+
a-tubulin[b]	(+)	(+)	−	−	(+)	(+)	−	−	+/−	+/−	+	+	+
a-actin	+	−	(+)	(+)	(+)	−	(+)	(+)	−	−	+	+	+
a−α-actin	+	−	+	(+)	(+)	−	(+)	(+)	−	−	+	+	+
a−myosin	+	−	+	−	+	−	+	−	−	−	+	+	+
a-vinculin	+	?	−	+	+	?	−	+	−	−	−	−	+
a-clathrin	nd	nd	nd	nd	nd	nd	nd	nd	nd	nd	nd	nd	+

AMLA, antimyolemmal staining; ASA, antisarcolemmal staining; Zb, Z-band-like staining; AFA, antifibrillary staining; ID, intercalated-disc-type stainin; pc, paracrystals after vinblastin treatment; net, filament net-like pattern; cap, cap structure after treatment with vinblastin 10 μg/ml; a-, anti.

[a] Sources: a-laminin (Medac); a-desmin, a-vimentin, a-keratin, α-tubulin, a-α-actinin, a-vinculin (Amersham); a-desmin (Boehringer Mannheim); a-actin, a-myosin (from patients with heart muscle disease with high titre positive serum and positive ELISA); a-actin (Enzo NY).

[b] Glutaraldehyde-borhydride fixation for the preservation of T tubules is recommended.

[c] Z-band-negative by commercially available a-laminin monoclonal antibody, positive by a polyclonal a-laminin antibody kindly provided by Dr. Timpl (Martinsried).

a-Vimentin and a-desmin antibodies can be distinguished best by using different cell lines for analysis; Hep 2 cells stain for desmin only, whereas BHK-21 cells stain for desmin and vimentin.

b d

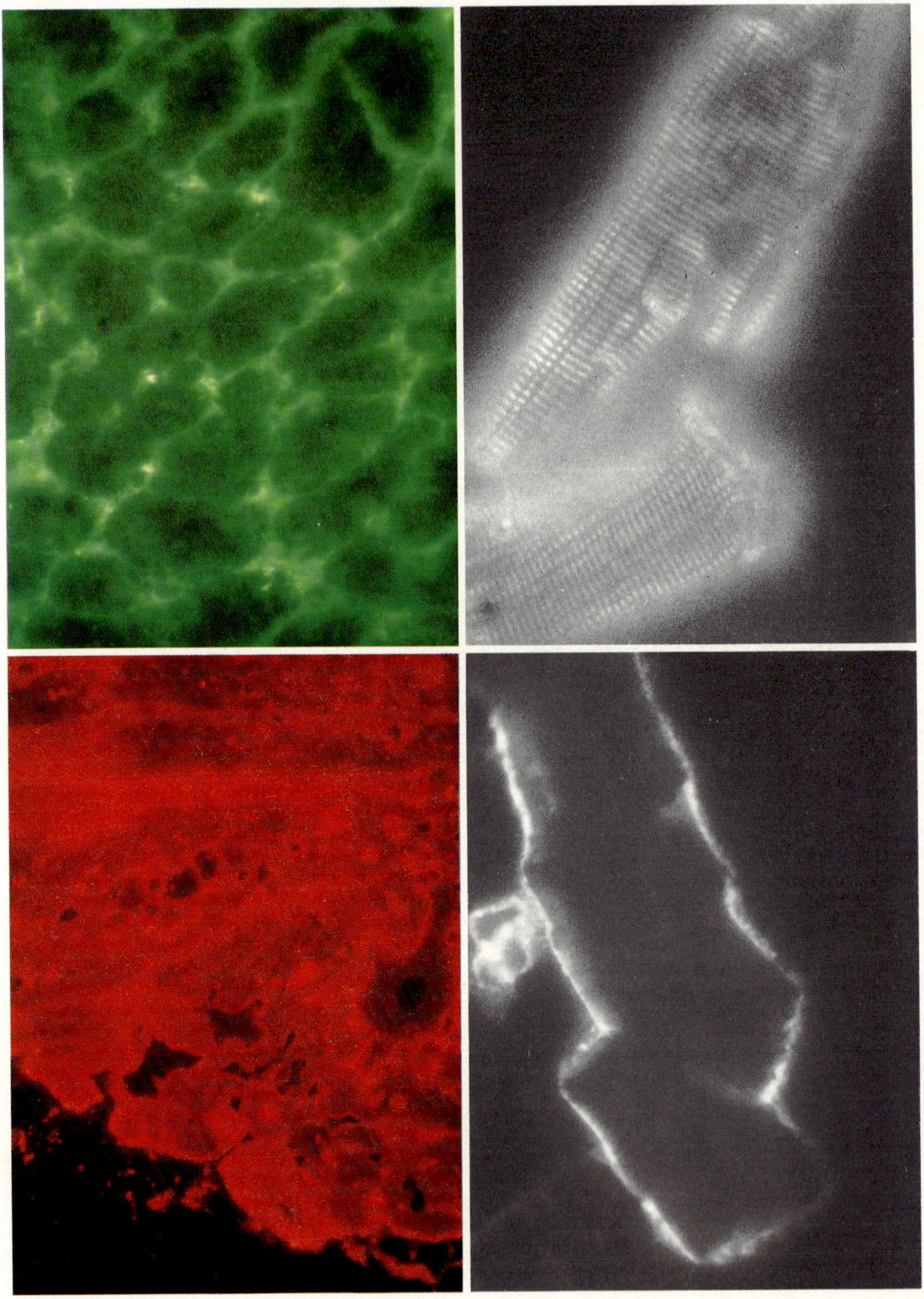

a c

f

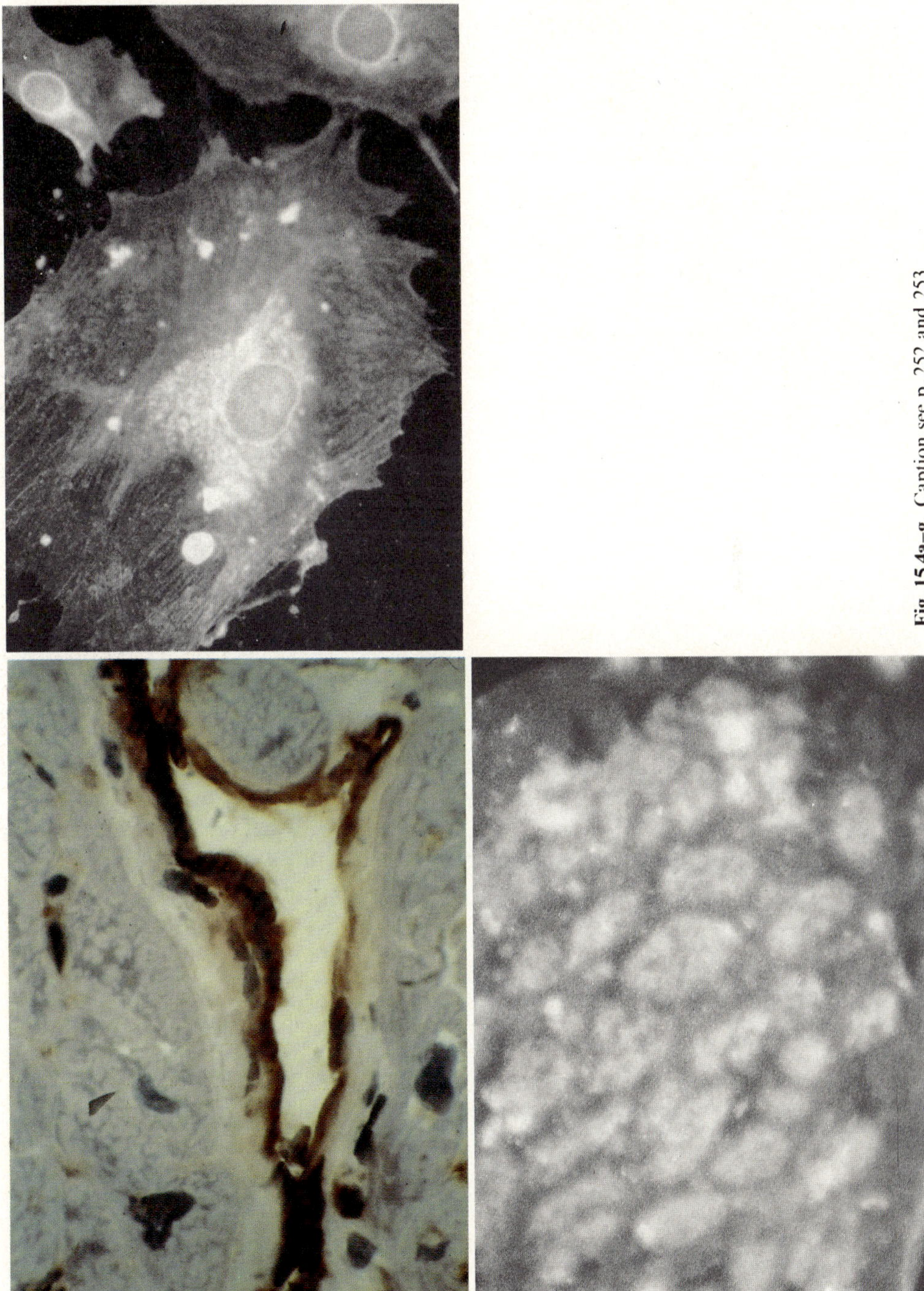

e

g

Fig. 15.4a–g. Caption see p. 252 and 253

Table 15.6. Circulating antibodies to the serocolemma, the extracellular matrix and intermediate filaments in healthy controls, myocarditis and perimyocarditis, pericarditis and dilated cardiomyopathy

References	*n*	AMLA (homol)	ASA (homol)	ALA	A-Fibron	Z-bands	A-Actin	A-Myosin
(a) Healthy controls								
Maisch et al. [168, 169]	200	31	35	nd	nd	5	5	5
Maisch et al. [156]	45	16	18	20	nd	nd	nd	nd
Obermayer et al. [197]	25	20	20	nd	nd	0	nd	nd
de Scheerder et al. [46a]	40	10	5	nd	nd	nd	5	3
Klein et al. [122]	nd	nd	nd	nd	nd	nd	nd	nd
Schultheiß et al. [224]	nd	nd	nd	nd	nd	nd	nd	nd
(b) Myocarditis and perimyocarditis								
de Scheerder et al. [46a]	12	110	12	nd	nd	nd	58	67
Klein et al. [122]	nd	nd	nd	nd	nd	nd	nd	nd
Maisch et al. [154, 156, 157]								
Viral myocarditis (adults) [168, 186]	44	79–90	75–90	nd	nd	15	7	10–50
Idiopathic myocarditis	144	59	45	nd	nd	nd	0	23
Maisch et al. [179]								
children		100	100	nd	nd	0	0	0
Maisch et al. [181]	132	nd	nd	30–35	nd	nd	nd	nd
Obermayer et al. [197]	25	64	72	nd	nd	16	0	4
Schultheiß [220, 223]	29	nd	nd	60	20	nd	nd	nd
(c) Pericarditis								
de Scheerder et al. [46a]	10	60	60	nd	nd	nd	10	10
Maisch et al. [160] Tuberculous pericarditis	10	100	100	nd	nd	0	8	67
Maisch et al. [160] uremic pericarditis	41	30–83	50–100	nd	nd	0	0	0
Obermayer et al. [197] idiopathic pericarditis	10	80	50	nd	nd	0	nd	nd
(d) Dilated cardiomyopathy								
Klein et al. [122]	nd	nd	nd	nd	nd	nd	nd	nd
Maisch et al. [49]	79	9	10	nd	nd	nd	4	20
Maisch et al. [171]	30	33	42	nd	nd	nd	10	33
Schultheiß et al. [224]	51	nd	nd	72	nd	nd	nd	nd
Obermayer et al. [197]	36	42	31	nd	nd	8	0	8

Fig. 15.4. a Demonstration of bound antisarcolemmal antibodies (IgG, C3 fixation, IgA) in the endomyocardial biopsy specimen of a 42-year-old male with post-viral (previous Coxsackie virus myocarditis) dilated heart muscle disease. The immunoglobulin binds to sarcolemma and interstitial space. (× 800; anti-human IgG, Medac; dilution 1:1000; TRICT-labelled Fa2 fragments). **b** The identity of bound and circulating (FITC-labelled) antisarcolemmal antibodies can be demonstrated in the same patient with a double sandwich technique. (× 800; anti-human IgG, Medac; dilution 1:1000; Fab2 fragments; serum dilution 1:320, **c** Demonstration of antimyolemmal antibodies of the same patient with an isolated intact human atrial cardiocyte. (× 1200; FITC-labelled anti-human IgG, Medac; dilution 1:1000; Fab2 fragments; serum dilution 1:320).

Table 15.6 (continued). *Abbreviations:* AMLA, antimyolemmal antibody; ASA, antisarcolemmal antibody; ALA, antilaminin antibody; A-, anti-; Fibron, fibronectin; ADA, anti-intercalated disc antibody; ANT, anti-nucleotide translocator; AEA, antiendothelial antibody; Bar, beta-adrenoceptor.

A-Tubulin	AIDA	A-Desmin	A-Vimentin	ANT	A-M7	AEA	A-BAR	A-Collagen I	III	IV	V
0	0	0	0	nd	nd	17	nd	nd	nd	nd	nd
nd	nd	nd	nd	nd	nd	nd	nd	nd	nd	nd	nd
0	nd	4	0	nd	nd	nd	nd	nd	nd	nd	nd
nd	nd	nd	nd	nd	nd	12	nd	5	5	5	5
nd	nd	nd	nd	nd	0	nd	nd	nd	nd	nd	nd
nd	nd	nd	nd	nd	nd	nd	nd	nd	nd	nd	nd
nd	nd	nd	nd	nd	nd	91	nd	35	40	35	35
nd	nd	nd	nd	nd	13	nd	nd	nd	nd	nd	nd
0	0	nd	nd	nd	nd	80	nd	nd	nd	nd	nd
9	0	nd	nd	nd	nd	40	nd	nd	nd	nd	nd
0	0	nd	nd	nd	nd	91	nd	nd	nd	nd	nd
nd	nd	nd	nd	nd	nd	nd	nd	nd	nd	nd	nd
0	nd	0	0	nd	nd	72	nd	nd	nd	nd	nd
nd	nd	nd	nd	nd	nd	nd	nd	30	40	35	35
nd	nd	nd	nd	nd	nd	70	nd	nd	nd	nd	nd
0	nd	nd	nd	nd	nd	42	nd	nd	nd	nd	nd
0	nd	nd	nd	nd	nd	20–50	nd	nd	nd	nd	nd
nd	0	0	0	0	nd	nd	nd	nd	nd	nd	nd
nd	nd	nd	nd	nd	30	nd	nd	nd	nd	nd	nd
2	nd	nd	nd	nd	nd	13	nd	nd	nd	nd	nd
2	nd	nd	nd	nd	nd	45	nd	nd	nd	nd	nd
nd	nd	nd	nd	nd	nd	nd	nd	12	24	6	24
nd	nd	0	0	nd	nd	31	nd	nd	nd	nd	nd

d Antimyosin antibodies in a 51-year-old patient with severe left ventricular dysfunction (ejection fraction 42%) after myocarditis 7 years previously. (× 1200; anti-human IgG, Medac; dilution 1:1000; Fab2 fragments; serum dilution 1:40). **e** De novo expression of major histocompatibility complex (MHC) class II antigens at the vascular endothelium in a 29-year-old woman with severe heart failure due to lymphocytic myocarditis. Cytomegalovirus DNA could be demonstrated by in situ hybridisation. **f** Antiendothelial antibodies as demonstrated with an isolated human endothelial cell from a HUVE cell culture. (× 1200; anti-human IgG, Medac; dilution 1:1000; Fab2 fragments; serum dilution 1:160). **g** Anti-Purkinje fibre antibodies in a 39-year-old woman with chronic myocarditis and recurrent third degree atrioventricular block. The patient died after 10 years of chronic disease from sudden cardiac death antibodies (Table 15.5a–d) are of pathogenetic relevance in autoreactive inflammatory myocardial diseases as well, or just an epiphenomenon in dilated cardiomyopathy, remains to be proven. Similarly Wallukat and Boewer [241] demonstrated beta-adrenoceptor antibodies that increased the beating frequency of isolated fetal heart cells. In contrast to the "beta-blocking" antibodies demonstrated by Limas and coworkers their functional assay permitted demonstration of a stimulatory antibody.

Bound Antimembrane Antibodies in Endomyocardial Biopsy Specimens

It has been clearly established that antimembrane antibodies not only circulate in the peripheral blood but are also bound to the sarcolemma and the interstitial tissue [77, 88, 157] in the endomyocardial biopsies of patients. It appears from our multicentre study [157] that apart from the regularly found IgG fixation, IgM, IgA and C3 or C1q fixation are of particular diagnostic value, indicating secondary immunopathogenesis in the course of an inflammatory or post-inflammatory process (Table 15.7).

Mitochondrial Proteins. Antibodies to mitochondrial proteins, which include the M7 protein [122, 123], its constituent sarcosin dehydrogenase (Berg, personal communication) and the antinucleotide translocator [220–223, 225, 228], were

Table 15.7. Immunohistological findings in endomyocardial biopsy: Würzburg multicentre study [from 157]

Clinical diagnosis	*n*	Trivalent	IgG	IgM	IgA	C3	C3 or IgM
Myocarditis (active/acute)	20	100[a,b]	90[a,b]	55[a,b]	70[a,b]	70[a,b]	85[a,b]
Perimyocarditis (active/acute)	20	100[a,b]	100[a,b]	95[a,b]	90[a,b]	90[a,b]	100[a,b]
Status post-myocarditis (no cardiomegaly)	22	100[a,b]	95[a,b]	32[a]	32[a]	36[a]	45[a]
Status post-perimyocarditis (no cardiomegaly)	15	73[a]	60[a]	13	7	33[a]	40[a]
Postmyocarditic heat muscle disease (cardiomegaly)	28	79[a]	75[a]	18	36[a]	61[a,b]	75[a]
Dilated cardiomyopathy (idiopathic)	50	60[a]	56[a]	48[a,b]	8	12	48a
Dilated heart muscle disease with increased alcohol intake	20	60[a]	60[a]	15	25[a]	35[a]	40[a]
Non-cardiac controls	17	12	12	0	0	0	0
Coronary artery disease	100	43[a]	41[a]	11	20[a]	3	14

[a] $p < 0.05$ by chi-squared analysis when compared with non-cardiac controls.
[b] $p < 0.05$ by chi-sequared analysis when compared with coronary artery disease.

demonstrated in patients with myocarditis and dilated cardiomyopathy (Table 15.6b, d). The latter has also been shown to interfere with the energy metabolism of the myocardial cell in experimental animals in vitro. A large body of evidence has been accumulated that further defines this cardiac autoantigen both immunologically and biochemically. Kühl et al. [125, 126] proposed that the antinucleotide translocator antibody may cross-react with the calcium channel. Schwimmbeck et al. [228], using synthetic peptides, demonstrated cross-reactivity between peptides from the adenine nucleotide translocator of the inner mitochondrial membrane and peptides from Coxsackie virus B3, substantiating also the hypothesis of molecular mimicry.

Antibodies to Myosin, Other Fibrils, the Cytoskeleton and the Extracellular Matrix. Antibodies to fibrils (Table 15.6a–d), particularly antibodies to myosin and actin, have been described in human and murine myocarditis. The latter were extensively reviewed by Beisel et al. [14]. Initially they were described in trypanosomiasis [2] and rheumatic fever [37, 38]. The sequence of myosin-cross-reactive epitopes of streptococcal M protein has been elucidated [39]. The pathogenetic relevance of antimyosin antibodies in viral heart disease is, however, still a matter for investigation. Cross-reactivity to Coxsackie virus proteins is less likely but not entirely excluded; cross-reactivity to mitochondrial proteins has been postulated but not conclusively demonstrated. Since fibrils lie intracellularly, antibodies directed to them are more likely to be a secondary phenomenon than a primary event, except for sequence homologies to sarcolemmal proteins not yet demonstrated. These sequence homologies have been elegantly demonstrated by means of monoclonal antibodies to streptococcal cell wall proteins by Dale and Beachey [39] and Cunningham et al. [37, 38].

Further non-organ-specific but defined antigens include desmin, (found in myocytes), vimentin (a marker of fibroblasts and histiocytes), collagen (particularly type III), fibronectin, myosin and actin (reviewed by [158]).

Table 15.6a–d give an overview of our present knowledge on circulating autoantibodies to cardiac epitopes in healthy control patients, in patients with myocarditis, perimyocarditis and pericarditis and in patients with dilated heart muscle disease.

Proteins found in many cells of the body, such as the microfilaments and intermediate filaments, the macrofilaments, or the extracellular matrix constituents, may evoke non-organ-specific immune responses separate from species-specific or individually unique epitopes, such as the constituents of the major histocompatibility complex, and from organ-specific autoreactivity. The tissue-specific epitopes seem to be of greater importance in immune diseases restricted to the myocardium, whereas in systemic disease, in which the myocardium may also be involved, these or non-specific proteins (e.g. parts of the cytoskeleton, the extracellular matrix and the microfilaments) could also be involved. Low titres of antibodies to extracellular matrix components have been described fairly frequently in endomyocardial biopsy [77, 125, 126, 154, 158], and less frequently circulating in the serum of patients with myocarditis [197].

The Vascular Endothelium. There is also renewed interest in the vascular endothelium, which plays a key role as a boundary zone between the circulating blood and cardiac tissue in immunological reactions that also involve the heart. Increased expression of class I and II antigens of the major histocompatibility complex (Fig. 15.4e) were found in myocarditis [87, 97]. Another form of involvement of the endothelial cells in the secondary immune response recently focused on antiendothelial antibodies, which may be cytolytic to living cultured human endothelial cells. These antibodies were demonstrated to be bound to the endomyocardial biopsy speciments of patients with biopsy-proven myocarditis, and to be circulating in the peripheral blood of the patients as cytolytic autoantibodies. They can be demonstrated specifically on isolated human endothelial cells (Fig. 15.4f). In rejection they may be involved in vasculitis and even in early graft sclerosis [183].

The Cardiac Conducting Tissue. Both viral processes [104] and autoreactive mechanisms [143, 172, 173] have been postulated to be involved in disturbances of cardiac conducting tissue in addition to the established causes such as coronary artery disease, hypertension, diabetes mellitus and progressive degeneration.

The immunopathogenesis of congenital heart block in neonates whose mothers have latent or manifest connective tissue disease and right bundle branch block associated with dermatomyositis or polymyositis is a well-established hypothesis that attributes relevance to anti-Ro or anti-La antibodies [143]. However, the true significance of circulating Purkinje cell antibodies (Fig. 15.4e) in either chronic heart block or bundle branch block is controversial [143, 172, 173, 198].

New data indicate a tenfold increased risk of developing sick sinus syndrome for patients with antisinus node antibodies, and a two- to three fold increased risk of acquiring an atrioventricular block for patients with antiatrioventricular node antibodies compared with age-mached control subjects without rhythm disturbances [173].

Previous myocarditis and rheumatic fever are predisposing factors for the existence of circulating antibodies directed against the conducting tissue in patients with sick sinus syndrome and atrioventricular block [173]. The new concept of the immunopathogenesis of tissue conduction disorders may also be applied to myocarditis and post-myocarditic heart diseases. It indicates that not only the myocardium but also the cardiac conducting system can be the target in secondary immunopathogenesis.

Circulating Immune Complexes

As has been shown in infective endocarditis, in myocarditis circulating immune complexes may be present at the time of the myocarditic viral illness in the majority of patients [89] and be in part responsible for some of the systemic features during this viral illness (e.g. proteinuria or erythrocyturia and even myalgia). Immune complex deposition can be seen in endomyocardial biopsy specimens of patients. On light microscopy it cannot easily be distinguised from bound antiendothelial antibodies by indirect immunofluorescence. Vasculitic changes in the myocardium have been described, but they are rare events in conventional haematoxylin/eosin stained preparations.

Autoreactivity: Horror Autotoxicus or Natural Event? A Perspective

Figure 15.5 schematically summarises the present view on antiviral and autoreactive processes in myocarditis. It is evident that humoral autoreactivity is much better analysed in humans than are the lymphocyte-, granulocyte- or macrophage-mediated processes.

Autoreactivity is the paradoxical facet of immunoreactivity that is needed when a host encounters infection, aging cells or tumor cells [24, 230]. The interaction between a viral or a microbial agent in inflammatory diseases is complex, but the immune response to the invading pathogen is the major host mechanism that determines the severity of the infective disorder, its course, its self-limitations, and its progression to post-infectious autimmunity. We have come a long way from Paul Ehrlich's "horror autotoxicus" and Jerne's [107] "forbidden clones" to a better understanding of autoreactive processes. Autoreactive T and B cells are most probably part of the individual's immune

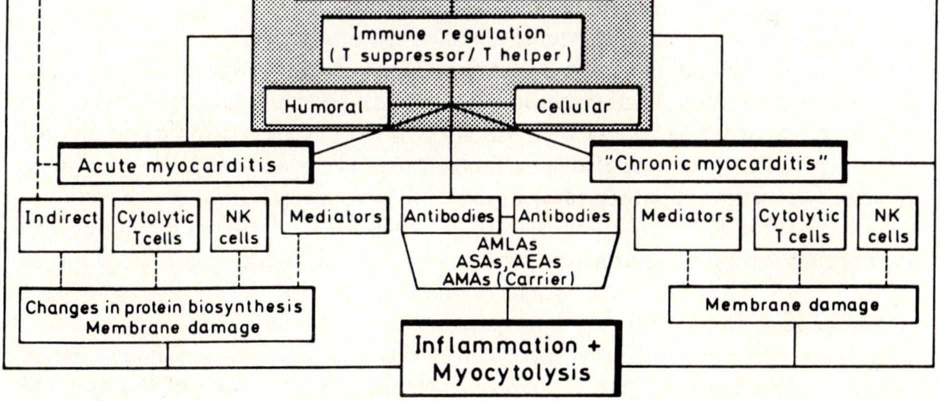

Fig. 15.5. Present status of antiviral and anticardiac autoreactivity in myocarditis and viral heart disease. [From 158]

repertoire. Autoantibodies, if low in titre or possible directed to foreign epitopes, are a very natural event [10, 158]. They may occur independently of infection, may belong more often to the lgM than to the lgG subclass and may demonstrate extensive cross-reactivity to other tissues. This is no rule, however, since there are numerous exceptions to it.

After a viral infection with cardiotropic agents the extent of the initial immune response in inflammatory myocardial, pericardial and endocardial disease is also influenced by the genetically fixed "aggressive" properties of the invading agent and the genetic composition of the host, which modulates regulator and effector organs. If antigenic mimicry is a pathogenetic principle in autoimmune disorders of the heart, mimicry should also most likely involve non-tissue-specific proteins and the previously mentioned antigenic binding sites or heat shock proteins that have come to our attention in trauma and sepsis.

It may well be that further investigations will demonstrate yet another immunoglobulin belonging to the microheterogeneity of antimembrane or anticardiac antibodies. Their mere presence may be of interest as a biographic or even prognostic marker. Their pathogenetic impact must be derived from the toxic properties that they exert on isolated resting [165, 168] or stimulated adult myocytes [49].

Animal Models

Introduction

Myocarditis remains a disease of many unresolved questions. In the clinical setting the diagnosis is hard to establish. Endomyocardial biopsies can be obtained safely from the myocardium, but the sensitivity is only about 50% for detecting an inflammatory infiltrate suggestive of myocarditis. Other diagnostic tools such as the electrocardiogram, echocardiogram and serological tests can support the diagnosis, but are never sufficient to establish it.

In most cases the exact time of onset of the disease remains unclear. The causative agent is rarely identified, although newer techniques such as in situ hybridisation or the polymerase chain reaction may eventually prove to be very helpful in this respect. Pathogenetic mechanisms remain to be fully elucidated, although valuable knowledge has been gained by several studies. Therapeutic trials have therefore been hampered by low numbers of patients being unquestionably diagnosed as having myocarditis and the lack of exact knowledge about the aetiology, pathogenesis or stage of the disease, and the results have been inconclusive so far.

In view of these problems animal models have been developed, of which Coxsackie virus B3-induced myocarditis in mice most closely resembles the human disease. Two major forms of the murine Coxsackie B3 myocarditis have been indentified: an acute or early form and a late form.

Early Phase Coxsackie Virus B3-Induced Murine Myocarditis

Acute Coxsackie virus B3-induced murine myocarditis reaches a peak of cardiac inflammation on day 7 after virus inoculation, although virus concentration in the heart is maximal on days 3 and 4. The disease subsides with scarring in the heart without noticeable inflammation after 15 days of the infection. Despite the fact that Coxsackie viruses are lytic to susceptible cells, the discrepancy between maximal virus titre and inflammation in the heart, as well as the histological feature of a polymorphonuclear and mononuclear infiltrate in the myocardium adjacent to necrotic myofibres, suggested a significant role of the immune system in the pathogenesis of the disease. The importance of T lymphocytes in mediating cardiac inflammation has subsequently been demonstrated. Using thymectomy and irradiation or anti-thymocyte serum for the depletion of T lymphocytes Woodruff [252], Wong et al. [250, 251] and Huber and co-workers [93, 94, 96] were able nearly to abolish cardiac lesions. Reconstituting the animals with functional splenocytes or lymph node cells reinstituted the disease. Further experiments showed that different T lymphocyte subpopulations are responsible for cardiac damage depending on the strain of mice used. In Balb/c mice the development of cardiac lesions is largely produced by Lyt2 + (CD8 +) cytolytic/suppressor T lymphocytes, whereas in DBA/2 mice myocarditis is exclusively mediated by L3T4 + (CD4 +) helper T cells. In A/J mice the depletion of L3T4 + T cells mitigates the disease whereas eliminating Lyt2 + T lymphocytes enhances myocardial inflammation and necrosis presumably by removing suppressor cells. The elemination of both T lymphocyte subpopulations at the same time reduces cardiac inflammation and necrosis in all three strains of mice (Fig. 15.6).

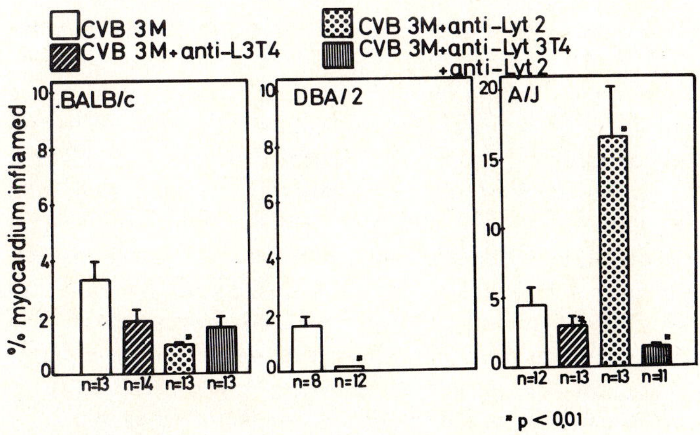

Fig. 15.6. Reduction of myocardial inflammation resulting from Coxsackie virus B3 (CVB3) by different antilymphocyte antibodies (anti-L3T4, anti-Lyt 2, anti-Lyt 3T4, anti-Lyt 2) in three different mouse strains(Balb/c, DBA/2, A/J)

In vitro studies revealed that T lymphocytes from Coxsackie virus B3-infected Balb/c mice exhibited strong cytotoxicity to cardiac myofibres. One subpopulation of these cytolytic T lymphocytes lyses Coxsackie virus B3-infected cardiac cells but not cells infected with another picornavirus, suggesting viral proteins are the antigenic determinants which are recognised by these cells. These cells are of the L3T4+ (CD4+) phenotype and recognise antigen in combination with class II proteins of the major histocompatibility complex. Another T lymphocyte population induced in the course of Coxsackie virus B3 infection kills non-infected cardiac myocytes. These autoimmune T cells are Lyt2+ (CD8+) lymphocytes. Proteins of the virus receptor or in its proximity may be the target antigens for these cells. Recently a third population of cytotoxic T lymphocytes has been identified. It reacts to epitopes which occur in metabolically disturbed cells and which can be induced by different picornaviruses as well as chemical substances, e.g. actinomycin D. This cell line may be of importance for the pathogenesis of chronic (recurring) myocarditis either by subsequent infections with other viruses or by exposure of the individual to chemical substances.

In the acute phase of Coxsackie virus B3 infection the activity of natural killer cells increases considerably. In this model of murine myocarditis natural killer cells have a protective function, because their depletion by specific antibodies leads to an aggravation of myocardial lesions. This may—at least in part—be due to a marked increase in cardiac virus concentrations.

T-lymphocyte-mediated immune reactions do not explain all forms of early myocarditis. A humoral immunopathogenesis of the disease has been described in DBA/2 mice. Upon infection with Coxsackie virus B3 these mice generate anti-cardiocyte antibodies of the IgM and IgG isotype and benefit from complement depletion by cobra venom factor. In contrast Balb/c mice, in whom cytotoxic T cells induce cardiac damage, demonstrate anti-cardiocyte antibodies exclusively of the IgM immunoglobulin class and do not improve with complement removal. This finding supports the idea of humorally mediated early myocarditis.

Antigenic mimicry between viral antigens and cardiac myofibres may hence be another pathogenetic principle. A cross-reaction of Coxsackie B3 proteins and isolated cardiocytes has been shown by immunoabsorption studies. Later Segusa et al. [229] generated a monoclonal antibody reacting to normal human myocardium and Coxsackie virus B4. Huber et al. [96] found a monoclonal antibody binding to Coxsackie virus B3 and several other murine tissues. Injecting this antibody into a Coxsackie virus B3-infected mouse enhances myocarditis tremendously, supporting the idea of a pathogenetic role of cross-reacting antibodies. Whether cross-reacting antibodies of this type play a role in the humorally mediated immunopathogenesis of early myocarditis in DBA/2 mice remains to be determined and is the subject of further studies.

Expression of class I and class II antigens of the major histocompatibility complex (MHC) is necessary for the action of cytotoxic lymphocytes. In experimental Coxsackie virus B3 myocarditis the expression of class I as well as class II antigens increases markedly and reaches a high level 5 days after viral infection. Whereas class I antigens are detectable on cardiac myofibres as well as on cardiac interstitial cells and endothelial cells, class II antigens could only be demonstrated on endothelial cells and some interstitial cells.

Late Phase Coxsackie Virus B3-Induced Murine Myocarditis

In late Coxsackie virus B3-induced myocarditis in mice different pathogenetic mechanisms seem to be operative. Histologically this phase is dominated by a mononuclear infiltrate in the heart and the concomitant demonstration of heart-specific antibodies. The late type of myocarditis starts from day 9 and persists up to 45 days. The presence of replicating Coxsackie virus B3 is not responsible for ongoing disease, since it is cleared from the myocardium after 15 days in most of the mouse strains. The demonstration of heart-specific autobodies is a hallmark of the development of late myocarditis. Two different types of antigen specificities, recognised by these antibodies, have been identified: one is the sarcolemma of heart muscle cells, the other cardiac myosin. In further studies anti-sarcolemmal antibodies proved to be a very sensitive and specific indicator of late phase myocarditis whereas cardiac myosin was the main immunopathogenetic antigen.

Sensitisation to this intracellularly located protein is thought to take place during cell necrosis induced by the virus or cytotoxic T lymphocytes in early myocarditis and is a common event. Many strains of inbred mice develop antibodies to this antigen. The isotype of anti-myosin antibodies, however, determines the course of Coxsackie virus B3 myocarditis. Whereas mice susceptible to late phase myocarditis produce highly specific anti-cardiac myosin antibodies of the IgG isotype, strains of mice resistant to this form of the disease generate antibodies of the IgM type only, that are also reactive to other types of myosin. Immunising mice, susceptible to late phase myocarditis with cardiac myosin but not skeletal myosin caused severe myocarditis resembling Coxsackie virus B3-induced late phase myocarditis very closely [196,197].

Genetics of Enterovirally Induced Murine Myocarditis

Thus Coxsackie B3 induces two forms of myocarditis: an acute form of short duration and an ongoing late form. Whereas all strains of mice seem to be susceptible to early myocarditis the severity of myocardial inflammation varies greatly. Only some strains, however, are predisposed to develop late phase myocarditis. Host genetics have been shown to be responsible for these differences. In early myocarditis Beisel et al. [14,15] and Buie et al. [27] demonstrated that genes belonging to the major histocompatibility complex have great influence on the extent of myocardial lesions induced by Coxsackie virus B3 using strains of mice with different MHC antigens but identical background genes (congenic mice). Interestingly susceptibility to myocarditis caused by a second cardiotropic picornavirus or encephalomyocarditis virus is related to MHC haplotypes different from those associated with Coxsackie virus B3-induced disease in the same strain of mice [27].

Although all strains of mice mount comparable antiviral antibody titres the onset of the generation of neutralising antibodies is faster in mice with mild early myocarditis and later in strains with severe early disease. This different behaviour seems to be regulated by genes belonging to the MHC. Susceptibility to late phase autoimmune myocarditis, dependent on the generation of anti-sarcolemmal and anti-cardiac myosin antibodies, is controlled by the background genes not belonging to the MHC region. MHC genes, however, are relevant to the severity of this form of myocarditis because their composition again influences the strength of the autoantibody production. Genetics not only determine susceptibility and resistance to early and late phase enteroviral-induced myocarditis but are also responsible for different immunopathogenetic mechanisms. Early myocarditis in Balb/c mice is mediated largely by cytotoxic T lymphocytes belonging to the CD8+ subpopulation. Their depletion by an anti-CD8 monoclonal antibody leads to protection from myocardial inflammation. In DBA/2 mice pathomorphology can be abolished by the administration of anti-CD4 monoclonal antibodies, stressing the importance of these lymphocytes for the development of the disease. F1 hybrid animals of these two strains are only protected from myocarditis if both monoclonal antibodies are administered simultaneously. Back-crossing F1 hybrid mice with either parental strain yields 50% protection from myocarditis on administration of one monoclonal antibody. This is to be expected if the respective immunopathogenetic mechanisms are inherited by means of a single gene [90].

Other Experimental Models

A number of antigen-induced or adjuvant models of myocarditis have been used to demonstrate cross-reactivity of streptococci to cardiac tissue. More importantly they have also demonstrated that by immunisation with cardiac membranes or whole heart extracts humoral and cellular effector mechanisms can be induced—e.g. in rabbits specific anticardiac lymphocytes can be generated [182], in rats humoral autoreactivity is a common phenomenon, [59, 60] and even giant cell myocarditis can be induced in experimental animals [101].

Future Expectations for Experimental Animal Models

Although Coxsackie virus B3-induced myocarditis in mice seems to resemble the disease in humans in many respects it is still unclear how close this model is to the situation in humans. Furthermore studies so far have almost all dealt with picornavirus-induced murine myocarditis. Many other infectious agents, however, have been implicated in inflammatory heart muscle disease and cardiomyopathy in patients. It may be desirable to develop other models of myocarditis in different animals with different causative agents in order to verify, correct and supplement the knowledge gained so far.

Animal models should be very helpful in clarifying questions as yet unanswered. In situ hybridisation has shown that the Coxsackie virus genome can be detected in the heart at times when replicating virus is no longer present in the tissue and clinical symptoms of an acute infection and histological signs of acute cardiac inflammation have long subsided. The relevance of persisting enteroviral genomes in the myocardium to the development of ongoing cardiac disease and dilated cardiomyopathy remains to be elucidated. The identification and characterisation of antigens in the heart, targeted by cytotoxic lymphocytes and (autoantibodies) is still incomplete. There are data that suggest that sarcolemmal proteins, cardiac myosin, the adenine nucleotide translocator and the cellular virus receptor are important antigenic structures for humoral and cellular immune reactions. Nevertheless do other studies support the idea of many more epitopes relevant for the disease. Knowing the antigens may bring forward quick and non-invasive ways to diagnose inflammatory heart disease and to monitor the course of the disease. Finally animal models should be used to further dissect out genetic and environmental predisposing factors for the development of myocarditis and dilated cardiomyopathy which cannot easily be assessed in man.

Summary and Conclusions

Animal models of enterovirally induced myocarditis have provided valuable knowledge about aetiology, pathogenesis and different clinical courses of the disease. They stress the importance of cellular and humoral immune pathomechanisms for the development of cardiac lesions. Susceptibility and resistance to overt early myocarditis and late phase autoimmune myocarditis are under the control of MHC genes and non-MHC (background) genes. This resembles at least in part the human situation, which appears to be more a B-lymphocyte-controlled viral heart disease, in which antigenic mimicry plays an important role. Both the antiviral and the anticardiac immune response makes use of cellular and humoral effector mechanisms which are controlled by immunoregulatory T helper and T suppressor cells (Fig. 15.6). The clinical and histological picture of acute or chronic myocarditis is the end result of the inflammation induced by macrophages, natural killer cells, T lymphocytes, mediators and autoantibodies.

References

1. Abelmann WH, Kowalski HJ, McNeely WF (1954) Cardiovascular studies during acute infectious hepatitis. Gastroenterology 27: 61–66
2. Acosta AM, Sadigursky M, Santos-Bush CA (1983) Anti-striated muscle antibody activity produced by *Trypanosoma cruzi*. Proc Soc Exp Biol Med 172: 364–374
3. Adams CW (1959) Post-viral myopericarditis associated with the influenza virus: report of eight cases. Am J Cardiol 4: 56–67
4. Ahvenainen EK (1952) Inclusion disease or generalized salivary gland virus infection: report of five cases. Acta Pathol Microbiol Scand 93 Suppl: 159–167
5. Ainger LE, Lawyer NG, Fitch CW (1966) Neonatal rubella myocarditis. Br Heart J 28: 691–697
6. Alvarez FL, Neu N, Rose NR, Craig SW, Beisel KW (1987) Heart-specific autoantibodies induced by coxsackievirus B: identification of heart autoantigens. Clin Immunol Immunopathol 43: 12–23
7. Anderson JL, Carlquist JF, Hammond EH (1982) Deficient natural killer cell activity in patients with idiopathic dilated cardiomyopathy. Lancet 2: 1124–1127
8. Anderson T, Foulis MA, Grist NR, Landsman JB (1951) Clinical and laboratory observations in a smallpox outbreak. Lancet 1: 1248–1252
9. Aretz Ht, Billingham ME, Edward WD (1987) Myocarditis: a histological definition and classification. Am J Cardiovasc Pathol 1: 3–13
10. Avrameas S (1986) Natural autoreactive B cells and autoantibodies: the know thyself of the immune system. Ann immunol (Paris) 137: 150–153
11. Banatvala JE (1983) Coxsackie B virus infections in cardiac disease. In: Waterson AP (ed) Recent advances in clinical virology vol. 3. Churchill Livingstone, Edinburgh, pp 99–115
12. Banatvala JE, Bryant J, Schernthaner G, Borkenstein M, Schober E, Brown D, de Solva LM, Mensa MA, Silink M (1985) Coxsackie B, mumps, rubella and cytomegalovirus-specific lgM responses in patients with juvenile onset insulin-dependent diabetes mellitus in Britain, Austria and Australia. Lancet 1: 1409–1412
13. Beisel KW (1989) Immunogenetic basis of myocarditis: role of fibrillary antigens. Springer Semin Immunopathol 11: 31–42
14. Beisel KW, Chow LH, Booth BJM, Nesbitt MN, McManus BM (1989) Linkage of susceptibility to autoimmune-based viral myocarditis with Tcra and Myhc-a loci on murine chromosome 14 (Abstr). Circulation 80 Suppl 2: 2673
15. Beisel K, Wolfgram L, Herskowitz A, Rose N (1991) Differences in severity of Coxsackievirus B3-induced myocarditis among H-2 congenic mouse strain. In: Skameme E (ed) Genetic control of host resistance to infection and malignancy, vol 3. Liss, New York, pp 195–205
16. Bell EJ, Grist NR (1968) Coxsackie virus infections in patients with acute cardiac disease and chest pain. Scott Med J 13: 47–51
17. Bengtsson E, Örndahl G (1954) Complications of mumps with special reference to the incidence of myocarditis. Acta Med Scand 149: 381–388
18. Berkovich S, Rodriguez-Torres R, Lin TS (1968) Virologic studies in children with acute myocarditis. Am J Dis Child 115: 207–212
19. Besteri RB (1989) Cardiac involvement in the acquired immune deficiency syndrome. J Cardiol 22: 143–146
20. Billingham ME, Mason JW (1984) Endomyocardial biopsy changes in myocarditis treated with immunosuppressives. In: Bolte H-D (ed) Viral heart disease. Springer, Berlin Heidelberg New York, pp 200–210
21. Bodey GP, Wertlake PT, Douglas G, Levin RH (1965) Cytomegalic inclusion disease in patients with acute leukemia. Ann Intern Med 62: 899–906
22. Bolte HD, Schultheiss P, Cyran J, Goss F (1980) Binding of immunoglobulins in the myocardium biopsy. In: Bolte H-D (ed) Myocardial biopsy. Springer, Berlin Heidelberg New York, pp 85–92
23. Bowles NE, Richardson PJ, Olsen EGJ, Archard LC (1986) Detection of Coxsackie B

virus-specific RNA sequences in myocardial biopsy samples from patients with myocarditis and dilated cardiomyopathy. Lance 1: 1120–1123

24. Boyden SV (1963) Natural antibodies and the immune response. Adv Immunol 5: 1–7
25. Bresnihan B, Jasin ME (1977) Suppressor function of peripheral blood mononuclear cells in normal individuals and in patients with systemic lupus erythematosus. J Clin Invest 59: 106–116
26. Bugher JC (1951) The pathology of yellow fever. In: Stoker GK (ed) Yellow fever. McGraw-Hill, New York, pp 137–163
27. Buie C, Lodge PA, Herzum M, Huber SA (1987) Genetics of Coxsackie virus B3 and encephalomyocarditis virus-induced myocarditis in mice. Eur Heart J 8 Suppl J: 389–401
28. Bülowius H, Maisch B, Klopf D, Schmier K, Hiby A, Schunk D, Kochsiek K (1983) Lymphozytensubpopulationen Bei akuter Perimyokarditis, sekundären und primären dilatativen Herzmuskelerkrankungen. Z Kardiol 72 Suppl 1: 16
29. Burch GE, Giles TG (1972) The role of viruses in the production of heart disease. Am J Cardiol 29: 231–240
30. Caldera R, Sarrut S, Mallet R, Rossier A (1961) Existe- t-il des complications cardiaques de la vaccine? Sem Hop Paris 37: 1281–1284
31. Cambridge G, MacArthur CGC, Waterson AP, Goodwin JF, Oakley C (1979) Antibodies to Coxsackie B viruses in congestive cardiomyopathy. Br Heart J 16: 692–696
32. Cambridge G, Campbell-Blay G, Wilmhurst P, Coltart DJ, Stern CMM (1983) Deficient "natural" cytotoxicity in patients with congestive cardiomyopathy (Abstr). Br Heart J 49: 623
33. Cannell DE (1928) Myocardial degenerations in yellow fever. Am J Pathol 4: 431–443
33a. Cheetham HD, Hart J, Coghill NF, Fox Z (1970) Rabies with myocarditis, two cases in England. Lancet I: 921–922
34. Christian HA (1951) Nearly ten decades of interest in idiopathic pericarditis. Am Heart J 42: 645–651
35. Coltman CA Jr (1962) Influenza myocarditis: report of a case with observations on serum glutamic oxaloacetic transaminase. JAMA 180: 204–208
36. Craighead JE, Huber SA, Martin WB (1991) Murine cytomegalovirus myocarditis. Eur Heart J 12 Suppl D: 69–72
37. Cunningham MW, Swerlick RA (1986) Polyspecificity of antistreptococcal murine monoclonal antibodies and their implication in autoimmunity. J Exp Med 164: 998–1004
38. Cunningham MW, Hall NK, Krisher KK, Spanier AM, (1986) A study of anti-group a streptococcal monoclonal antibodies cross-reactive with myosin. J Immunol 136: 293–298
39. Dale JB, Beachey EH (1986) Sequence of myosin-crossreactive epitopes of streptococcal M protein. J Exp Med 164: 1785–1789
40. Dalgaard JB (1957) Fatal myocarditis following smallpox vaccination. Am Heart J 54: 156–158
41. Daly K, Richardson PJ, Olsen EGJ, Morgan-Capner P, McSorley C, Jackson G, Jewitt DE (1984) Acute myocarditis: role of histological and virological examination in the diagnosis and assessment of immunosuppressive treatment. Br Heart J 51: 30–35
42. Das SK, Callen JP, Doson VN, Cassidy JT (1971) Immunoglobulin binding in cardiomyopathic hearts. Circulation 44: 612–621
43. Das SK, Petty RE, Meengs WA, Tubergen DG (1980) Studies of cell-mediated immunity in cardiomyopathy. In: Sekiguchi M, Olsen EGJ (eds) Cardiomyopathy. University of Tokyo Press, Tokyo, pp 375–377
44. De Crombrugghe B, Liau G, Setoyama C, Schmidt A, McKeon C, Mudry M (1985) Structural and foundational studies on interstitial collagen genes. In: Evered D, Whelan J (eds) Fibrosis. Pitman, London, pp 20–32
45. Deck WG, Palacios IF, Fallon JT, Aretz HT, Mills J, Lee DCS, Johnson RA (1985) Active myocarditis in the spectrum of acute dilated cardiomyopathies. N Engl J Med 342: 885–897
46. Dell A, Antone SM, Gauntt CJ, Crossley CA, Clark WA, Cunningham MW (1991) Autoimmune determinants of rheumatic carditis: localization of epitopes in human cardiac myosin. Eur Heart J 12 Suppl D: 158–162
46a. De Scheerder, de Buyzere M, Algoed L, de Lange M, de Langhe J, Bogaert AM, Clement DL

(1987) Characteristics anti-heart antibody patterns in post-cardiac injury syndrome endocarditis and acute myocarditis. Eur Heart J 8 Suppl I: 237–238
47. Doerr W (1971) Morphologie der Myokarditis. Verh Dtsch Ges Inn Med 77:301–335
48. Dolgopol VB, Cragen MD (1948) Myocardial changes in poliomyelitis. Arch Pathol 46: 202–211
49. Drude L, Wiemers F, Maisch B (1991) Impaired myocyte function in vitro incubated with sera from patients with myocarditis. Eur Heart J 12 Suppl D: 36–38
50. Eckstein R, Mempel W, Bolte H-D (1982) Reduced suppressor cell activity in congestive cardiomyopathy and in myocarditis. Circulation 65: 1224–1229
51. Eghbali M, Czaja MJ, Chepko G, Hern MA, Seifter S, Blumenfeld OO (1987) Differential collagen gene expression in heart cells. Fed Proc 46: 2040
52. Eghbali ME, Egbali M, Robinson TF, Seifter S, Blumenfeld OO (1987) Role of fibroblasts in the accumulation of collagens in growing and adult rat hearts. J Mol Cell Cardiol 19 Suppl 4: 854
53. Fenoglio JJ Jr, Ursell PC, Kellogg CF, Drusin RE, Wiss MB (1983) Diagnosis and classification of myocarditis by endomyocardial biopsy. N Engl J Med 308: 12–18
54. Finland M, Parker F Jr, Barnes MW, Joliffe LS (1945) Acute myocarditis in influenza infections: two cases of non-bacterial myocarditis with isolation of virus from the lungs. Am J Med Sci 209: 455–468
55. Fletcher E, Brennan CF (1957) Cardiac complications of Coxsackie virus infection. Lancet 1: 913–915
56. Fletcher GF, Coleman MT, Feorius PM, Marine WM, Wenger NK (1968) Viral antibodies in patients with primary myocardial disease. Am J Cardiol 21: 6–14
57. Fowles RE, Bieber CP, Stinson EB (1978) Defective in vitro suppressor cell function in idiopathic congestive cardiomyopathy. Circulation 59: 483–491
58. Francesini R, Petillo A, Corazza M, Nizzo MC, Azzolini A, Gianrossi R (1983) Lymphocyte response in dilated cardiomyopathy. IRCS Med Sci 2: 1019–1021
59. Friedman I, Laufer A (1976) Electron microscopical studies of the effect of antiheart antibodies and complement on beating heart cells in culture. J Mol Cell Cardiol 8: 641–650
60. Friedman I, Laufer A, Ron N, Davies AM (1971) Experimental myocarditis: in vitro and in vivo studies of lymphocytes sensitized to heart extracts and group A streptococci. J Immunol 20: 225–232
61. Fuchs E, Hanukoglu C (1983) Unraveling the structure of the intermediate filaments. Cell 34: 332–342
62. Gardinger AJS, Short D (1973) Four faces of acute myopericarditis. Br Heart J 35: 433–442
63. Gauntt CJ, Goeny EK, Lutton CM, Pernandes G (1989) Role of natural killer cells in experimental murine myocarditis. Springer Semin Immunopathol 11: 51–59
64. Geisler N, Kaufman E, Weber K (1971) Protein chemical characterization of three structurally distinct domains along the protofilament unit of the desmin 10-mm filaments. Cell 30: 277–281
65. Giles C, Shuttleworth EM (1957) Postmortem findings in 46 influenza deaths. Lancet 2: 1224–1225
66. Giustra FX, Nilsson DC (1950) Myocarditis following measles. Am J Dis Child 79: 487–490
67. Godeney EK, Gauntt CJ (1987) Murine natural killer cells limit Coxsackievirus B3 replication. J Immunol 139: 913–918
68. Goldstein MA, Entman ML (1979) Microtubules in mammalian heart muscle. J Cell Biol 80: 183–189
69. Gore I, Kline IK (1968) Pericarditis and myocarditis. In: Gould SE (ed) Pathology of the heart and blood vessels, 3rd edn Thomas, Springfield, pp 731–759
70. Gore I, Saphir O (1947) Myocarditis: a classification of 1402 cases. Am Heart J 34: 827–830
71. Grist NR, Bell EJ (1969) Coxsackie viruses and the heart. Am Heart J 77: 295–300
72. Grist NR, Bell EJ (1974) A six year study of Coxsackie virus B infections in heart disease. J Hyg (Camb) 73: 165–174
73. Grody WW, Cheng L, Pang, M, Lewis W (1989) Direct infection of the heart by human immunodeficiency virus (HIV) (Abstr). Circulation 80 Suppl 2: 2644

74. Hackel DB (1953) Myocarditis in association with varicella. Am J Pathol 29: 369–379
75. Hallgren HM, Yunis EJ (1977) Suppressor lymphocytes in young and aged humans. J Immunol 118: 2004–2008
76. Hamburger WW (1938) The heart in influenza. Med Clin North Am 22: 111–121
77. Hammond EH, Menlove RL, Anderson JL (1988) Immunofluorescence microscopy in the diagnosis and follow-up of patients suspected of having inflammatory heart disease. In: Schultheiss HP (ed) New concepts in viral heart disease: virology, immunology and clinical management. Springer, Berlin Heidelberg New York pp 303–311
78. Harding SE, MacLeod KT, Jones SM, Vescovo G, Poole-Wilson PA (1991) Contractile responses of myocytes isolated from patients with cardiomyopathy. Eur Heart J 12 Suppl D: 44–49
79. Haskowa V, Holub M, Hasek J (1987) Changes in the microtubular skeleton of human lymphocytes produced by immunosuppressive substances. Czech Med 10: 164–169
80. Hauck AJ, Kearney DL, Edwards WS (1989) Evaluation of postmortem endomyocardial biopsy specimens from 38 patients with lymphocytic myocarditis: implications for role of sampling error. Mayo Clin Proc 64: 1235–1245
81. Hay ED (1981) Extracellular matrix. J Cell Biol 91: 205–217
82. Hay Ed (1982) Cell biology of extracellular matrix. Plenum, New York
83. Hengstenberg C, Rose M, Olsen E, Richardson PJ, Archard L, Yacoub M (1989) Immonological parameters in patients with different heart diseases (Abstr) Eur Heart J 10 Suppl: 27
84. Henson D, Mufson MA (1971) Myocarditis and pneumonitis with type 21 adenovirus infection: association with fatal myocarditis and pneumonitis. Am J Dis Child 121: 433–422
85. Herskowitz A, Beisel KW, Wolfgram LJ, Rose NR (1985) Coxsackievirus B3 murine myocarditis: wide pathologic spectrum in genetically defined inbred strains. Hum Pathol 16: 671–678
86. Herskowitz A, Wolgram LJ, Rose NR, Beisel KW (1987) Coxsackievirus B3 murine myocarditis: a pathologic spectrum of myocarditis in genetically defined inbred strains. J Am Cell Cardiol 9: 1311–1329
87. Herskowitz A, Neumann DA, Rose NR, Beschorner WE, Sell KI, Ansari AA, Baughman KL (1989) Histocompatibility (MHC) antigens in human myocarditis: new markers of immunemediated disease (Abstr). Circulation 80 Suppl 2: 2686
88. Herzum M, Maisch B (1989) Anti-viral and anti-myocyte antibodies in experimental myocarditis. Springer Semin Immunopathol 11: 69–76
89. Herzum M, Maisch B, Kochsiek K (1987) Circulating immune complexes in perimyocarditis and infective endocarditis. Eur Heart J 8 Suppl J: 323–326
90. Herzum M, Huber SA, Maisch B (1988) Coxsackie B3 myocarditis: genetic aspects of different immunopathogenic mechanisms in Balb/c and DBA/2 mices. Antigenic specificity of heart-reactive antibodies in DBA/2 mices. In: Schultheiss HP (ed) New concepts in viral heart disease. Springer, Berlin Heidelberg New York, pp 188–194
91. Hirschmann SZ, Hammer GS (1974) Coxsackie virus myopericarditis: a microbiological and clinical review. Am J Cardiol 34: 224–232
92. Hoagland RJ (1956) Cardiac involvement in infectious mononucleosis. Am J Med Sci 232: 252–257
93. Huber SA, Lodge PA (1984) Coxsackie B3 myocarditis: identification of different pathogenic mechanisms in DBA/2 and Balb/c mice. Am J Pathol 122: 284–291
94. Huber SA, Lodge PA (1984a) Coxsackievirus B3 myocarditis in BALB/c mice: evidence for autoimmunity to myocyte antigens. Am J Pathol 116: 21–29
95. Huber SA, Job LP, Woodruff JF (1980) Lysis of infected myofibres by Coxsackie virus B3 immune T-lymphocytes. Am J Pathol 98: 681–694
96. Huber SA, Simpson K, Weller A, Herzum M (1988) Immunopathogenic mechanisms in experimental myocarditis: evidence for autoimmunity to the virus receptor and antigenic mimicry between the virus and the myocardium. In: Schultheiss HP (ed) New concepts in viral heart disease. Springer Berlin Heidelberg New York, pp 179–187

97. Hufnagel G, Maisch B (1989) MHC antigen expression in endomyocardial biopsies in patients with myocarditis and dilated cardiomyopathy (Abstr). Eur Heart J 10 Suppl: 28
98. Hufnagel G, Pfeifer U, Maisch B (1987) Immunohistological investigation in suspected cardiac sarcoidosis. Eur Heart J 8: Suppl J 59–62
99. Hynes RO (1985) Molecular biology of fibronectin. Annu Rev Cell Biol 1:67–79
100. Hynes RO, Yamada S (1982) Fibronectins: multifunctional nodular glycoprotein. J Cell Biol 95:369–376
101. Izumi T, Kodama M, Shibata A (1991) Experimental giant cell myocarditis induced by cardiac myosin immunization. Eur Heart J 12 Suppl D: 166–168
102. Jacobs B, Matsuda Y, Deodhar S (1979) Cell-mediated cytotoxicity to cardiac cells of lymphocytes from patients with primary myocardial disease. Am J Clin Pathol 72: 1–4
103. James TN (1983) Myocarditis and cardiomyopathy. N Engl J Med 308: 39–41
104. James TM, Umamura K (1981) Virus-like particles associated with intracardiac ganglionitis in two cases of sudden unexpected death. Jpn Heart J 22: 447–454
105. Javett SN, Heymann S, Mundel B, Peler WL, Lurie HJ, Gear J, Measroch V, Kirsch Z (1956) Myocarditis in new born infant: a study of an outbreak associated with Coxsackie group B virus infection in a maternity home in Johannesburg. J Padiatr 48: 1–22
106. Jennings RC (1966) Coxsackie group B fatal neonatal myocarditis associated with cardiomegaly. J Clin Pathol 19: 325–327
107. Jerne NK (1955) The natural selection theory of antibody formation. Proc Natl Acad Sci USA 41: 849–857
108. Kandolf R, Hofschneider PH (1989) Viral heart disease. Springer Semin Immunopathol 11: 1–13
109. Kandolf R, Ameis D, Kirschner P, Canu A, Hofschneider PH (1987) In situ detection of enteroviral genomes in myocardial cells: an approach to the diagnosis of viral heart disease. Proc Natl Acad Sci USA 84: 6272–6276
110. Kaplan MH (1967) Multiple nature of the cross-reactive relationships between antigens of group A streptococci and mammalian tissue. In: Trentin JJ (ed) Cross-reaction, antigens and neoantigens. Williams and Wilkins, Baltimore, pp 48–55
111. Katz AM, Messineo FC, Herbette L (1985) Membrane damage in the pathogenesis of cardiomyopathies. J Mol Cell Cardiol Suppl 2: 17: 11–17
112. Kawai C, Matsumori A, Kitaura Y, Takatsu T (1978) Viruses and the heart: viral myocarditis and cardiomyopathy. In: Yu PN, Goodwin JF (eds) Progress in cardiology. Lea and Febiger, Philadelphia, pp 141–162
113. Kawai S, Okada R (1987) A histopathological study of dilated cardiomyopathy: with special reference to clinical and pathological comparisons of the degeneration-predominant type and fibrosis-predominant type. Jpn Circ J 51: 654–660
114. Kefalides NA, Alper R, Clarc CC (1979) Biochemistry and metabolism of basement membranes. Int Rev Cytol 61: 67–75
115. Kibrick S, Benirschke K (1956) Acute aseptic myocarditis and meningoencephalitis in the newborn child infected with Coxsackie virus group B, type 3. N Engl J Med 255: 883–889
116. Kipkie GF, McAuley JSM (1954) Acute myocarditis occurring in bulbar poliomyelitis. Can Med Assoc J 70: 315–317
117. Kirsner AB, Hess EV, Fowler NO (1973) Immunologic findings in idiopathic cardiomyopathy. Am Heart J 86: 625–630
118. Kishimoto C, Crumpacker CS, Abelman WH (1988) Ribavirin treatment of murine coxsackievirus B myocarditis with analyses of lymphocyte subsets. J Am Coll Cardiol 12: 1334–1342
119. Kishimoto C, Crumpacker CS, Abelman WH (1988) Prevention of murine Coxsackie B3 viral myocarditis and associated lymphoid organ atrophy with recombinant human leukocyte interferon alpha. Cardiovasc Res 22: 732–738
119a. Klappacher G, Pacher R, Woluszczuk W, Glogar D (1991) Increased release of neopterin and tumor necrosis factor alpha into the serum of patients with primary dilated cardiomyopathy (Abstr). Eur Heart J 12 Suppl: 315

120. Klappacher G, Pacher R, Woluszczuk W, Glogar D (1991) Elevated circulating levels of β2-microglobulin in primary dilated cardiomyopathy (Abstr). Eur Heart J 12 Suppl: 316
121. Klein J, Stanek G, Bittner R, Horvat R, Holzinger C, Glogar D (1991) Lyme borreliosis as a cause of myocarditis and heart muscle disease. Eur Heart J 12 Suppl D: 73–75
122. Klein R, Maisch B, Kochsiek K, Berg PA (1984) Demonstration of organ specific antibodies against heart mitochondria (anti-M7) in sera from patients with some forms of heart disease. Clin Exp Immunol 58: 283–292
123. Klein R, Spiel L, Kleemann U, Hassenstein P, Berg PA (1987) Relevance of antimitochondrial antibodies (anti-M7) in cardiac disease. Eur Heart 8: J Suppl J 223–226
124. Kline IK, Saphir O (1960) Chronic pernicious myocarditis. Am Heart J 59: 681–684
125. Kühl U, Ulrich G, Schultheiss H-P (1987) Cross-reactivity of antibodies to the ADP/ATP translocator of the inner mitochondrial membrane with the cell surface of cardiac myocytes. Eur Heart J 8 Suppl J: 219–222
126. Kühl U, Ulrich G, Melzner B, Schöber, B, Morad M, Schultheiss HP (1989) Characterization of autoantibodies against of Ca^{2+}-channel inducing cytotoxicity by enhancement of calcium permeability. 7th International Congress of Immunology, July 30–Aug 5, Berlin
127. Kurnick JT, Leary C, Palacios IF, Fallon JT (1987) Culture and characterization of lymphocytic infiltrates from endomyocardial biopsies of patients with idiopathic myocarditis. Eur Heart J 8 Suppl J: 135–139
128. Kysal A, Haverich A, Heublein B, Kemnitz J, Gerogh A (1981) C-*myc* oncogene expression in myocytes in heart allografts. 7th International Congress of Immunology, July 30–Aug 5, Berlin
129. Laake H (1951) Myocarditis in poliomyelitis. Acta Med Scand 140: 159–169
130. Lazarides E (1976) Two general classes of cytoplasmic actin filaments in tissue culture cells: the role of tropomyosin. J Supramol Struct 5: 531–539
131. Lazarides E (1978) The distribution of desmin (100-Å) filaments in primary cultures of embryonic chick cardiac cells. Exp Cell Res 11: 265–269
132. Lazarides E (1980) Intermediate filaments as mechanical integrators of cellular space. Nature 283: 249–256
133. Leatherbury L, Chandra RS, Shapiro SR, Perry LW (1988) Value of endomyocardial biopsy in infants, children and adolescents with dilated or hypertrophic cardiomyopathy and myocarditis. J Am Coll Cardiol 12: 1547–1554
134. Lerner AM, Wilson FM (1973) Virus myocardiopathy. Prog Med Virol 15: 63–91
135. Leroay EC (1985) Collagen disposition in autoimmune disease: the expanding role of the fibroblast in human fibriotic disease. In: Evered D, Whelan J (eds) Fibrosis. Pitman, London, pp 196–204
136. Leslie KO (1988) Progressive interstitial collagen deposition in Coxsackievirus B3-induced murine myocarditis (Abstr). International Symposium on inflammatory Heart Disease, July 27–31, Snowmass
137. Lewis W (1989) AIDS: cardiac findings from 115 biopsies. Prog Cardiovasc Dis 32: 207–215
137a. Lie JT (1988) Myocarditis and endomyocardial biopsy in unexplained Heart failure: a diagnosis in search of a disease. Ann Intern Med 109: 525–528
138. Limas CJ, Goldenberg IF (1987) Autoantibodies against cardiac beta-adrenoceptors in human dilated cardiomyopathy. Circulation 76 Suppl 4: 262–269
139. Limas CJ, Goldenberg IF, Limas C (1989) Autoantibodies against beta-adrenoceptors in human idiopathic dilated cardiomyopathy. Circ Res 64: 97–103
140. Lodge PA, Herzum M, Olszewski J, Huber SA (1987) Coxsackie B-3 myocarditis: acute and chronic forms of the disease caused by different immunopathogenic mechanisms. Am J Pathol 128: 455–463
142. Longson M, Cole FM, Davies C (1969) Isolation of Coxsackie virus group B, type 5, from the heart of a fatal case of myocarditis in an adult. J Clin Pathol 22: 654–658
143. Lotze U, Maisch B (1989) Humoral immune response to cardiac conducting tissue. Springer Semin Immunopathol 11: 409–422

144. Lowry PJ, Edwards CW, Nagle RE (1982) Herpes-like virus particles in myocardium of patient progressing to congestive cardiomyopathy. Br Heart J 48: 501–504
145. Lowry PJ, Thompson RA, Littler WA (1983) Humoral immunity in cardiomyopathy. Br Heart J 50: 390–394
146. Lowry PJ, Thompson RA, Littler WA (1984) Humoral and cellular mechanisms in congestive cardiomyopathy (Abstr). Br Heart J 51: 109
147. Ludden TE, Edward JE (1949) Carditis in poliomyelitis: an anatomic study of thirty-five cases and review of the literature. Am J Pathol 25: 357–381
148. Lundgren E, Terracio L, Borg TK (1985) Adhesion of cardiac myocytes to extracellular matrix components. Basic Res Cardiol 80 Suppl 1: 69–76
149. Maisch B (1984) Cytolytic serum activity in patients with carditis. In: Bolte HD (ed) Viral heart disease. Springer, Berlin Heidelberg New York, pp 121–130
150. Maisch B (1984) Diagnostic relevance of humoral and cell-mediated immune reactions in patients with acute myocarditis and congestive cardiomyopathy. In: Chazov EL, Smirnov VN, Organov RG (eds) Cardiology. Plenum, London, pp 1327–1338
151. Maisch B (1984) Humorale immunologische Effecktormechanismen bei Perimyokarditis. Internist (Berlin) 25: 155–164
152. Maisch B (1985) Rickettsial perimyocarditis: a follow up study. Heart Vessels 2: 55–59
153. Maisch B (1985) Surface antigens of adult heart cells and their use in diagnosis. Basic Res Cardiol 80 Suppl 1: 47–52
154. Maisch B (1986) Immunologic regulator and effector functions in perimyocarditis, post-myocarditic heart muscle disease and dilated cardiomyopathy. Basic Res Cardiol 81 Suppl 1: 217–242
155. Maisch B (1987) Immunological mechanisms in human cardiac injury. In: Spry JE (ed) Immunology and molecular biology of cardiovascular disease (Current status of clinical cardiology). MTP, London, pp 225–252
156. Maisch B (1987) The sarcolemma as antigen in the secondary immunopathogenesis of myopericarditis. Eur Heart J 8 Suppl J: 155–165
157. Maisch B (1988) The use of myocardial biopsy in heart failure. Eur Heart 9 Suppl H: 59–71
158. Maisch B (1989) Autoreactivity to the cardiac myocyte, connective tissue and the extracellular matrix in heart disease and postcardiac injury. Springer Semin Immunopathol 11: 369–396
159. Maisch B, Drude L (1991) Pericardioscopy: a new diagnostic tool in inflammatory diseases of the pericardium. Eur Heart J 12 Suppl D: 2–6
160. Maisch B, Kochsiek K (1983) Humoral immune reactions in uremic pericarditis. Am J Nephrol 3: 264–271
161 Maisch B, Wendl J (1989) Cytomegalovirus DNA in endomyocardial biopsies of patients with (peri)myocarditis (Abstr). Eur Heart J 9 Suppl 1: 1000
162. Maisch B, Berg PA, Schuff-Werner P, Kochsiek K (1979) Clinical significance of immunopathological findings in patients with postpericardiotomy syndrome. I. Relevance of antibody pattern. Clin Exp Immunol 38: 189–197
163. Maisch B, Berg PA, Schuff-Werner P, Kochsiek K (1979) Clinical significance of immunpathological findings in patients with postpericardiotomy syndrome. II. The significance of serum inhibition and rosette inhibitory factors. Clin Exp Immunol 38: 198–203
164. Maisch B, Berg PA, Kochsiek K (1980) Immunological parameters in patients with congestive cardiomyopathy. Basic Res Cardiol 75: 221–222
165. Maisch B, Trostel-Soeder R, Berg A, Kochsiek K (1981) Assessment of antibody mediated cytolysis of adult cardiocytes isolated by centrifugation in a continuous gradient of Percoll in patients with acute myocarditis. J Immunol Methods 44: 159–169
166. Maisch B, Maisch S, Kochsiek K (1982) Immune reactions in tuberculous and chronic constrictive pericarditis. Am J Cardiol 50: 1007–1013
167. Maisch B, Mayer E, Kochsiek K (1982) Nachweis zirkulierender Immunkomplexe bei kardialen Erkrankungen. Verh Dtsch Ges Inn Med 88: 624–627
168. Maisch B, Trostel-Soeder R, Stechermesser E, Berg PA, Kochsiek K (1982) Diagnostic relevance of humoral and cell-mediated immune reactions in patients with acute viral myocarditis. Clin Exp Immunol 48: 533–545

169. Maisch B, Deeg P, Liebau G, Kochsiek K (1983) Diagnostic relevance of humoral and cytotoxic immune reactions in patients with primary and secondary heart muscle disease. Am J Cardiol 52: 1072–1078
170. Maisch B, Mayer E, Schubert U, Berg PA Kochsiek K (1983) Immune reactions in infective endocarditis. Relevance of circulating immune complexes, of serum inhibition factors, of lymphocytotoxic reactions, and of antibody dependent cellular cytotoxicity against cardiac target cells. Am Heart J 106: 338–344
171. Maisch B, Büschel G, Izumi T, Eigel P, Regitz V, Deeg P, Pfeifer U, Schmaltz A, Herzum M, Kochsiek K (1985) Four years of experience in endomyocardial biopsy: an immunohistologic approach. Heart Vessels Suppl 1: 59–67
172. Maisch B, Lotze U, Schneider J, Kochsiek K (1985) Antibodies to human sinus node in sick sinus syndrome. New Trend Arrhythmias 1: 417–421
173. Maisch B, Lotze U, Schneider J, Kochsiek K (1986) Antibodies to human sinus node in sick sinus syndrome. PACE 9: 1101–1109
174. Maisch B, Bauer E, Thometzek P, Herzum M, Kochsiek K (1987) Autoreactive immune mechanisms in infective endocarditis. Eur Heart J 8 Suppl J: 311–318
175. Maisch B, Cirsi M, Gehrke J, Kirschner A (1987) Lectin binding sites of the sarcolemma and surrounding interstitial tissue. Eur Heart J 8 Suppl 5: 175
176. Maisch B, Dienesch C, Wendl I (1987) Effect of leukotrienes on isolated vital cardiac cells: an in vitro model of cardiocytotoxic mediators in inflammation? Eur Heart J 8 Suppl J: 463–465
177. Maisch B, Hauck H, Königer U, Endter S, Klopf D, Schmier U, Schmier K (1987) Suppressor cell activity in (peri)myocarditis and infective endocarditis. Eur Heart J Suppl 8: 147–153
178. Maisch B, Hufnagel G, Bauer E, Haverich A, Schäfers HJ, Kemnitz J, Borst HG (1987) Value of immunohistological and immunoserological monitoring in cardiac transplantation. Eur Heart J 8 Suppl J: 29–34
179. Maisch B, Schwab D, Bauer E, Sandhage K, Schmaltz AA (1987) Antimyolemmal antibodies in myocarditis in children. Eur Heart J 8 Suppl J: 167–173
180. Maisch B, Selmayer N, Brugger E, Ertl G, Eilles C, Heinrich J, Gerhard W, Hufnagel G, Schmidt M, Kochsiek K (1987) Cardiac sarcoidosis: clinical and immunoserological study. Eur Heart J 8 Suppl J: 63–71
181. Maisch B, Wedeking U, Kochsiek K (1987) Quantitative assessment of antilaminin antibodies in myocarditis and perimyocarditis. Eur Heart J 8: Suppl J 233–235
182. Maisch B, Wittner B, Wiethölter H (1987) Experimental myocarditis in rabbits: cellular effector mechanisms. Eur Heart J 8 Suppl J: 425–432
183. Maisch B, Weyerer O, Hufnagel G, Hengstenberg, Schönian U, Haverich A, Kochsiek K (1989) The vascular endothelium as target of humoral autoreactivity in myocarditis and rejection. Z Kardiol 78: 95–99
184. Maisch B, Crombach C, Schönian U(1991) Cytomegalovirus infection as a cause of viral myocarditis (Abstr) Eur Heart J 12 Suppl: 228 (A1216)
185. Maisch B, Outzen H, Roth D, Hiby A, Herzum M, Hengstenberg C, Hnufagel F, Schönian U, Kochsiek K (1991) Prognostic determinants in conventionally treated myocarditis and perimyocarditis: focus on antimyolemmal antibodies. Eur Heart J 12 Suppl D: 76–80
185a. Maisch B, Schönian U (1992) Assessment of cytomegalovirus-DNA in endomyocardial biopsies of patients with myococarditis. Circulation 86 (Suppl I): 793 Abstr. 3157
186. Maisch B, Bauer E, Cirsi M, Thometzek P (1993) Cytolytic cross-reactive antibodies directed against the cardiac membrane of adult human myocytes in Coxsackie B myocarditis: analysis by Western blot, immunofluorescence test and antibody-mediated cytolysis of cardiocytes. Circulation (in press)
187. Mall G, Klingel K, Albrecht M, Seemann M, Rieger P, Kandolf R (1991) Natural history of coxsackievirus B3-induced myocarditis in ACA/Sn mice: viral persistence demonstrated by quantitative in situ hybridization histochemistry. Eur Heart J 12 Suppl D: 121–123
188. Mason JW, Billingham ME, Ricci DR (1980) Treatment of acute inflammatory myocarditis assisted by endomyocardial biopsy. Am J Cardiol 45: 1037–1044

189. Maut K (1963) Mort subité due à une myocardité focale suivant une vaccination contre la variole. Ann Med Leg 43: 1–3
190. McManus BM, Galinit CJ, Cassung RS (1988) Immunopathologic basis of myocardial injury. Cardiovasc Clin 18: 163–184
191. Mills AS, Hastillo A, Hess ML (1984) Lymphocytic infection of he myocardium in idiopathic dilated cardiomyopathy: underestimation of myocarditis with endomyocardial biopsy (Abstr). Circulation 70 Suppl 2: 401
192. Monif GRG, Lee CW, Hsiung GD (1967) Isolated myocarditis with recovery of ECHO type 9 virus from the myocardium. N Engl J Med 277: 1353–1355
193. Moore CM, Henry J, Benzing G, Kaplan S (1969) Varicella myocarditis. Am J Dis Child 118: 899–902
194. Mues B, Brisse B, Zwaldo G, Ghemann H, Bender F, Sorg C (1989) Myocarditis diagnosis: use of monoclonal antibodies to macrophages in immunocytology. 7th International Congress of Immunology, July 30–Aug 8, Berlin
195. Neu N, Beisel K, Traystman M, Rose N, Craig SW (1987) Autoantibodies specific for the cardiac myosin isoform are found in mice susceptible to coxsackie virus B3-induced myocarditis. J Immunol 138: 2488
196. Neu N, Rose NR, Beisel KW, Herskowitz A, Gurri-Glass G, Craig SW (1987) Cardiac myosin induces myocarditis in genetically presdisposed mices. J Immunol 138: 2488–2492
197. Obermayer U, Scheidler J, Maisch B (1987) Antibodies against micro- and intermediate filaments in carditis and dilated cardiomyopathy: are they a diagnostic marker? Eur Heart J 8: Suppl J, 181–186
198. Obiassi M, Brucato A, Meroni PL, Vismara A, Lettin M, Poloni F, Finzi A, Fenini MG, Rossi L (1987) Antibodies to cardiac Purkinje cells: further characterization in autoimmune disease and atrioventricular heart block. Clin exp Immunol 42: 141–148
199. Oceasohn R, Adelson L, Kaji M (1959) Clinicopathologic study of thirty-three fatal cases of Asian influenza. N Engl J Med 260: 509–518
200. Osborn M (1984) Summary: intermediate filaments. Ann NY Acad Sci 455: 669
201. Parillo JE, Cunnion RE, Ebstein SE, Parker MM, Suffredini AV, Brenner M, Saer GL, Palmeri ST, Cannon RO, Alling D, Wittes JT, Ferrans VJ, Roderigues ER, Fauci AS (1989) A prospective, randomized, controlled trial of prednisone for dilated cardiomyopathy. N Engl J Med 321: 1061–1068
202. Paris S, Fosset M, Samuel D, Ailhaud G (1977) Chick embryo plasma membrane from cardiac muscle and cultured heart cells: isolation procedures and absence of fatty acid-activation enzymes. J Mol Cell Cardiol 9: 161–173
203. Perimann P, Perlmann H (1971) Cytotoxic lymphocytes: mechanisms of activation and target cell destruction. Int Arch Allergy 41: 36–39
204. Pollard TD (1976) Cytoskeletal function of cytoplasmic contracile protein. J Supramol Struct 5: 317–327
205. Ragosta M, Crabtree J, Sturner WQ, Thompson PD (1980) Report of the WHO/ISFC Task Force on the definition and classification of cardiomyopathies. Br Heart J 44: 672
206. Rose ML, Coles MI, Griffin RJ, Pomerance A, Yacoub MH (1986) Expression of class I and class II major histocompatibility antigens in normal and transplanted human heart. Transplantation 41: 776–782
207. Rose NR, Wolfgram LJ, Herskowitz A, Beisel KW (1986) Postinfectious autoimmunity: two distinct phases of coxsackievirus B3-induced myocarditis. Ann NY Acad Sci 475: 146–156
207a. Ross E, Armentrout SA (1962) Myocarditis associated with rabies: Report of a case. N Engl J Med 260: 1087–1089
208. Sack W, Scheurin H, Wachsmut ED (1975) Antikörper gegen Herzmuskelsarkolemm im Serum von Patienten mit primärer Cardiomyopathie. Klin Wochenschr 53: 103–111
209. Sainani GS, Krompotic E, Slodki SJ (1968) Adult heart disease due to the Coxsackie virus B infection. Medicine (Baltimore) 47: 133–147
210. Sampson CC (1959) Varicella myocarditis: report of case. J Natl Med Assoc 51: 138–139
211. Samsonov M, Nassonov E, Kostin S, Samko A, Alexandrova L, Masenko V, Naumov V, Mareev V, Shevlyagin S, Zhadanov V (1991) Serum neopterin: possible immunological marker

of myocardial inflammation in patients with dilated heart muscle disease. Eur Heart J 12 Suppl D: 147–150

212. Samuel JL, Rappaport K, Mercadie JJ, Lompre AM, Sartore S, Triban C, Schiaffina S, Schwartz K (1983) Distribution of myosin isozymes with single cardiac cells. Circ Res 52: 200–209
213. Samuel JL, Schwartz K, Lompre AM, Delcayre C, Marotte F, Swynghedauw B, Rapparot L (1983) Immunological quantitation and localizatiom of tubulin in adult rat heart isolated myocytes. Eur J Cell Biol 31: 99–103
214. Saphir O, Amromin GD, Yokoo H (1956) Myocarditis in viral (epidemic) hepatitis. Am J Med Sci 231: 168–176
215. Schaper J, Froede R, Bleese N, Lüthe N, Schaper W (1987) Veränderungen der Ultrastruktur und des Zytoskeletts in explantierten menschlichen Herzen. Z Kardiol 77 Suppl 1: 82
216. Schaper J, Froede, Buck A, Bleese N (1989) Impaired myocardial ultra-structure and cytoskeleton in cardiomyopathic human myocardium. In: Schultheiss H-P (ed) New concepts in viral heart disease. Springer, Berlin Heidelberg New York, pp 295–302
217. Schönian U, Maisch B (1989) Cellular ELISA for antimyolemmal antibodies (AMLA) in DCM and myocarditis (Abstr). 7th International Congress of Immunology, July 30–Aug 8, Berlin
218. Schönian U, Crombach M, Maisch B (1991) Does CMV infection play a role in myocarditis? New aspects form in-situ hybridization. Eur Heart J 12 Supl D: 65–68
219. Schramm P (1986) Rarissima, I, TAUNUS-VERLAG 4
220. Schultheiss HP (1987) The mitochrondrium as antigen in inflammatory heart disease. Eur Heart J 8 Suppl J: 203–210
221. Schultheiss HP (1989) the significance of autoantibodies against the ADP/ATP carrier for the pathogenesis of myocarditis and dilated cardiomyopathy: clinical and experimental data. Springer Semin Immunopathol 11: 15–30
222. Schultheiss HP, Bolte HD (1985) Immunological analysis of autoantibodies against the adenine nucleotide translocator in dilated cardiomyopathy. J Mol Cell Cardiol 17: 603–617
223. Schultheiss HP, Kühl U (1987) Charakterisierung verschiedener Autoantikörper gegen myokardiale Matrixproteine by Myokarditis und dilativer Kardiomyopathie. Klin Wochenschr 65: Suppl 9: 263
224. Schultheiss HP, Bolte HD, Schwimmbeck P (1984) Autoantibodies against the adenine nucleotide translocator in myocarditis and dilated cardiomyopathy. In: Bolte HD (ed) Viral heart disease. Springer, Berlin Heidelberg New York, pp 131–143
225. Schulze K, Becker BF, Strauer B, Schultheiss HP (1990) Antibodies to ADP/ATP carrier— an autoantigen in myocarditis and dilated cardiomyopathy—impair cardiac function. Circulation 81: 959–969
226. Schwartz P, Piper HM, Spahr R, Hütter JF, Spiekermann PF (1985) Development of new intercellular contracts between adult cardiac myocytes in culture. Basic Res Cardiol 80 Suppl 1: 75–79
227. Schwarz RS (1986) Are natural autoantibodies real? Ann Immunol (Paris) 137: 156–158
228. Schwimmbeck PL, Schultheiss HP, Strauer BE (1989) Identification of a main autoimmunogenic epitope of the adenine nucleotide translocator which cross-reacts with coxsackie B3 virus: use in the diagnosis of myocarditis and dilatative cardiomyopathy (Abstr), Circulation 80 Suppl 2: 2642
229. Segusa J, Prabhakar BS, Essani K, McClintock PR, Fukuda Y, Ferrans VJ, Notkins AL (1986) Monoclonal antibody to coxsackievirus B4 reacts with myocardium. J Infect Dis 153: 372–373
230. Seligman M (1986) The origin and nature of autoantibodies: introduction. Ann Immunol (Paris) 137: 149–150
231. Senécal J-L, Fortin S, Roussin A, Joyal F (1987) Anticytoskeletal autoantibody to microfilament anchorage sites recognizes novel focal contact proteins. J Clin Invest 80: 778–785
232. Shanes Gahli J, Billingham ME, Ferrans VJ, Fenoglio JJ, Edwards WD, Tsai CC, Saffitz JE, Isner J, Furner S, Subramanian R (1987) Interobserver variability in the pathologic interpretation of endomyocardial biopsy results. Circulation 75: 401–405
233. Sylvest E (1934) Epidemic myalgia: Bornholm disease. London, Oxford

234. Szarman A, Terranova VP, Rennard SI, Fiodart J-M, de Datima Lima M, Scheinman JI, Martin GR (1982) Antibodies to laminin in Chagas' disease. JE p Med 155: 1161–1169
235. Tatter D, Gerad PW, Silverman AH, Wang C, Peterson HE (1964) Fatal varicella pancarditis in a child. Am J Dis Child 108: 88–93
236. Tazzari PI, Gobbi M, Zauli D, Tassinari A, Crespi C, Miserocchi F, Dinota A, Bandini G, Ricci P, Ura S (1987) Close association between antibodies to cytoskeletal intermediate filaments and chronic graft-versus-host disease. Transplantation 44: 234–237
236a. Thiede WH (1962) Cardiac involvement in lymphocytic choriomeningitis Arch Intern Med 109: 50–54
237. Thometzek P, Maisch B (1987) Antibodies cross-reactive to streptococci in infective endocarditis. Eur Heart J 8 Suppl J: 318–321
238. Timpl R (1979) Lamini: a glycorprotien from basement membranes. J Biol Chem 254: 9933–9937
239. Van Houten N, Huber SA (1989) Role of cytoxic T-cells in experimental myocarditis. Springer Semin Immunopathol 11: 61–68
240. Von Schroetter P (1899) Die Insuffizienz des Herzmuskels. Verh Congr Inn Med, 50: 17–23
241. Wallukat G, Boewer V (1988) Stimulation of chronotropic beta-adrenoceptors of cultured neonatal rat heart myocytes by the serum of gammaglobulin fraction of patients with dilated cardiomyopathy and myocarditis. In: Internationales Symposium: Herzinsuffizienz, Pathogenese und Differentialtherapie, Feb 28–March 2 Berlin. Universitätsverlag, Berlin (Book of Abstracts, A 24)
242. Waterson AP (1978) Virology investigation in congestive cardiomyopthy. Postgrad Med J 54: 505–509
243. Weber KT, Janicki JS, Pick R, Abrahams C, Shroff SG, Bashey RI, Chen RM (1987) Collagen in hypertrophied, pressure-overloaded myocardium. Circulation 75 Suppl 1: 1–9
244. Weiland DS, Donaldson KP, Isner JM (1984) How well does the endomyocardial biopsy represent the state of the heart? (Abstr) Circulation 70 Suppl 2: 501
245. Weinstein L, Shelokov A (1951) Cardiovascular manifestations in acute poliomyelitis. N Engl J Med 244: 281–285
246. Weiss MB, Ursell PC, Scala F, Frusin R, Genoglio JJ Jr (1982) Immunosuppression therapy in chronic forms of myocarditis (Abstr). Circulation 66 Suppl 2: 215
247. Wittner B, Maisch B, Kochsiek K (1983) Quantification of antimyosin antibodies in experimental myocarditis by a new solid-phase fluorometric assay. J Immunol Methods 64: 239–247
248. Wolfgram LJ, Beisel KW, Rose NR (1985) Heart-specific autoantibodies following murine coxsackievirus B3 myocarditis. J Exp Med 161: 1112–1121
249. Wolfgram LJ, Beisel KW, Herskowitz A, Rose NR (1986) Variations in the susceptibilty to coxsackievirus B3-induced myocarditis among different strains of mice. J Immunol 136: 1846–1852
250. Wong Y, Woodruff JJ, Woodruff JF (1977) Generation of cytolytic T-lymphocytes during Coxsackie virus B3 infection. I. Model and viral specificity. J Immunol 118: 1159–1164
251. Wong Y, Woodruff JJ, Woodruff JF (1977) Generation of cytolytic T-lymphocytes during Coxsackie virus B3 infections. II. Characterization of effector cells, and demonstration of cytotoxicity against viral infected myofibers. J Immunol 118: 1165–1169
252. Woodruff JF (1980) Viral myocarditis: a review article. Am J Pathol 101: 425–484
253. Yamada K, Akiyama S, Hasegawa T, Gasegawa E, Humphries M, Kennedy D, Nagata K, Urishihara H, Olden K, Chen W (1985) Recent advances in the research on fibronectin and other cell attachment proteins. J Cell Biochem 28
254. Yamakawa K, Fukuta S, Yoshinaga T, Umenoto S, Itagaki T, Kusukawa R (1987) Study of immunological mechanism in dilated cardiomyopathy. Jpn Circ J 51: 665–675
255. Yu Z, Sekiguchi M, Niroe M, Take M, Hirosawa K (1984) Histopathological findings of acute and convalescent myocarditis obtained by serial biopsy. Jpn Circ J 48: 1368–1371
256. Zinkemagel RM, Doherty PC (1974) Restriction of the in vitro T cell-mediated cytotoxicity in lymphocytic choriomeningitis within a syngeneic or semiallogeneic system. Nature 248: 701–702

CHAPTER 16

Enteroviral Heart Muscle Disease: Current Molecular Studies and Future Research

L. Cunningham, P. J. Richardson, and L. C. Archard

Current Investigations

Introduction (see Chaps. 2, 4, 5, 14 and 15)

Enterovirus infection, particularly with Coxsackie B virus serotypes, has been associated with heart muscle disease by serological studies and the use of mouse models. A study in Scotland by Grist and Bell [1] provided comprehensive serological data correlating enterovirus infection with myocarditis. However, the association of these viruses with dilated cardiomyopathy was less well established and was based mainly on the observation of high titres of neutralising antibody in cases of sudden onset disease (see below); this led to the proposal that dilated cardiomyopathy is a progression from an enteroviral myocarditis, itself a sequela of a common, frequently trivial or subclinical, enteric infection [2].

Isolation of infectious virus from patients with heart muscle disease is rare [3]. No enterovirus was isolated from, nor virus-specific antibodies detected by immunocytochemistry in endomyocardial biopsies from 70 patients with myocarditis or dilated cardiomyopathy [4], despite serological evidence of association with virus infection. Enterovirus-specific neutralising antibody is often found in patients with heart muscle disease, particularly in the early stages; Cambridge et al. [5] reported that 30% of 50 patients with dilated cardiomyopathy had elevated titres of enterovirus neutralising antibodies compared with only 2% of controls, and that particularly high titres were detected in patients with a short history of disease. Although many healthy individuals have neutralising antibodies indicative of previous enterovirus infection, 14 of 38 (36%) myocarditis patients were positive for Coxsackie B virus-specific IgM compared with none of 46 controls [6] and such IgM responses have been shown to persist for up to 6 months [7]. Coxsackie B virus-specific IgM responses in patients with end-stage dilated cardiomyopathy and undergoing cardiac transplantation have been reported: 28 of 86 (33%) such patients were positive for enterovirus IgM compared with 10 of 84 (12%) ischaemic controls, and IgM responses were detected up to 19 months before transplantation [8].

The development of animal models confirmed the ability of Coxsackie B viruses to induce both myocarditis and dilated cardiomyopathy. A myocarditic strain of Coxsackie B3 [9] induces inflammatory heart muscle disease in mice

[10]. A mouse model for dilated cardiomyopathy was also developed, but virus infection alone was not sufficient to produce the disease: however, infected mice placed under stress by being forced to exercise (swim) developed dilated cardiomyopathy [11]. Recent work in our laboratory demonstrates that host factors can influence the severity of infection with a particular enterovirus serotype. A sequenced cDNA clone of Coxsackie virus B3 [12] was reactivated in cultured cells to produce infectious virus which was used to infect Balb/c or SWR/J mice. A virus inoculum of $10^{2.5}$ PFU killed 50% of Balb/c mice but, while the similarly infected SWR/J mice developed myocarditis, the mortality rate was 0. These animal experiments show that CB3 can cause both myocarditis and dilated cardiomyopathy and that the latter may be a sequela of myocarditis with the involvement of other factors.

Molecular Hybridisation Studies

Molecular hybridisation probes were developed to detect enteroviral RNA sequences in samples of myocardium in circumstances where conventional techniques of virus isolation or the immunocytochemical demonstration of virus-specific antigens had been unsuccessful.

We have used an enterovirus group-specific cDNA hybridisation probe prepared by reverse transcription of genomic RNA from Coxsackie virus B2 and molecular cloning into plasmid pBR322. The region chosen was a 1 Kb fragment from within the viral RNA-dependent RNA polymerase gene, 3D. This region has been shown to be highly conserved among enteroviruses [13] and this was confirmed by nucleotide sequence analysis of our probe, which is 78% homologous with the analogous region of other Coxsackie B virus genomes and 66%–68% homologous with that of poliovirus serotypes. The probe was excised from the plasmid vector, radiolabelled with phosphorus-32 by random oligonucleotide priming and used in quantitative slot blot hybridisations to search for enteroviral sequences in RNA extracted from endomyocardial biopsies or tissue from explanted hearts.

Total nucleic acid was extracted by proteolytic digestion in the presence of ionic detergent and human placental ribonuclease inhibitor, followed by phenol extraction and ethanol precipitation. RNA was selectively denatured with formaldehyde and immobilised onto duplicate nitrocellulose filters. One filter was hybridised with a radiolabelled control probe, 7B6 [14], to quantitate the amount of cellular RNA recovered from any particular sample and the duplicate filter was hybridised with the enterovirus group-specific probe. After hybridisation and stringent washing, the filters were autoradiographed using X-ray film and the degree of autoradiographic development determined by scanning densitometry. The total amount of RNA immobilised on the filter is proportional to the signal with the control probe 7B6 [15]. Control samples of cardiac muscle were included on each filter and the data for each sample are expressed as the ratio of the hybridisation signal with the enterovirus probe to that with the

Table 16.1. Detection of enterovirus RNA by molecular hybridisation in samples of myocardium from 170 patients with myocarditis or dilated cardiomyopathy or from 61 patients with other specific heart muscle diseases (total 231 patients)

	Endomyocardial biopsy samples						Explanted hearts			
Enteroviral RNA	Active or healing myocarditis		Healed myocarditis/ dilated cardio-myopathy		Controls		Dilated Cardiomyopathy		Controls	
	n	%	*n*	%	*n*	%	*n*	%	*n*	%
Positive	23	43	40	41	2	5	6	32	1	5
Negative	31		57		40		13		18	
Total	54		97		42		19		19	

control probe. Samples were considered positive for the presence of enteroviral RNA if this hybridisation index exceeded the mean of the negative controls plus three standard deviations ($p < 0.0015$).

Enteroviral RNA was detected in a proportion of samples of myocardium from all histologically proven grades of inflammatory disease [16–18] and from end-stage dilated heart muscle disease requiring cardiac transplantation [15]. To date we have examined biopsy samples of myocardium from 151 cases of histologically proven heart muscle disease. Enteroviral RNA was detected in 23 of 54 (43%) cases of histologically proven myocarditis and in 40 of 97 (41%) cases of dilated cardiomyopathy, compared with only 2 of 42 (5%) cases of specific heart muscle disease without a viral aetiology (such as amyloidosis, sarcoidosis, muscular dystrophy or alcoholic cardiomyopathy). Virus RNA was also detected in tissue from 6 of 19 (32%) explanted hearts from end-stage dilated cardiomyopathy patients compared with only 1 of 19 (5%) of the control group of patients transplanted for ischaemic heart muscle disease (Table 16.1). These data demostrate that enterovirus RNA can be detected in all histologically confirmed grades of heart muscle disease and that virus can persist in myocardium to end-stage dilated cardiomyopathy requiring transplantation. The data suggest that persistence of enterovirus after myocarditis disposes to the subsequent development of dilated cardiomyopathy. On the basis of previous investigations, it is unlikely that infectious virus could have been isolated or virus-specific antigens demonstrated in any such sample obtained after the initial inflammatory stage, which raises the question of the molecular basis of virus persistence.

Mechanism of Persistence

Molecular hybridisation demonstrates that enterovirus RNA can be present in myocardium after the healing stage of inflammatory heart muscle disease and can persist to end-stage dilated cardiomyopathy. We have used single-strand-specific RNA probes to investigate the mechanism of viral persistence. The enterovirus group-specific cDNA probe described above was re-cloned into a riboprobe vector, downstream of an SP6 transcriptional promoter, allowing synthesis of radiolabelled, single-stranded RNA probes. By cloning the fragment in either orientation, probes complementary to either the positive, genomic strand or the negative, template strand of enteroviral RNA can be produced to study the process of infection in vitro or in clinical samples.

It is well established that during productive, cytolytic infection by enteroviruses, synthesis of viral RNA is asymmetric and the viral RNA-dependent RNA polymerase preferentially copies the negative, template strand [19]. We used single-strand-specific RNA probes to confirm this observation and found that positive strand synthesis exceeds negative strand synthesis by more than 100 to 1 [20]. Our studies on myocardium from non-inflammatory heart muscle disease showed that enteroviral RNA was present in positive:negative ratios ranging from less than unity to near normal values (Fig. 16.1) [21]. We used the same single-stranded RNA probes to detect enteroviral sequences in skeletal muscle biopsy samples from patients with postviral fatigue syndrome, a chronic post-inflammatory disease which has some analogies with dilated cardiomyopathy and may be found in association with it. Again, we found that positive and negative strands of enteroviral RNA were present in similar amounts, in contrast to the asymmetric synthesis seen in a productive infection [20]. These data suggest that persistence of enterovirus in either cardiac or skeletal muscle results from the selection of mutants defective in the control of virus RNA replication, presumably during the initial inflammatory stage of disease when virus replicates productively and cytolytically. Enteroviruses accumulate sequence mutations with high frequency during replication because of the error rate of the viral

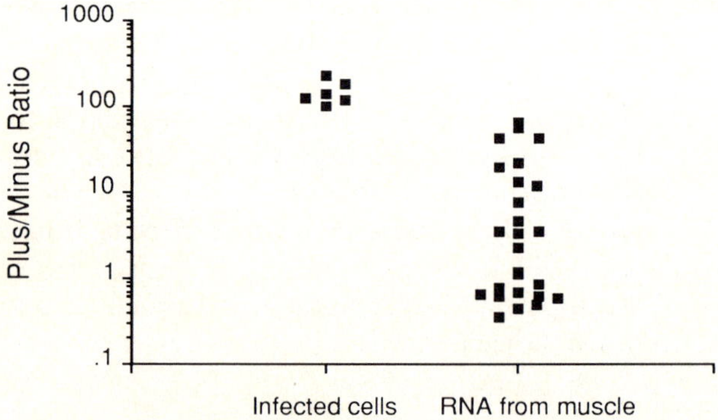

Fig. 16.1. Detection of enterovirus RNA using single-stranded riboprobes specific for either the genomic, sense (+) or the template, antisense (−) strand of viral RNA. The data are expressed as the relative abundance of positive to negative strands of viral RNA. Values are shown for infected cells and from tissue from non-inflammatory heart and skeletal muscle disease. The data demonstrate that persisting enterovirus infection in vivo is associated with an aberration in the control of viral RNA synthesis

RNA-dependent RNA polymerase and these mutations could result in changes in the specificity of the viral polymerase or in its affinity for its proposed recognition sequence.

Coxsackie B Serology

To determine whether the persistence of virus in myocardium elicits a humoral immune response, sera from 88 patients with myocarditis or dilated cardiomyopathy were tested for the presence of Coxsackie B1-to B5- specific IgM by an M antibody capture enzyme-linked immunoadsorbent assay (ELISA). A chi-squared test of mutual independence of the variables in a 3D contingency table showed no correlation between the presence of enteroviral RNA in endomyocardial biopsies and the occurrence of Coxsackie B virus-specific IgM in either the myocarditis group (41 patients) or the dilated cardiomyopathy group (47 patients; Table 16.2). However, specific serology was not performed for other enteroviruses such as the Coxsackie A and ECHO viruses which may be involved in heart muscle disease and the genomic RNA of which would be detected by the group-specific hybridisation probe. The examination of tissue for virus RNA sequences remains mandatory to establish the true incidence of enteroviral heart muscle disease.

Prognostic Significance of Enterovirus Persistence

We conducted a prospective investigation of the prognostic significance of persisting enterovirus infection of myocardium in patients with some grade of myocarditis or dilated cardiomyopathy. This study involved 123 patients of mean age 44.9 years (range 6–70) and mean duration of symptoms 13.9 months (range

Table 16.2. The presence of Coxsackie B1- to B5-specific IgM was determined by an M-antibody capture ELISA for enterovirus positive and negative patients in both the myocarditis and dilated cardiomyopathy groups. A chi-squared test of mutual independence of the variables in a 3D contingency table was performed. The expected and observed values are very similar, showing the variables are independent of one another. There is no correlation between presence of enteroviral RNA and Coxsackie B-specific IgM in either group of patients

	Myocarditis		Dilated cardiomyopathy		
	Enteroviral RNA +ve	Enteroviral RNA −ve	Enteroviral RNA +ve	Enteroviral RNA −ve	
IgM-positive	1	4	3	2	Observed
	1.06	3.6	1.21	4.13	expected
IgM-negative	6	30	10	32	Observed
	8.26	28.08	9.47	32.19	Expected

$\chi^2 = 4.56$, $p = 0.34$.

1–99) during a mean follow-up period of 25.2 months (range 11–50). Routine clinical assessment included history of preceding viral illness and other aetiological factors including chronic excessive alcohol consumption, exposure to other toxins, and systemic disease known to be related to heart muscle disease. Cardiac catheterisation with left ventriculography and, where indicated, coronary arteriography was performed to exclude significant coronary artery disease. Endomyocardial biopsy samples were subjected to histological, histochemical and ultrastructural evaluation and classified according to the Dallas criteria; in addition probing by molecular hybridisation was done to detect the presence of enteroviral RNA.

Three patients were found to have amyloid heart muscle disease and 4 others were lost to follow-up. Of the remaining 116, 40 (34%) were positive for enterovirus RNA in myocardial biopsy samples and 76 were negative. One enterovirus-positive and 3 enterovirus-negative patients underwent cardiac transplantation and are excluded from further consideration. Of the remainder, 10 of 39 (26%) of the virus-positive group compared with only 2 of 73 (3%) of the virus-negative group died during the follow-up study. There was no significant difference in the two groups in clinical variables including history of heart failure, arrhythmia, chest pain, emboli, ethanol abuse, viral illness, age at presentation, cardiothoracic ratio, left ventricular end-diastolic filling pressure or reduced ejection fraction. However, patients positive for the presence of enteroviral RNA in myocardium presented with a shorter duration of symptoms (mean 7.8 months) than clinically similar patients who were enterovirus-negative (mean 14.9 months; $p < 0.05$). Survival curves illustrate the significantly increased mortality in the enterovirus-positive group ($p = < 0.001$; Fig. 16.2). The detection of persisting enterovirus RNA sequences in myocardial biopsy samples is the most significant predictor of reduced survival ($p < 0.001$), even when compared with reduced ejection fraction ($p < 0.01$; Table 16.3).

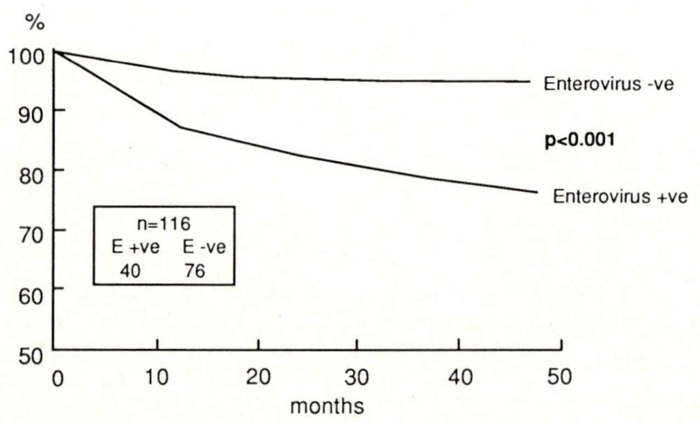

Fig. 16.2. Survival curves for patients with histologically confirmed heart muscle disease. Of 116 patients 40 were positive for enteroviral RNA in endomyocardial biopsy sample at the time of diagnosis and 76 were negative

Table 16.3. Predictors of survival in follow-up (mean 25.2 months) of 116 patients with myocarditis or dilated cardiomyopathy

Prognostic factor	*p* value
Detection of persisting enterovirus RNA in myocardium by molecular hybridisation	<0.001
Reduced ejection fraction	<0.01
Cardiac failure	<0.05
Bundle branch block	<0.05
Duration of symptoms	NS
Arrhythmias	NS
History of viral illness	NS
Cardiothoracic ratio	NS
Left ventricular end-diastolic filling pressure	NS

NS, not significant

Future Research

A number of obvious problems remain to be resolved. First, there is no correlation between detection of enteroviral RNA sequences in myocardium using a group-specific hybridisation probe and the detection of Coxsackie B virus-specific IgM. Does this reflect the inability of the persisting infection to elicit a humoral immune response or the involvement of a different enteroviral serotype? Second, it is clear that enteroviruses, which normally replicate productively and cytolytically, can persist focally in myocardium to end-stage dilated heart muscle disease without generating gross histopathology. What is the molecular mechanism of persistence and is more than one mechanism involved? Third, whatever the molecular mechanism of enteroviral persistence in myocardium, what is the pathogenetic link between virus persistence, myocardial dysfunction and the development of dilated heart muscle disease? Finally, given that enterovirus persistence in myocardium disposes to the development of dilated cardiomyopathy with a poor prognosis, what rational basis is there for therapy?

Molecular Epidemiology

From a clinical perspective, it may be advantageous to determine the type of the persisting virus. Thus, if a patient has serological evidence of enterovirus infection and enteroviral RNA is detected in myocardium, it would be important to know whether the same virus was involved and to differentiate between the involvement of polio, Coxsackie A or B serotypes or ECHO viruses in the development of heart muscle disease. Although all groups of human enteroviruses have been associated by reterospective serology with some form of heart muscle disease [9] the group most commonly associated is that of the Coxsackie B viruses. However,

Table 16.4. A comparison of the percentage sequence homologies of a 3′ fragment in the region of the RNA-dependent RNA polymerase gene of various enteroviruses

	B1	B2	B3	B4	A9	A21	PV1	PV3
B1	—	78	84	82	90	67	69	67
B2	78	—	78	78	78	68	66	69
B3	84	78	—	81	84	69	68	69
B4	82	78	81	—	79	67	68	67
A9	90	78	84	79	—	68	66	66
A21	67	68	69	67	68	—	81	81
PV1	69	66	68	68	66	81	—	82
PV3	67	69	69	67	66	81	82	—

B1–B4, A9 and A21 are serotypes of Coxsackie virus; PV1 and PV3 are serotypes of poliovirus

most molecular studies have used group-specific probes which detect conserved subgenomic sequences rather than a Coxsackie B virus-specific probe to detect viral RNA in samples of heart muscle. Although from a molecular viewpoint enteroviruses are similar in their replication strategies and differ only in tissue tropisms and the antigenic nature of their capsid proteins, we must consider the value of using type- or even serotype-specific probes to identify the particular viruses involved in heart muscle disease. The homology between enterovirus serotypes in the RNA sequence encoding the 3D polymerase gene is particularly high, as would be expected in a gene the function of which is essential to viral replication (Table 16.4). The 5′ non-coding region, which appears to control RNA replication and translation of viral proteins, is also highly conserved (Table 16.5). Subgenomic probes directed against these regions are therefore group-specific.

In contrast, homology between serotypes is lower in the genes which code for the viral proteins which determine immunological response. VP1 is the major capsid protien determining serotype; type-specific probes derived from this area

Table 16.5. A comparison of the percentage sequence homologies of the 5′ non-coding region of various enteroviruses

	B1	B3	B4	A9	A21	PV1	PV3
B1	—	ND	ND	85.5	66.9	ND	ND
B3	ND	—	84.4	86.4	75.9	70	ND
B4	ND	84.4	—	83.6	71.4	71.4	71.1
A9	85.5	86.4	83.6	—	70	ND	69.9
A21	66.9	75.9	71.4	70	—	81.3	82.3
PV1	ND	70	71.4	ND	81.3	—	82
PV3	ND	ND	71.1	69.9	82.3	82	—

B1–B4, A9 and A21 are serotypes of Coxsackie virus; PV1 and PV3 are serotypes of poliovirus; ND, no data of the genome have been produced as cloned sequences or, where the nucleotide sequence of the region is known, as synthetic oligonucleotide probes. An alternative approach is to use the polymerase chain reaction (PCR) to amplify a defined region within VP1 and to sequence the resulting fragment. This approach is limited by the sequence data currently available; although all three poliovirus serotypes have been fully sequenced, only 3 of 6 Coxsackie B virus sequences, 2 of 23 Coxsackie A virus sequences and no complete ECHOvirus sequences have been published.

Mechanism of Persistence

Although persisting virus is defective in the control of RNA replication as described above, we do not know the precise nature of the defect which causes this abnormal situation in vivo. Recent work on poliovirus has shown that the secondary structure of the first 100 base pairs of the 5′ non-coding region of the genomic strand of viral RNA are important in controlling RNA replication. Mutations in this region which alter intragenomic base pairing result in reduced production of positive-strand RNA and so alter the positive: negative strand ratios [22]. This may be similar to the mutation presumed to generate this effect in vivo. This hypothesis may be tested using the polymerase chain reaction to amplify this region and so determine sequence changes present in clinical isolates. Computer analysis may predict differences in secondary structure resulting from changes between the protoype 5′ non-coding sequence and this region in clinical isolates. A similar strategy can be used to identify mutations in other viral genes, the products of which are involved directly in RNA replication. The most important of these is the RNA-dependent RNA polymerase 3D and, as viral RNA replication cannot take place without this activity, a mutation may alter its enzymatic activity. The mechanism of priming RNA replication is still not fully understood, but a sequence mutation in the primer binding site could alter the ability of the polymerase to copy one strand rather than the other.

As well as alteration of the control of RNA replication, there may be other mutations which permit virus persistence in vivo without attracting an inflammatory response. Changes in translation or processing of viral proteins may result in reduced amounts of viral proteins, perhaps undetectable by conventional immunological methods, which in turn result in assembly of insignificant numbers of infectious progeny virus particles. Additionally, mutations in the viral capsid proteins, against which neutralising antibodies are normally directed, could result in defective virus unable to bind to cell surface receptors and so to infect neighbouring cells.

A major question in viral persistence is to what extent, if at all, viral proteins are translated and processed. If high molecular weight viral RNA is synthesised as similar amounts of positive and negative strands, it is likely that much of this is present as double-stranded RNA and that translation of viral proteins by cellular ribosomes would be inhibited from such a double-stranded template.

Comparative studies on enteroviral protein expression in productive or persistent infection are complicated by the fact that the reactivity of diagnostic and clinical sera is directed mainly against epitopes on the major capsid protein VP1 and so detect only this protein in immunoblots (our unpublished data). The levels of expression of other capsid and non-structural proteins are therefore difficult to determine by this approach. One solution to this problem is to express individual viral proteins from subgenomic cDNA clones and to raise polyclonal sera to them (R. Kandolf, personal communication). Antibodies produced in this way can be titrated against viral proteins to produce an antibody mixture which detects all viral gene products with equal affinity and can be used to compare viral gene expression in productive or persistent infection.

An existing mouse model allows the mechanism of persistence to be investigated by two approaches. The first is to take a full length, reactivatable Coxsackie B virus cDNA clone and to introduce specific sequence mutations in vitro. This approach has been used previously in investigations of the molecular basis of neurovirulence in poliovirus and a full length, infectious cDNA Coxsackie B3 virus clone is available [12]. Cultured cells are transfected with the mutated construct and the reactivated mutants used to infect murine hosts: comparison of the mutant and parent strains shows the phenotypic effect of that particular mutation. The second approach is to analyse "natural" mutations in an animal model such as that of Reyes et al. [11] which mimics viral persistence in the clinical situation. Sequence changes in genomic RNA of the persisting virus can then be determined after amplification by PCR and compared with that of the prototype.

Pathogenetic Mechanism

The mechanism by which persisting enterovirus infection of cardiac myocytes results in dysfunction and dilatation of the whole organ is unknown. In addition to the value of the basic research, elucidation of the pathogenetic mechanism may provide a basis for development of rational therapies for enteroviral heart muscle disease.

It is clear from in situ hybridisation with an enterovirus group-specific probe that persisting viral RNA sequences are localised in widely distributed foci, each involving only a small number of cardiac myocytes [18]. The key question is how virus persistence in a small proportion of myocytes results in global dysfunction. Although there are virtually no experimental data to support them, there are three major hypotheses which are the object of current investigations.

Firstly, it is common experience in experimental virology that persistent infection of specialised cell types results in the loss of specific functions and that such cells revert to a "housekeeping" phenotype involving the expression of essential genes only. For example neuroblastoma cells in culture persistently infected with lymphocytic choriomeningitis virus (LCMV) of mouse continue to grow normally but have aberrations in the synthesis and degradation of acetylcholine [23]. Similarly, in a persistently LCMV-infected mouse strain, C3H, the mice are hypoglycaemic and growth-retarded. Studies on pituitary cells showed that these effects were caused by a decrease in transcription of the gene encoding growth hormone to one sixteenth of the mRNA level in uninfected animals. This was unique to pituitary growth hormone as the messengers for other proteins, such as thyroid stimulating hormone and actin, were transcribed at normal levels. The mechanism of this selective translational inhibition of specialised gene function resulting from persistent virus infection is not known. Similarly, a diabetogenic strain of Coxsackie virus B4 was still detectable in mouse pancreatic beta cells 8 weeks post-infection and resulted in reduced levels of expression of preproinsulin mRNA leading to hypoglycaemia [24]. It is possible that persistent enterovirus infection of cardiac cells affects the expression of cellular genes encoding essential functions such as contractile or cytoskeletal proteins. The effect of persistent enterovirus on cardiac gene expression is currently being investigated by 2D electrophoretic gel separation of proteins from normal or diated myocardium (M. Dunn, personal communication). Identification of proteins the expression of which varies between normal and that in cardiac tissue persistently infected with enterovirus may provide clues to the mechanism of pathogenesis.

Secondly, it has been proposed that some diffusible product of persistently infected cells may have a remote effect on non-infected myocytes and modify their function leading to dysfunction of the whole ventricle. There are no data to support this concept and the nature of such a product has not been specified.

Thirdly, it is clear that cardiac myocytes are networked in terms of electrical conduction. We have proposed that perturbation of cell membrane function, which is common in persistent virus infection, may allow a small number of infected cells to disrupt the contractility of the whole organ. Again, there are no experimental data to support this hypothesis.

Potential Therapy

The association between enterovirus infection of myocardium and the development of dilated heart muscle disease has been established and the question remains as to what can be done to prevent or treat the disease. A specific anti-Picornaviral drug exists (WIN 51711: Fig. 16.3a) which acts by stabilising the virion capsid by binding to a hydrophobic pocket in the structural protein VP1. This prevents virus uncoating during penetration into the cell, leaving intact virions in endosomes where they are degraded by cellular enzymes [25]. Because the drug acts by interfering with virus uncoating, it may be useful in inflammatory heart muscle disease generated by productive infection. However, it seems unlikely that this agent would be therapeutic in dilated heart muscle disease resulting from persisting infection with a replication-defective enterovirus which seems not to assemble infectious progeny.

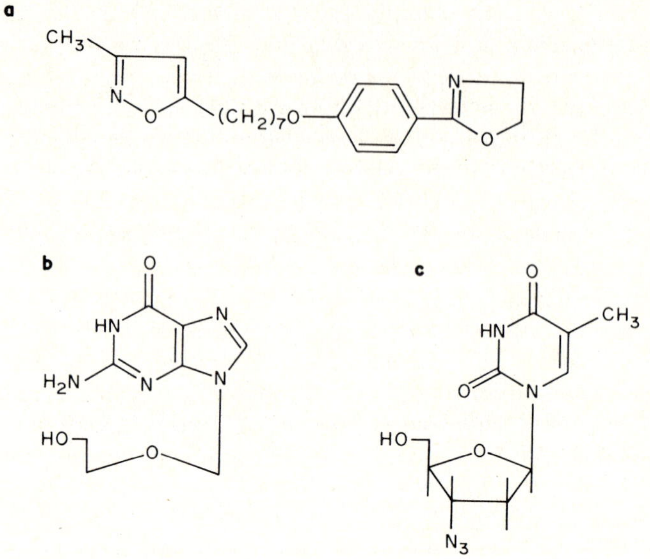

Fig. 16.3 a–c. Antiviral agents: **a** WIN 51711; **b** acyclovir; **c** zidovudine

Enterovirus persistence in myocardium in dilated cardiomyopathy appears to involve at least the continuing synthesis of virus RNA, mediated by the viral RNA-dependent RNA polymerase. A therapeutic strategy which may be appropriate to this situation is the use of nucleoside analogues to inhibit the acitvity of this virus-specific enzyme. Development of such antiviral drugs involves identifying a unique step in the replication cycle of a virus. Probably the best known and most commonly used antiviral drug is acyclovir (9-[(2-hydroxyethoxy) methyl] guanine), a guanosine analogue which is active against herpes simplex virus (HSV). Its selective activity against HSV results from its preferential phosphorylation by the viral thymidine kinase (TK) and its subsequent incorporation into DNA resulting in chain termination. Similarly, the activity of zidovudine (3′-azido-2′,3′-dideoxythymidine) against human immunodeficiency virus (HIV) results from phosphorylation of the analogue by reverse transcriptase, an enzyme unique to retroviruses, and its incorporation into proviral DNA [26].

In the case of enteroviral infection of heart, it is likely that the viral RNA continues to be replicated for years after the onset of symptoms, although no viral antigens are detected. We propose that the natural choice of target for an anti-Picornaviral drug effective in persistent infection would be the viral RNA-dependent RNA polymerase which is unique to this group of viruses. By analogy with the examples above, an ideal drug would be a chain-terminating nucleoside which the viral enzyme binds preferentially to its natural substrate. As with the other antiviral nucleoside analogues, it could be expected that resistant mutants would emerge in long-term therapy.

Conclusions

Much progress has been made in establishing a viral aetiology of both inflammatory and dilated heart muscle disease since the original observations of a serological association between enterovirus infection and these diseases. Molecular methods have established that enterovirus RNA can be detected in samples of myocardium from all stages of histologically proven disease in a progression from myocarditis to dilated cardiomyopathy. Virus persistence in late-stage disease appears to result from the generation of replication-defective mutants during the initial, inflammatory stage. Virus-specific gene products seem not to be translated and processed normally, nor is infectious progeny virus assembled, resulting in the inability to detect persisting virus by conventional techniques of isolation or immunochemistry. Enterovirus persistence in myocardium appears to be the most significant predicator of poor prognosis in patients with dilated cardiomyopathy.

Although some data are available concerning the molecular mechanism of virus persistence, essentially nothing is known of the pathogenetic mechanism by which persisting infection results in the development of dilated heart muscle disease and this remains a major area of investigation.

The development of specific antiviral therapy will be facilitated by a clearer understanding of the molecular mechanisms of persistence and pathogenesis which, it is hoped, will emerge from future research.

Acknowledgements. We would like to thank Hong Yi Zhang and Colette Freeke for the use of unpublished data.

References

1. Grist NR, Bell EJ (1974) A six year study of Coxsackie virus B infections in heart disease. J Hyg 73: 165–172
2. Goodwin JF (1983) Myocarditis as a possible cause of cardiomyopathy. In: Just H, Schuster HP (eds) Myocarditis. Cardiomyopathy. Springer, Berlin Heidelberg New York, pp 7–11
3. Grist NR, Bell EJ (1978) Enteroviruses in human disease. In: Melnick JL (ed) Progress in medical virology. Karger, Basel, pp 114–157
4. Morgan-Capner P, Richardson PJ, McSorley C, Daly K, Pattison JR (1984) Virus investigations in heart muscle disease. Springer, Berlin Heidelberg New York, pp 95–115
5. Cambridge G, MacArthur CGC, Waterson AP, Goodwin JF, Oakley CM (1979) Antibodies to Coxsackie B viruses in primary congestive cardiomyopathy, Br Heart J 41: 13–23
6. El-Hagrassy MMO, Banatvala JE, Coltart DJ (1980) Coxsackie B specific IgM responses in patients with cardiac and other disease. Lancet 2: 1160–1162
7. McCartney RA, Banatvala JE, Bell EJ (1986) Routine use of mu-antibody-capture ELISA for the serological diagnosis of Coxsackie B virus infections. J Med Virol 19: 205–212
8. Muir P, Nicholson F, Tilzey AJ et al. (1989) Chronic relapsing pericarditis and dilated cardiomyopathy: serological evidence of persistent enterovirus infection. Lancet 1: 804–807

9. Woodruff JF (1980) Viral myocarditis: a review. Am J Pathol 101: 425–484
10. Huber SA, Lodge PA, Job LP (1984) The role of virus and immune mediated cardiocyte injury in Coxsackie B3 induced myocarditis In: Bolte HD (ed) Viral heart disease. Springer, Berlin Heidelberg New York, pp 64–73
11. Reyes MP, Ho KL, Smith FE, Lerner AM (1981) A mouse model of dilated type cardiomyopathy due to Coxsackie B3 virus. J Infect Dis 144: 232–236
12. Klump WM, Bergmann I, Muller BC, Ameis D, Kandolf R (1990) Complete nucleotide sequence of infectious Coxsackievirus B3 cDNA: two initial 5′ uridine residues are regained during plus-strand RNA synthesis. J Virol 64: 1573–1583
13. Stalhandske PO, Lindberg M, Pettersson U (1984) Replicase gene of Coxsackievirus B3. J Virol 51: 742–746
14. Kaczmarek L, Calabretta B, Baserga R (1985) Expression of cell-cycle-dependent genes in phytohemagglutinin-stimulated human lymphocytes. Proc Natl Acad Sci USA 82: 5375–5379
15. Bowles NE, Rose ML, Taylor P et al. (1989) End-stage dilated cardiomyopathy: persistence of enterovirus RNA in myocardium at cardiac transplantation and lack of immune response. Circulation 80: 1128–1136
16. Bowles NE, Richardson PJ, Olsen EG, Archard LC (1986) Detection of Coxsackie-B-virus-specific RNA sequences in myocardial biopsy samples from patients with myocarditis and dilated cardiomyopathy. Lancet 1: 1120–1123
17. Archard LC, Richardson PJ, Olsen EG, Dubowitz V, Sewry C, Bowles NE (1987) The role of Coxsackie B viruses in the pathogenesis of myocarditis, dilated cardiomyopathy and inflammatory muscle disease. Biochem Soc Symp 53: 51–62
18. Kandolf R, Amies D, Kirschner P et al. (1987) In situ detection of enteroviral genomes in myocardial cells by nucleic acid hybridization: an approach to the diagnosis of viral heart disease. Proc Natl Acad Sci USA 84: 6272–6276
19. Rotbart HA, Abzug MJ, Murray RS, Murphy NL, Levin MJ (1988) Intracellular detection of sense and antisense enteroviral RNA by in situ hybridization; J Virol Methods 22: 295–301
20. Cunningham L, Bowles NE, Lane RJ, Dubowitz V, Archard LC (1990) Persistence of enteroviral RNA in chronic fatigue syndrome is associated with the abnormal production of equal amounts of positive and negative strands of enteroviral RNA. J Gen Virol 71: 1399–1402
21. Archard LC, Bowles NE, Cunningham L, Freeke CA, Olsen EGJ, Rose ML, Meany B, Why HJF, Richardson PJ (1991) Molecular probes for detection of persisting enterovirus infection of human hearts and their prognostic value. Eur Heart J 12 (Suppl D): 56–59
22. Andino R, Rieckhof GE, Baltimore D (1990) A functional ribonucleoprotein complex forms around the 5′ end of poliovirus RNA. Cell 63: 369–380
23. Oldstone MB (1989) Viral alteration of cell function. Sci Am 261: 42–48
24. Chatterjee NK, Nejman C (1988) Insulin mRNA content in pancreatic beta cells of Coxsackie virus B4-induced diabetic mice. Mol Cell Endocrinol 55: 193–202
25. Otto MJ, Fox MP, Fancher MJ, Kuhrt MF, Diana GC, McKinlay MA (1985) In vitro activity of WIN 51711: a new broad spectrum antipicornavirus drug. Antimircrob Agents Chemother 27: 883–886
26. Hirsch MS, Kaplan JC (1990) Antiviral agents. In: Fields BN (ed) Virology. Raven Press, New York, pp 90: 441–468

CHAPTER 17

The Molecular Genetics of Familial Hypertrophic Cardiomyopathy

H. Watkins, C. E. Seidman, and W. J. McKenna

Inheritance Patterns in Hypertrophic Cardiomyopathy (see also Part III)

Ever since its initial description, hypertrophic cardiomyopathy has been identified as a condition which is frequently inherited in a familial fashion. Teare's original account in 1958 [1] describes nine cases of sudden death which include a brother and sister from the same family. The subsequent report [2] of the three generation pedigree of the family of these two siblings showed hypertophic cardiomyopathy segregating in a manner consistent with an autosomal dominant trait. Demonstration of a Mendelian form of inheritance implied that familial hypertrophic cardiomyopathy (FHC) was the result of a single gene disorder. This conclusion was supported by a number of clinical reports, from the early 1960s onwards, of single pedigrees showing autosomal dominant transmission of FHC [3–7].

Thereafter, attempts were made to screen systematically the first degree relatives of patients with hypertrophic cardiomyopathy to determine modes of inheritance. Over the last three decades methods used for the investigation of this condition have evolved, as have the diagnostic criteria, and the resulting data must be interpreted in context. In the 1960s and early 1970s hypertrophic cardiomyopathy was characterised by the presence of a dynamic left ventricular outflow tract gradient. Patients and their families were screened by clinical examination, electrocardiography, chest radiography and haemodynamic investigation [8]. Thus, Emanuel et al. [9] concluded from these investigations, supplemented by operative and autopsy findings where available, that hypertrophic cardiomyopathy was familial in 30%–50% of cases. Some of their data suggested that in addition to the autosomal dominant mode of inheritance, some families appeared to exibit a recessive pattern of inheritance, i.e. both parents of one or more affected siblings were diagnosed as being normal, and the disease was not seen in offspring.

When M-mode echocardiography became widely available the presence of asymmetric septal hypertrophy in individuals without features of obstruction was revealed [10, 11]. A higher proportion of the first degree relatives screened were found to be affected and up to 90% [12] of index cases were considered to have familial disease. Demonstration of previously unsuspected disease in parents or offspring also revealed that families that had appeared to show recessive inheritance were in fact carrying a dominantly expressed gene [13]. Having excluded those studies that precede the use of echocardiography, there are no convincing reports in the literature of autosomal recessive transmission of FHC.

The advent of 2D echocardiography revealed a still broader spectrum of manifestations in this condition [14–16]. While the majority of patients have asymmetric septal hypertrophy, hypertrophy may be concentric or confined to the left ventricular free wall, posterior wall, or apex and rarely to the right ventricle. These studies revealed that the striking diversity of clinical manifestations may be as great within a given family as it is between unrelated families [17, 18]. Family screening studies using 2D echocardiography thus give the best assessment of the inheritance patterns in FHC available to date. However, variations in findings still result from differences in selection of probands and precise criteria used in interpretation of the clinical investigations [19]. Two comprehensive surveys are those of Marón et al. [20] and Greaves et al. [21], whose findings are similar. Familial disease was identified in 56% and 67%, respectively, of the families of probands who had at least three available first degree relatives. It should be noted that this may be an underestimate because a number of relatives could not be studied and in some instances sporadic hypertrophic cardiomyopathy was assumed. In these studies, and others, it is striking that the observed incidence of familial disease increases with increasing numbers of family members studied.

In assessing a member of an FHC family it is appropriate to have a low threshold for making the diagnosis. In practice, the demonstration of any unexplained hypertrophy of the left and/or right ventricle, whether it is asymmetric, concentric or localised, established the diagnosis in a family member. A variety of electrocardiographic abnormalities, though they may be non-specific, are very sensitive indicators of disease in such individuals, who have *a priori* odds of 1 in 2 of carrying the disease gene. The use of these criteria is strongly supported by the results of the genetic analyses discussed below, where the clinical diagnoses have been independently confirmed by demonstration of the genotype.

Sporadic Disease

As discussed above, estimates of the proportion of hypertrophic cardiomyopathy that occurs in the absence of a family history have varied with diagnostic modality. Studies based on clinical and haemodynamic evaluation of FHC showed an apparent familial involvement in one third of all cases, the remainder being labelled "sporadic" [22, 23]. In contrast, most authorities would now consider the majority of cases to be familial, although a significant minority appear to be sporadic. It should be noted that in almost all studies of the prevalence of familial transmission in hypertrophic cardiomyopathy a number of relatives could not be studied and a sporadic pattern was assumed [20, 21].

As the number of individuals studied increases in a family the likelihood of finding familial disease increases. No sporadic disease was found in 13 families that had over six first degree relatives available for study [21], suggesting that the incidence of sporadic disease has been exaggerated by inclusion of unrecognised FHC.

A number of potential mechanisms exist whereby affected individuals can appear to have sporadic disease. An incorrect diagnosis of sporadic disease can be made in an autosomal dominant single gene disorder if there is incomplete penetrance, such that an apparently normal parent actually bears a sub clinical form of the condition. Equally, this can result from unrecognised instances of non-paternity. Additionally, apparently sporadic cases will occur if there is a high new mutation rate. The probability of the disease trait being passed to any offspring is 1 in 2, and so this will not always manifest in subsequent generations, particularly where the family is small.

In contrast, true sporadic cases must occur through aetiologically distinct mechanisms, which might include both environmental and genetic processes. For example, environmental influences might perhaps act on a genetic background conferring susceptibility; such a genetic predisposition could result from the influences of many genes. Alternatively, another possible mechanism is that of a somatic mutation during embryogenesis (possibly affecting the same gene as the inherited form of the disease) which affects the heart but not the germ-line. At present, the origins and frequency of sporadic cases of hypertrophic cardiomyopathy are unknown. Although there have been few formal comparisons of individuals with sporadic disease with those with familial disease, no obvious differences in clinical features have been reported.

Gene Penetrance and Phenotypic Expression

There remain areas of difficulty in establishing the diagnosis of hypertrophic cardiomyopathy. Frequently there is a delay in appearance of the morphological manifestations of the disease until after adolescence [24]. This is illustrated by the variation of prevalance of hypertrophic cardiomyopathy in first degree relatives when categorised by age, as has been seen in all family studies. For example, ten Cate et al. [13] report the prevalence of the disease by echocardiographic criteria to be 52% in parents and 41% in siblings but only 20% in children of their 33 index cases. Inclusion of children in family studies has led in the past to underestimation of the proportion of familial disease and the erroneous conclusion that inheritance can be by recessive transmission.

Even within an adult population, penetrance may not be complete. It is clear that the severity of disease manifestation is very variable, even within a family, sometimes to the extent that an individual who must be carrying the disease gene may appear normal [25]. However, very few documented instances exist where there are no abnormalities at all on electrocardiographic or echocardiographic examination. In theory, a numerical estimate of penetrance can be calculated from a comparison of the observed incidence of disease among first degree relatives with the expected incidence—which is 50% for an autosomal dominant trait. In practice, such a figure is hard to obtain with any reliability because of the relative small sample sizes and the variation in the sensitivity of the diagnostic criteria used in published series. For the purposes of the genetic linkage analyses detailed below, an estimate for penetrance of $P = 0.95$ was used for family members of 16 years or older. Other problem areas relate to the limitations of a diagnosis of exclusion. Coexistent hypertension, obesity or the physiological hypertrophic response to athletic training frequently make definitive diagnosis impossible. These issues have long underscored the need to develop a molecular marker for this disease.

Mendelian inheritance in FHC implies the presence of an identical gene defect in all affected members of a given family. This does not, however, dictate that the defect need be the same in unrelated families with FHC. Either a different mutation within the same gene or a mutation in another gene could be responsible. The variable expression which is characteristic of FHC is a frequent finding in single gene disorders and hence does not predict the presence of more than one gene. Moreover, some aspects of the phenotype vary as much within families, where a single gene defect must be common to all members, as between families [17]. Differences of expression presumably result from interaction with the environment and/or other genes carried by the individual. There is evidence that at least some part of this effect is environmental in origin, in that three pairs of monozygotic twins with hypertrophic cardiomyopathy have been reported, each with widely differing degrees of clinical severity in the two twins [25–27].

Genetic Analysis

Recent advances in molecular biological techniques have led to the successful identification of the precise gene defects responsible for a number of important inherited conditions, including some where there was no prior knowledge of any defect at the protein level. Such "reverse genetics" can be accomplished by way of several different approaches. Most productive has been the use of linkage analysis to map a disease gene to a specific chromosomal locus. For example, linkage analysis has been used to identify the genetic loci of Huntington's disease, cystic fibrosis, Duchenne muscular dystrophy and adult polycystic kidney disease. Identification of close genetic linkage led to the subsequent identification of the gene itself in both Duchenne muscular dystrophy and cystic fibrosis.

Additional strategies that can be used in the first instance, or once linkage has been established, are the examination of candidate genes for mutations in affected individuals and the matching of cytogenetic abnormalities (e.g. chromosomal deletions) with inheritance of the disease trait within a pedigree. Examples of these applications are the demonstration of mutations in the rhodopsin gene when examined as a candidate gene for retinitis pigmentosa, and the localisation of the gene for familial polyposis coli to chromosome 5, where it was associated with a deletion in one family.

Reports of associations of FHC with other syndromes suggest some potential genetic loci for involvement, while at the same time suggesting the presence of genetic heterogeneity. Hypertrophic cardiomyopathy, or a clinically similar phenotype, is recognised in association with some familial conditions the genetic loci for which have been mapped: neurofibromatosis (chromosome 17) [28, 29], Freidreich's ataxia (chromosome 9) [30], aniridia with catalase deficiency (chromosome 11) [31] and hereditary spherocytosis (chromosome 14) [32, 33]. It is also seen in association with Noonan syndrome, a condition the gene for which remains unmapped. None of these loci, however, are known to involve genes with cardiac expression which would be considered as candidates for FHC. It is also apparent that many of the hypertrophic phenotypes described in these syndromes show features only partly consistent with the diagnosis of FHC, and it seems likely that these syndromes represent different aetiologies sharing a final common pathway of pathological expression.

There have also been reports that suggest either genetic linkage of FHC with the major histocompatibility (HLA) locus on chromosome 6 [34, 35], or association of obstructive forms of hypertrophic cardiomyopathy with specific HLA-DR alleles [36]. However, subsequent studies have excluded linkage with the HLA locus in large pedigrees [37] and in sibling pair analyses [38] and have failed to demonstrate any disease association with HLA haplotype [39].

Linkage Mapping

In the absence of any apparent candidate genes or of any known cytogenetic anomaly in FHC, the approach that was adopted, and that proved successful, was the use of linkage analysis. Linkage analysis involves the detection of "co-segregation" of a disease trait with a DNA polymorphism of known chromosomal location. If a particular marker gene is situated close to the disease gene on a given chromosome, then a polymorphism at this site will tend to be inherited with the disease trait in a family pedigree. Where a marker gene and a disease gene are separated by some distance (even if on the same chromosome) they will tend to become separated by cross-overs, or recombinations, during meiosis. Thus the extent of co-inheritance, or co-segregation, defines the closeness of linkage.

The polymorphic markers used were restriction fragment length polymorphisms (RFLPs), identified by a series of DNA probes, that together construct a genetic linkage map spanning the human genome [40]. Natural variations in DNA sequence, mostly in non-coding regions of the genome, result in differences in the sites of cleavage of the DNA by sequence-specific bacterial restriction enzymes. Genomic DNA from different individuals will yield fragments of different lengths when incubated with a specific restriction enzyme; the varied fragments can be separated by agarose gel electrophoresis. These are then transferred to a filter (a process known as a Southern blot) and identified by hybridisation with radiolabelled DNA probes which selectively bind to homologous sequences in the region of the polymorphic restriction site. RFLPs are inherited according to classical Mendelian patterns and so a particular polymorphism can easily be traced through a family pedigree, identifying which of each of a pair of chromosomes is inherited from which parent.

A large French-Canadian family (family A, Fig. 17.1), previously studied by Pare et al. [4], was selected for further evaluation [41]. Based on previous clinical assessments and/or post-mortem examination, 24 deceased individuals had FHC. All surviving members over the age of 16 were assessed by clinical examination, electrocardiography and 2D echocardiogram and Doppler study. Of these, 20 were judged to be affected by demonstration of unexplained left and/or

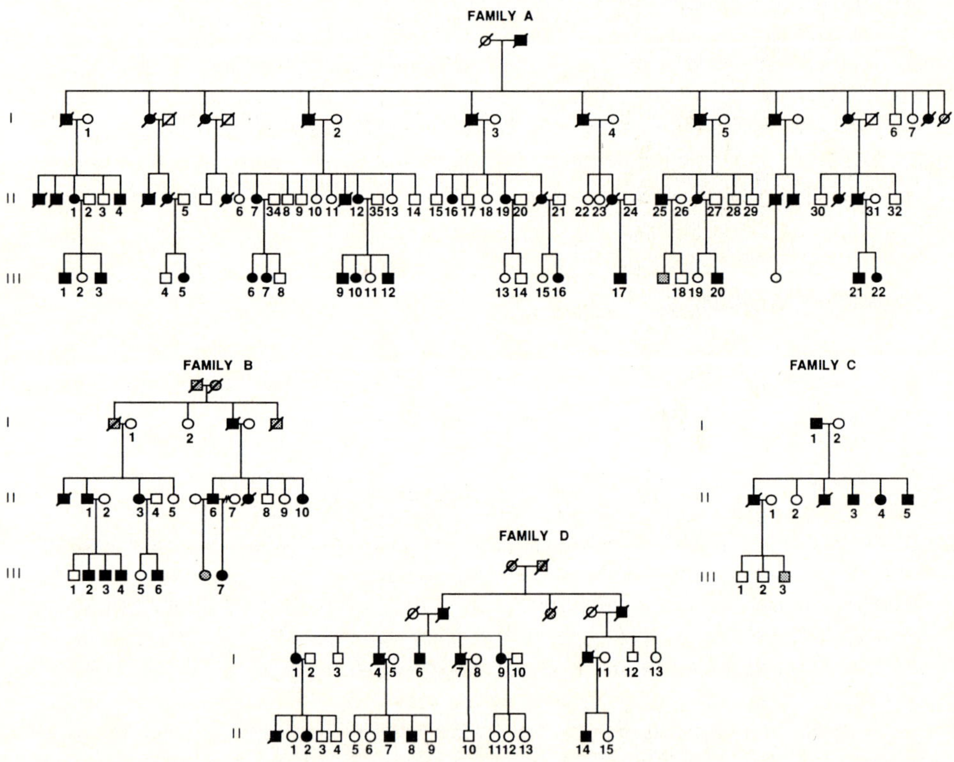

Fig. 17.1. Pedigrees of the families used in linkage analyses. Disease status is indicated by shading: affected, *filled symbols*; unaffected, *open symbols*; unknown, *stippled symbols*. Deceased family members are marked with a *slash*. Individual BII-6 was divorced from individual BII-7 (*double slashes*). (Reproduced from [42], the *Journal of Clinical Investigation*, 1990, 86: 993–999, by copyright permission of the American Society for Clinical Investigation).

right ventricular hypertrophy and 54 judged to be unaffected. Blood samples were obtained from each family member and continuous lymphoblastoid cell lines established as a source of DNA. Linkage analyses were performed with DNA probes, selected randomly from a panel of probes which identify polymorphic loci spaced throughout the genome, until one was found which identified a polymorphism that co-segregated with disease. A DNA probe identifying an RFLP previously mapped to chromosome 14 (probe L436) revealed two alleles which were co-inherited with the phenotypic presence or absence of FHC (Fig. 17.2). There were no recombinations (cross-overs in meiosis).

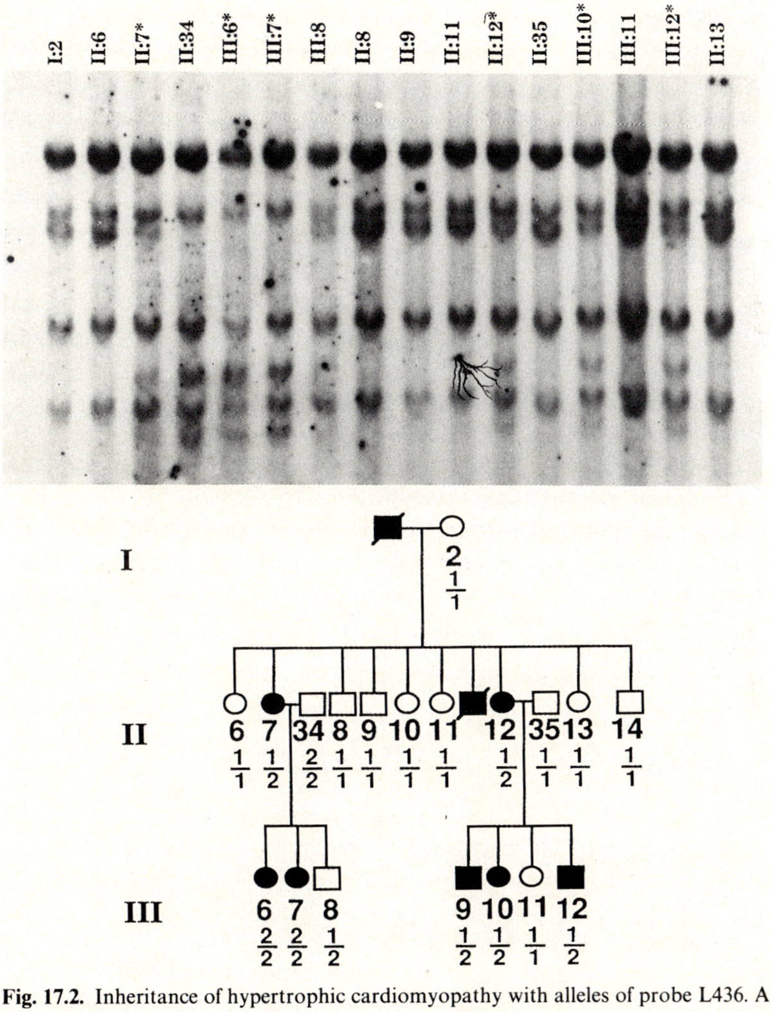

Fig. 17.2. Inheritance of hypertrophic cardiomyopathy with alleles of probe L436. A Southern blot performed with probe L436 in part of family A is shown and the alleles present in each individual are indicated on the pedigree below. Allele 1 designates a 4.2 kilobase band, allele 2 designates a pair of bands at 2.2 and 1.8 kilobases. Hypertrophic cardiomyopathy is seen to segregate with allele 2: all affected individuals inherit allele 2 from their affected parent

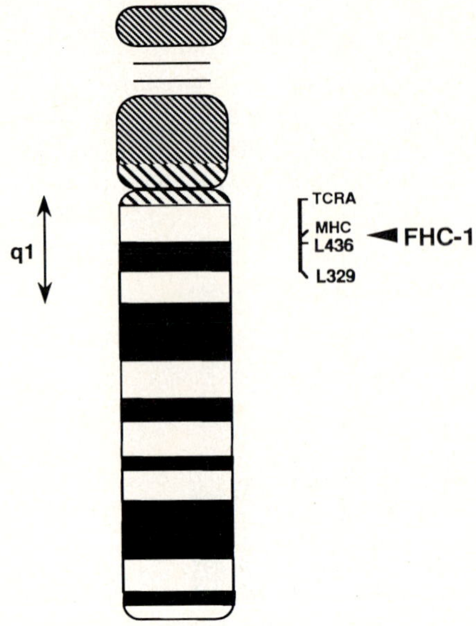

Fig. 17.3. Cytogenetic map of chromosome 14 showing assignment of FHC-1 locus. The conventional banding pattern on Giemsa staining is shown, with band q1 indicated. A genetic linkage map of the probes used is aligned with the cytogenetic map. The relative positions of the probe loci are from [48]. The L436 locus has been assigned by chromosomal in situ hybridisation. (Adapted from information appearing in NEJM, Jarcho et al. 1989, Mapping a gene for familial hypertrophic cardiomyopathy to chromosome 14q1. N Engl J Med 321: 1372–1378 [41]).

The statistical significance of the linkage was assessed by calculation of a LOD score. This is the logarithm of the probability of observing co-segregation of two loci, assuming that they are genetically linked, divided by the probability of detecting co-segregation if they are unlinked, i.e. by random chance. The LOD score generated for this data was +11.28 at a recombination distance of 0. This is equivalent to odds of greater than 100 billion to 1 in favour of the gene for FHC in this family being linked to this locus on chromosome 14. Subsequent chromosomal in situ hybridisation studies have confirmed the linkage assignment of this locus to a region of the long arm of chromosome 14, designated as 14q11-12. The chromosome 14q11-12 locus for this disease has been designated FHC-1 (Fig. 17.3).

Genetic Heterogeneity

The mapping of the gene for FHC in this family provided a basis for determining whether additional genetic loci can cause this disorder independently in unrelated families. To investigate whether a gene at this chromosomal locus was responsible for disease in other families with FHC, 62 members from three additional families were studied using the same protocol [42]. The clinical manifestations of FHC in these families were typical of the condition; no significant differences in signs or symptoms were detected between the families. Linkage analyses were performed using three probes which identify polymorphisms at 14q1, to determine whether alleles at these loci are inherited with

Map Distance (cM)	-10	-7	-3	0	1	3	6	12	Probability
Family A	10.85	11.64	12.39	13.13	13.07	12.67	10.70	10.42	>.99
Family B	3.62	3.88	4.14	4.39	4.29	4.17	3.07	2.69	>.99
Family C	-0.27	-0.67	-1.35	-4.65	-2.60	-1.62	-1.07	-0.14	<.0001
Family D	-0.92	-1.18	-1.54	-2.08	-2.14	-2.32	-3.26	-1.42	<.0085

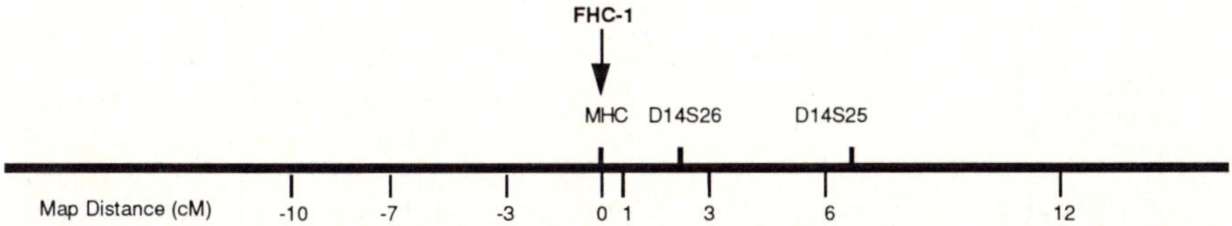

Fig. 17.4. Multipoint linkage analyses in families A, B, C and D from Fig. 17.1 demonstrating genetic heterogeneity. LOD scores for each family are shown at various map distances (in centimorgans) from the FHC locus with the probability of linkage to this locus. Families A and B are shown to be linked to this locus on chromosome 14q1, while families C and D are shown not to be linked. A schematic map of chromosome 14q1 is shown; the locus D14S26 is identified by probe L436; D14S25 is identified by probe L329. (Reproduced from [42], the *Journal of Clinical Investigation*, 1990, 86: 993–999, by copyright permission of the American Society for Clinical Investigation)

disease status. Of the three new families, one (family B, Fig. 17.1) was found to exhibit tight linkage to the chromosome 14q1 locus, with no recombinants in 13 informative meioses. The two other families (C and D, Fig. 17.1), however, yielded significant negative LOD scores, excluding linkage to the chromosome 14 locus (Fig. 17.4). This confirms the presence of genetic heterogeneity, and implies the presence of one or more additional loci for FHC.

Subsequent linkage studies have independently confirmed the linkage to FHC-1. Heijtmancik et al. [43] report the results of linkage analyses with the 14q1 probes in nine unrelated families which, with their linkage date pooled, generate a net LOD score of +5.6. However, in the light of the demonstrated genetic heterogeneity it may not be valid to pool unrelated families; those families which were essentially uninformative could equally be linked to a different disease locus. In two of the families there are cross-overs which imply non-linkage to chromosome 14q1. Other linkage data in support of the existence of alternative loci for FHC include the recent report of a family that shows co-segregation of FHC with a fragile site on chromosome 16 [44], and a report from a Japanese group [45] suggesting linkage to chromosome 18, again with a cumulative LOD score derived from a collection of small families.

One of the limitations of genetic linkage studies is that the majority of smaller families fail to generate significant LOD scores, particularly as so often some members are uninformative for any given RFLP. (If an affected parent by chance has the same RFLP allele on both chromosomes it is not possible to determine which chromosome is passed on to each offspring, i.e. to determine whether the polymorphism segregates with disease status or not). To achieve a statistically significant LOD score in favour of linkage generally requires in the region of ten informative meioses, i.e. genotype analyses of individuals whose parents have also been studied and have passed on different alleles at a given locus. In practice, this usually necessitates the availability of three generations of any family and good fortune with the degree of heterozygosity identified by the probes used.

Demonstration of Mutations in the Cardiac Myosin Heavy Chain Genes: A Molecular Basis for FHC

The localisation of the disease locus to this region of chromosome 14 suggested candidate genes that might be involved in the pathogenesis of FHC. Most provocative of these were the alpha and beta cardiac myosin heavy chain (MHC) genes, which have been mapped to 14q11.2-q13[46,47]. Myosin is a major component of the contractile apparatus in muscle, and exists in numerous isoforms. These cardiac isoforms of the heavy chains are expressed at high levels in the myocardium, with beta chain dimers being predominant in the adult ventricle in man. Myosin heavy chain gene expression is altered in rodent models of cardiac hypertrophy. The cardiac myosin heavy chains were therefore studied to look for linkage to FHC. The two cardiac myosin heavy chain genes are tandemly arranged within 4 kilobases of each other; each gene is composed of 40 exons (sections of coding sequence) distributed over 30 kilobases of DNA and codes for a 220 kilodalton polypeptide. A DNA probe, derived from the cardiac beta myosin heavy chain gene, was shown to be closely linked to disease status in the two families whose disease maps to chromosome 14q1[48].

During genetic linkage analysis of the FHC-1 locus with the myosin probe, a novel restriction fragment was identified in the cardiac MHC genes of all affected members of family B[49]. This fragment was not seen in any of 200 other unrelated individuals. To determine the molecular basis of the mutation resulting in thils novel variant, the alpha and beta cardiac MHC genes from these affected individuals were compared with those found in unaffected individuals. Cloned fragments of the two genes were examined by restriction mapping, comparing the arrangement of known restriction enzyme sites. Both rearranged and duplicated fragments were seen in the digests. Analysis of the novel fragment by restriction mapping and sequencing revealed a hybrid gene composed of alpha cardiac MHC sequence fused to beta cardiac MHC sequence. The fusion point is located in exon 27 and occurs without any concomitant deletion or frameshift of the coding sequence. As the alpha and beta genes are arranged in tandem and are highly homologous in structure and sequence, this mutation presumably was caused by an unequal cross-over event in meiosis. The result is that the disease-related allele in this family consists of a normal alpha cardiac MHC gene and a normal beta cardiac MHC gene, as well as the additional alpha/beta hybrid gene which would be expected to encode a novel cardiac MHC polypeptide.

To confirm the hypothesis that this mutation is related to the presence of disease in these individuals, an analysis was undertaken of the MHC genes in the original family that showed linkage to the FHC-1 locus (family A) [50]. The cardiac MHC genes from affected and unaffected members were compared by restriction mapping, but no gross rearrangements were observed. Fine structure restriction mapping of overlapping clones of both the alpha and beta genes was performed with 20 restriction enzymes. This revealed six previously unidentified RFLPs. Of these, only one segregated with disease, was not found in unaffected individuals and was located in coding sequence. This was a restriction fragment length polymorphism in the beta gene, which was present in every affected individual in this family, but not seen in 100 unrelated individuals (Fig. 17.4). This polymorphism was mapped to exon 13 of the beta cardiac MHC gene. Sequencing revealed it to be due to a single base pair substitution: adenine is substituted for guanine, resulting in the conversion of an arginine residue to a glutamine residue (Fig. 17.5). The significance of this missense mutation is supported by the resulting change in amino acid net charge from +1 to 0, which is likely to cause regional alterations in peptide conformation. Moreover, the arginine residue at this site is conserved in myosin heavy chain isoforms from other species. Such evolutionary conservation must denote this region as being one of particular functional importance (Fig. 17.6).

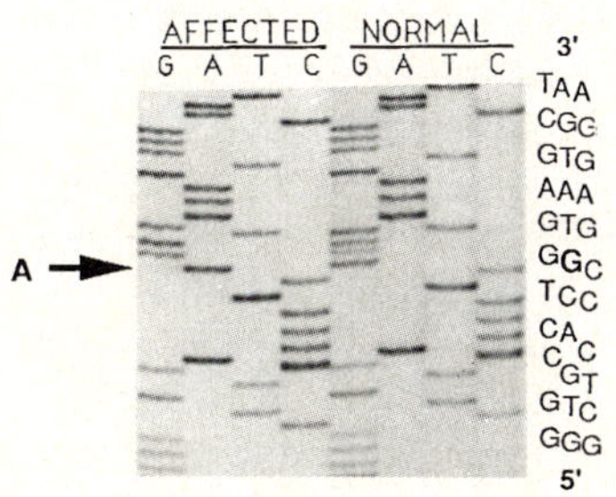

A

```
Unaffected   luAlaAspLysSerAlaTyrLeuMetGlyLeuAsnSerAlaAspLeuLeuLysGlyLeuCys
             TCCAGAGGCTGACAAGTCTGCCTACCTCATGGGGCTGAACTCAGCCGACCTGCTCAAGGGGCTGTGC  10154
Affected     ...................................................................

Unaffected   HisProArgValLysValGlyAsnGluTyrValThrLysGlyGlnAsnValGlnGln
             CACCCTCGGGTGAAAGTGGGCAATGAGTACGTCACCAAGGGGCAGAATGTCCAGCAGGTGGGTCCAT  10221
Affected     .......A...........................................................
             Gln
```

B

Fig. 17.5A, B. Nucleotide and amino acid sequences showing the exon 13 missense mutation in family A. **A** A DNA sequencing gel shows the missense mutation, identified by an *arrow*, which converts a G in the normal sequence to an A in the cloned DNA from an affected member of family A. **B** The predicted amino acid sequence encoded by exon 13 is presented in the three-letter code for amino acids. The region covered by the sequence shown in A is *overlined*. The G to A substitution converts the normal arginine residue to glutamine in the affected individuals. [From 50]

```
                            FHC-1 A  ......................Q................

               cardiac β (human)  EADKSAYLMGLNSADLLKGLCHPRVKVGNEYVTKGQSVQQ
                 cardiac β (rat)  ........................................
                cardiac α (rat)  D...................................T.D.
embryonic skeletal muscle (human)  V.T.T........S....A..F..............T.D.
  embryonic skeletal muscle (rat)  V...T......M.S....A..F..............T.D.
        skeletal muscle (rabbit)  V...A...QT..T.....A.KY............  D...
             embryonic (chicken)  V...A.............A..Y..............T...
        smooth muscle (chicken)  A.Q.VCA...I.VT.FTRSILT..I...RDV.Q.A.TKE.
            nonmuscle (chicken)  A.Q.VSH.L.I.VT.FTR.ILT..I...RD..Q.A.TKE.
               C. elegans unc54  ..E.ASNMY.IGCEEF..A.TK......T.W.S...NCE.
               C. elegans my1a  ..ERACNMY.IDVVQF..A.VS......T.W.S...N.D.
               C. elegans my2a  D.ERA.KCF.ID.EEF..A.TR........W.N...KIE.
               C. elegans my3a  D.LNA.AML.IQAEEF..A.TK......T.W.N...NLE.
                D. Melanogaster  .GGRVSK.F.CDT.E.Y.N.LK..I.....F.TQ.RN...
                 A. castellanii  .LNIA.E.L.VSA.G.KA..LS..I.A...W..RALNKPK
```

Fig. 17.6. Comparison among species of myosin heavy chain amino acid sequences encoded by exon 13. The normal human beta cardiac MHC sequence of exon 13 is shown along the top line in the single-letter code. The corresponding residues in other MHC peptides are shown below; where they are identical they are represented by *dots*. Areas of complete conservation between these species are boxed. The mutated glutamine (Q) of family A is identified above, designated FHC-1a; the arginine (R) it replaces is seen to be one of those residues that is completely conserved. [From 50]

The demonstration of unique mutations in two unrelated families with FHC, which are not present in unaffected individuals, demonstrates that defects in the cardiac MHC genes can cause FHC. Further information about the way in which mutations perturb MHC function will be obtained by analysis of additional FHC-causing mutations. In addition, it is of paramount clinical importance to know the proportion of all hypertrophic cardiomyopathy that results from MHC mutations and to know whether most families have unique (i.e. new) mutations or whether there is a preponderance of particular mutations within the FHC population.

This information is becoming available through the use of techniques for screening the coding sequence of genes to detect abnormalities. Until automated sequencing techniques are available genes such as the MHC genes are too large to make direct sequencing a realistic or accurate means of identifying new mutations in many individuals. Moreover, the majority of all disease-causing mutations occur in the coding sections (exons) of a gene—which in this instance represent only one fifth of the total sequence (Fig. 17.7). By studying in fine detail the coding sequence of the MHC genes from one affected representative of each family, a large number of families with FHC can be screened for mutations. In this way, even single base pair substitutions can be identified with relative efficiency. We are developing techniques that allow rapid and systematic screening of the entire coding sequence of beta cardiac MHC gene to detect mutations. DNA from individuals from unrelated families with FHC is amplified

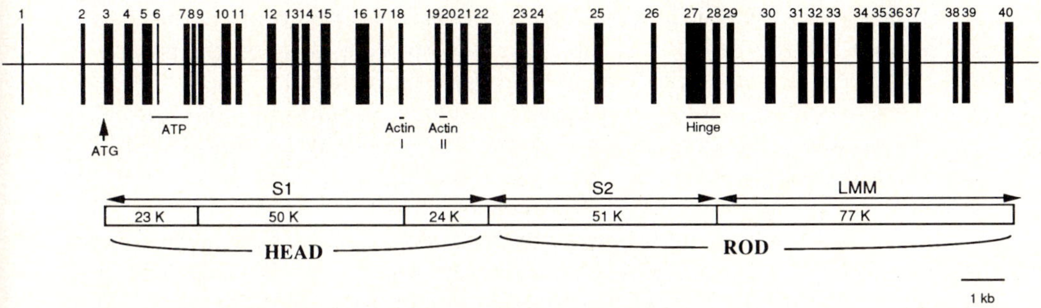

Fig. 17.7. A representation of the beta cardiac MHC gene. The 40 exons which comprise the coding sequence are indicated by *boxes*. Exons encoding ATPase and actin binding activities, associated with the head region of the myosin heavy chain polypeptide, are identified. Several proteolytic fragments that can be obtained by digestion are shown, along with the demarcation between the globular head and the rod. [Adapted from 50]

by the polymerase chain reaction and examined by ribonuclease protection analysis. Using this approach a missense mutation in exon 9 was identified in a conserved residue of the beta MHC gene in a further family [51]. This missense mutation, which results in the conversion of an arginine to a glutamine residue, was present in all clinically affected adult members. Genetic diagnosis based on detection of the mutation in this family made preclinical diagnosis in children possible for the first time.

Future Directions

Once a complete screen of the beta MHC gene has been completed in a group of families the proportion of disease attributable to MHC mutations will be known and the distribution and diversity of the responsible mutations will be revealed. In families with defined mutations genetic diagnosis will be immediately available—allowing diagnosis in presymptomatic children and in those adults difficult to diagnose clinically. Longitudinal studies following the natural history of the disease in pre-symptomatic subjects are under way and prospective, controlled studies of possible therapeutic interventions will be feasible. If particular mutations are predominant, or a particular region of the gene is most frequently involved, then it will be possible to create tailored diagnostic probes to identify these, thus making DNA diagnosis simpler and practicable as a screening test in individual cases (as is the situation with the cystic fibrosis gene).

It will soon be possible to create a new classification of FHC by genetic type. Families can be categorised as to whether the mutation involves the myosin heavy chain gene or an alternative locus, and subdivided by type and location of precise mutation within the domains of the MHC gene. Each subtype will be examined for correlation with clinical features and natural history of the disease in the hope that this will identify clinically useful information about the prognosis and relative risk of complications in the different groups.

Understanding of the different genetic origins of families with FHC may also predict associated abnormalities not otherwise apparent at the clinical level. The beta isoform of cardiac myosin heavy chain is also expressed in skeletal muscle, particularly in type 1 fibres (slow twitch oxidative fibres) [52]. Those FHC families with beta MHC mutations might be expected to have subclinical skeletal muscle abnormalities, in contrast to those with non-beta MHC mutations. It is known that in a proportion of individuals with FHC there are myopathic abnormalities on electromyography and histopathological examination and that these are indeed confined to type 1 fibres [53]. These abnormalities may identify those families with beta MHC mutations. It has already been shown that transcripts of beta cardiac myosin heavy chain gene can be detected in blood lymphocytes and used to screen for mutations causing FHC. Prenatal screening would permit longitudinal study of the disease [51].

The finding of MHC missense mutations in hypertrophic cardiomyopathy appears to parallel the findings in one of the animal model systems used to investigate disordered MHC function. In the nematode *C. elegans*, missense mutations in a skeletal MHC gene are clustered in two regions of the globular head and are associated with a dominant phenotype of body wall paralysis [54]. The dominant expression is explained by a "poison polypeptide" mechanism, whereby structurally flawed copies of the myosin heavy chain polypeptide are incorporated into myosin filaments and then prevent normal assembly and function. In contrast, null mutations in the *C. elegans* MHC, which cause complete disruption or failure of expression of one copy of the gene, produce a recessive phenotype. As recent technology has generated means of creating transgenic animals, it is now possible to insert the missense mutations which cause FHC in man into this, and other, animal models to study their effects at a biochemical and histopathological level.

Analysis of the diversity of the mutations that can cause this condition will provide insight into the functional domains of the MHC molecules and may suggest other contractile protein elements as candidates for disease-causing mutations in the "unlinked" families. It is anticipated that the defect in those families not linked to the MHC locus will involve a gene, or genes, for the cardiac isoforms of other contractile proteins which closely associate with the myosin heavy chains. There are therefore many possible candidates, most of which occur in more than one isoform—for example myosin light chains, actin, troponin and tropomyosin.

Finally, demonstration of the molecular basis of FHC raises the posibility that other inherited cardiomyopathies might also result from mutations in cardiac myosin or other contracile proteins. Just as many clinically diverse haemolytic anaemias can arise from mutations in the alpha and beta haemoglobin genes, and either Duchenne or Becker muscular dystrophy can result from different types of mutations in the dystrophin gene, familial forms of restrictive or dilated cardiomyopathy may be found to share similarities of molecular aetiology with FHC.

In the majority of genetic conditions mapped by reverse genetics the gene ultimately identified as the site of the mutation has been a previously unknown one and the characteristics and role of the protein product have not been immediately apparent. This has been the case with both Duchenne muscular dystrophy and cystic fibrosis. In contrast, in FHC, the first primary cardiac disease to be characterised at the molecular level, the defect occurs in a particularly well-known and much-studied gene. It is in part because of this that the findings in FHC are quickly expanding in clinical and scientific impact in the ways discussed. Knowledge of the role of the defective beta MHC protein and of the mechanisms that control expression of both the beta and alpha MHC isoforms may ultimately lead to therapeutic manipulations that will intervene in the development of this condition.

References

1. Teare D (1958) Asymmetrical hypertrophy of the heart in young adults. Br Heart J 20: 1–8
2. Hollman A, Goodwin JF, Teare D, Renwick JW (1960) A family with obstructive cardiomyopathy (asymmetrical hypertrophy). Br Heart J 22: 449–456
3. Brent LB, Aburano A, Fisher DL, Moran TJ, Myers JD, Taylor WJ (1960) Familial muscular subaortic stenosis, an unrecognised form of "idiopathic heart disease", with clinical and autopsy findings. Circulation 21: 167–180
4. Pare JAP, Fraser RG, Pirozynski WJ, Shanks JA, Stubington D (1961) Hereditary cardiovascular dysplasia: a form of familial cardiomyopathy. Am J Med 31: 37–62
5. Wood RS, Taylor WJ, Wheat MV, Schreibler GL (1962) Muscular subaortic stenosis in childhood: report of occurrence in three siblings. Paediatrics 30: 749–758
6. Horlick L, Petrovich NJ, Bolton CF (1966) Idiopathic hypertophic subvalvular stenosis: a study of a family involving four generations. Clinical, hemodynamic and pathologic observations. Am J Cardiol 17: 411–418
7. Haughland H, Ohn O-J, Boman H, Thorsby E (1986) Hypertrophic cardiomyopathy in three generations of a large Norwegian family: a clinical, echocardiographic and genetic study. Br Heart J 55: 168–175
8. Goodwin JF, Hollman A, Cleland WP, Teare D (1960) Obstructive cardiomyopathy simulating aortic stenosis. Br Heart J 22: 403–414
9. Emanuel R, Withers R, O'Brien K (1971) Dominant and recessive modes of inheritance in idiopathic cardiomyopathy. Lancet 2: 1065–1067
10. Abbasi AS, MacAlpin RN, Eber LM, Pearce ML (1972) Echocardiographic diagnosis of idiopathic hypertrophic cardiomyopathy without outflow obstruction. Circulation 46: 897–904
11. Henry WL, Clark CE, Epstein SE (1973) Asymmetric septal hypertrophy (ASH): echocardiographic identification of the pathognomonic anatomical abnormality of IHSS. Circulation 47: 225–233
12. Clark CE, Henry WL, Epstein SE (1973) Familial prevalence and genetic transmission of idiopathic hypertrophic subaortic stenosis. N Engl J Med 289: 709–714
13. Ten Cate FJ, Hugenholtz PG, van Dorp WG, Roelandt J (1979) Prevalence of diagnostic abnormalities in patients with genetically transmitted asymmetric septal hypertrophy. Am J Cardiol 43: 731–737

14. Maron BJ, Gottdiener JS, Epstein SE (1981) Patterns and significance of distribution of left ventricular hypertrophy in hypertrophic cardiomyopathy: a wide angle, two dimensional echocardiographic study of 125 patients. Am J Cardiol 48: 418–428
15. Shapiro L, McKenna WJ (1983) Distribution of left ventricular hypertrophy in hypertrophic cardiomyopathy: a two-dimensional chocardiographic study. J Am Coll Cardiol 2: 437–444
16. McKenna WJ, Kleinebenne A, Nihoyannopoulos P, Foale R (1988) Echocardiographic measurement of right ventricular wall thickness in hypertrophic cardiomyopathy: relation to clinical and prognostic features. J Am Coll Cardiol 11: 351–358
17. Ciro E, Nichols PF, Maron BJ (1983) Heterogeneous morphologic expression of genetically transmitted hypertrophic cardiomyopathy: two-dimensional echocardiographic analysis. Circulation 67: 1227–1233
18. Maron BJ, Bonow RO, Cannon RO, Leon MB, Epstein SE (1987) Hypertrophic cardiomyopathy: interrelations of clinical manifestations, pathophysiology, and therapy. N Engl J Med 316: 780–789, 844–852
19. Autore C, Fragola PV, Picelli A, Maccari AM, Ruscitti G, Cannata D, Sangiori M (1988) Equivocal and borderline myocardial hypertrophy in relatives of patients with hypertrophic cardiomyopathy: possible implications in genetics of the disease. Cardiology 75: 348–356
20. Maron BJ, Nichols PF, Pickle LW, Wesley YE, Mulvihill JJ (1984) Patterns of inheritance in hypertrophic cardiomyopathy: assessment by M-mode and two-dimensional echocardiography. Am J Cardiol 53: 1087–1094
21. Greaves SC, Roche AH, Neutze JM, Whitlock RM, Veale AM (1987) Inheritance of hypertrophic cardiomyopathy: a cross-sectional and M mode echocardiographic study of 50 families. Br Heart J 58: 259–266
22. Braunwald E, Lambrew CT, Rockoff SD, Ross J, Morrow AG (1964) Idiopathic hypertrophic subaortic stenosis. I. A description of the disease based upon an analysis of 64 patients. Circulation 30 Suppl 4: 3–119
23. Frank S, Braunwald E (1968) Idiopathic hypertrophic subarotic stenosis: clinical analysis of 126 patients with emphasis on natural history. Circulation 37: 759–788
24. Maron BJ, Spirito P, Wesley YE, Arce J (1986) Development and progression of left ventricular hypertrophy in children with hypertrophic cardiomyopathy. N Engl J Med 315: 610–614
25. Epstein ND, Lin HJ, Fananapazir L (1990) Genetic evidence of dissociation (generational skips) of electrical from morphologic forms of hypertrophic cardiomyopathy. Am J Cardiol 66: 627–631
26. Littler WA (1972) Twin studies in hypertrophic cardiomyopathy. Br Heart J 34: 1147–1151
27. Reid JM, Houston AB, Lundmark E (1989) Hypertrophic cardiomyopathy in identical twins. Br Heart J 62: 384–388
28. Fitzpatrick AP, Emanuel RW (1988) Familial neurofibromatosis and hypertrophic cardiomyopathy. Br Heart J 60: 247–251
29. Barker D, Wright E, Nguyen K et al. (1987) Gene for von Recklinghausen neurofibromatosis is in the pericentromeric region of chromosome 17. Science 236: 1100–1102
30. Child JS, Perloff J, Bach P, Wolfe AD, Perlman S, Kark RAP (1986) Cardiac involvement in Friedreich's ataxia: a clinical study of 75 patients. J Am Coll Cardiol 7: 1370–1378
31. Gilgenkrantz S, Vigneron C, Gregoire MJ et al. (1982) Association of del(11)(p15.1p12), aniridia, catalase deficiency and cardiomyopathy. Am J Med Genet 13: 39–49
32. Moiseyev VS, Korovina EA, Polotskaya EL, Poliyanskaya IS, Yazdovsky VV (1987) Hypertrophic cardiomyopathy associated with hereditary spherocytosis in 3 generations of one family. Lancet 2: 853–854
33. Kimberling WJ, Taylor RA, Chapman RG, Lubs HA (1978) Linkage and gene localization of hereditary spherocytosis (HS). Blood 52: 859–867.
34. Matsumori A, Hirose K, Wakabayashi A et al. (1979) HLA and hypertrophic cardiomyopathy. Am heart J 97: 428–431
35. Kishimoto C, Kaburagi T, Takamaya S et al. (1983) Two forms of hypertrophic cardiomyopathy distinguished by inheritance of HLA haplotypes and left ventricular outflow tract obstruction. Am Heart J 105: 988–994

36. Matsumori A, Kawai C, Wakabayashi A et al. (1981) HLA-DRW4 antigen linkage in patients with hypertrophic obstructive cardiomyopathy. Am Heart J 101: 14–16
37. Haughland H, Ohm O-J, Boman H, Thorsby E (1986) Hypertrophic cardiomyopathy in three generations of a large Norwegian family. Br Heart J 55: 168–175
38. Zezulka A, MacKintosh P, Jobson S, Lowry P, Shapiro L (1986) Human lymphocyte antigens in hypertrophic cardiomyopathy. Int J Cardiol 12: 193–202
39. Gardin JM, Gottdiener JS, Radvany R, Maron BJ, Lesch M (1982) HLA linkage vs association in hypertrophic cardiomyopathy: evidence for the absence of an association in a heterogeneous caucasian population. Chest 81: 466–472
40. Donis-Keller H, Green P, Helms C et al. (1987) A genetic linkage map of the human genome. Cell 51: 319–337
41. Jarcho JA, McKenna WJ, Pare JAP, Solomon SD, Holcombe RF, Dickie S, Levi T, Donis Keller H, Seidman JG, Seidman CE (1989) Mapping a gene for familial hypertrophic cardiomyopathy to chromosome 14q1. N Engl J Med 321: 1372–1378
42. Solomon SD, Jarcho JA, McKenna WJ, Geisterfer-Lowrance A, Salerni R, Seidman JG, Seidman CE (1990) Familial hypertrophic cardiomyopathy is a genetically heterogeneous disease. J Clin Invest 86: 993–999
43. Hejtmancik JF, Brink PA, Towbin J, Hill R, Brink L, Tapscott T, Trakhtenbrolt A, Robert R (1991) Localization of gene for familial hypertrophic cardiomyopathy to chromosome 14q1 in a diverse US population. Circulation 83: 1592–1597
44. Ferraro M, Scarton G, Ambrosini M (1990) Cosegregation of hypertrophic cardiomyopathy and a fragile site on chromosome 16 in a large Italian family. J Med Genet 27: 363–366
45. Nishi H, Kimura A, Sasaki M et al. (1989) Localisation of the gene for hypertrophic cardiomyopathy to chromosome 18q (Abstr). Circulation 80: II–457
46. Saez LJ, Gianola KM, McNally EM, Feghali R, Eddy R, Shows TB, Leinwand LA (1987) Human cardiac myosin heavy chain genes and their linkage in the genome. Nucleic Acids Res, 15: 5443–5459
47. Matsuoka R, Yoshida MC, Kanda N, Kimura R, Osasa H, Takao A (1989) Human cardiac myosin heavy chain gene mapped within chromosomal region 14q11.2-q13. Am J Med Genet 32: 279–284
48. Solomon SD, Geisterfer-Lowrance AT, Vosberg H-P, Hiller G, Jarcho JA, Morton C, McBride WO, Mitchell AL, Bale AE, McKenna WJ, Seidman JG, Seidman CE (1990) A locus for familial hypertrophic cardiomyopathy is closely linked to the cardiac myosin heavy chain genes on chromosome 14 at q11-q12. Am J Hum Genet 47: 389–394
49. Tanigawa G, Jarcho JA, Kass S, Solomon SD, Vosberg HP, Seidman JG, Seidman CE (1990) A molecular basis for familial hypertrophic cardiomyopathy: an alpha/beta cardiac myosin heavy chain hybrid gene. Cell 62: 991–998
50. Geisterfer-Lowrance A, Kass S. Tanigawa G, Vosberg HP, McKenna WJ, Seidman JG, Seidman CE (1990). A molecular basis for familial hypertrophic cardiomyopathy: a beta cardiac myosin heavy chain gene missense mutation. Cell 62: 999–1006
51. Rosenzweig A, Watkins H, Hwang D-S, Miri M, McKenna WJ, Traill T, Seidman JG, Seidman CE (1991) Preclinical diagnosis of familial hypertrophic cardiomyopathy by genetic analysis of blood lymphocytes. N Engl J Med 325: 1753–1760
52. Saez LJ, Leinwand L (1986) Characterization of diverse forms of myosin heavy chain expressed in adult human skeletal muscle. Nucleic Acids Res 14: 2951–2969
53. Caforio ALP, Rossi B, Risaliti R et al. (1989) Type 1 fiber abnormalities in skeletal muscle of patients with hypertrophic and dilated cardiomyopathy: evidence of subclinical myogenic myopathy. J Am Coll Cardiol 14: 1464–1473
54. Bejsovec A, Anderson P (1990) Functions of the myosin ATP and actin binding sites are required for *C. elegans* thick filament assembly. Cell 60: 133–140

Subject Index

Printing: Mercedesdruck, Berlin
Binding: Buchbinderei Lüderitz & Bauer, Berlin